Integrative Veterinary Medicine

Integrative Veterinary Medicine

Edited by

Mushtaq A. Memon
Department of Veterinary Clinical Sciences
Washington State University
Pullman, Washington, USA

Huisheng Xie
Chi University
Reddick, Florida, USA

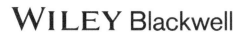

Registered Office
John Wiley & Sons, Inc., 111 River Street, Hoboken, NJ 07030, USA

For details of our global editorial offices, customer services, and more information about Wiley products visit us at www.wiley.com.

Wiley also publishes its books in a variety of electronic formats and by print-on-demand. Some content that appears in standard print versions of this book may not be available in other formats.

Library of Congress Cataloging-in-Publication Data
Names: Memon, Mushtaq Ahmed, editor. | Xie, Huisheng, editor.
Title: Integrative veterinary medicine / edited by Mushtaq A. Memon, Department of Veterinary Clinical Sciences,
    Washington State University, Atlanta, Georgia, Huisheng Xie, Chi University, Reddick, Florida.
Description: First edition. | Hoboken, NJ, USA : John Wiley & Sons, Inc., 2023. | Includes bibliographical references and index.
Identifiers: LCCN 2023000265 (print) | LCCN 2023000266 (ebook) | ISBN 9781119823520 (Hardback) |
    ISBN 9781119823537 (ePDF) | ISBN 9781119823544 (epub) | ISBN 9781119823551 (oBook)
Subjects: LCSH: Alternative veterinary medicine. | Integrative medicine.
Classification: LCC SF745.5 .V53 2023 (print) | LCC SF745.5 (ebook) | DDC 636.089/55--dc23/eng/20230215
LC record available at https://lccn.loc.gov/2023000265
LC ebook record available at https://lccn.loc.gov/2023000266

Cover Images: © Janice Huntingford; © Emily Mangan
Cover Design: Wiley

Set in 9.5/12.5pt STIXTwoText by Integra Software Services Pvt. Ltd, Pondicherry, India

SKY10048237_052223

Contents

List of Abbreviations

Acronyms (Abbreviations) for Specializations and Certifications

AVMA-Recognized Specializations

DACT	Diplomate American College of Theriogenologists
DACVP	Diplomate American College of Veterinary Pathologists
DACVS	Diplomate American College of Veterinary Surgeons
DACVECC	Diplomate American College of Veterinary Emergency and Critical Care
DACVIM	Diplomate American College of Veterinary Internal Medicine
DACVSMR	Diplomate American College of Veterinary Sports Medicine and Rehabilitation
CVFT	Certified Veterinary Food Therapist
CVPP	Certified Veterinary Pain Practitioner
CVTP	Certified Veterinary Tui-Na Practitioner
CVMMP	Certified Veterinary Medical Manipulation Practitioner
CVBMA	Certified Veterinary Balance Method Acupuncturist
EDO	Equine Diploma Osteopathy
FAAVA	Fellow American Academy of Veterinary Acupuncture
VHCM	Advanced Certification in Veterinary Chinese Herbal Medicine

Certifications

CCRT	Certified Canine Rehabilitation Therapist
CCRV	Certified Canine Rehabilitation Veterinarian
CAVCA	Certified by the American Veterinary Chiropractic Association
CDA	Certified Disk Arthroplasty surgeon
CERPV	Certified Equine Rehabilitation and Performance Veterinarian
CHPV	Veterinarians Certified in Hospice and Palliative Care
CTCVMP	Certified Traditional Chinese Veterinary Medicine Practitioner
CVA	Certified Veterinary Acupuncturist
CVC	Certified Veterinary Chiropractor
CVCH	Certified Veterinary Chinese Herbalist

About the Editors

Mushtaq A. Memon, BVSc, MSc, PhD, Dip ACT, CVA

Dr Memon is a Professor Emeritus at Washington State University (WSU); Courtesy Professor at University of Florida (UF); and Professor, Chi University, Reddick, Florida.

Dr Memon has 35 years' experience in teaching, clinical practice, and research. He received his veterinary education at Punjab University, Lahore, and MSc in animal reproduction from University of Agriculture, Faisalabad, Pakistan. He earned his PhD in Theriogenology in the United States from the University of Minnesota. This was followed by clinical training in Food Animal Medicine and Surgery at the University of Illinois and becoming a Diplomate, American College of Theriogenologists in 1984.

He has been a member of the veterinary school teaching faculties at Oklahoma State University, Louisiana State University, Tufts University, and Washington State University (1991–2016 retirement). He is an internationally recognized scholar; author of more than 120 publications, and has delivered 150+ presentations at international, regional, and local level.

As a clinical scientist and teacher, Dr Memon has received multiple teaching awards. He is a Fulbright Scholar and served as a Fulbright Ambassador for four years. He was instrumental in establishing the Fulbright Academy at WSU and currently serves as a Fulbright Specialist implementing focused projects in other countries. As Chair of the Curriculum Committee of WSU Veterinary College, Dr Memon became aware of a WSU graduate veterinarians' survey in which 60% of the responding veterinarians mentioned poor to no education was provided in complementary therapies. Comments on the survey noted 30% of the respondents had clients requesting these services (e.g., acupuncture, rehabilitation). Through courses and contact with Dr Xie and Chi University, followed by a six-month sabbatical in the Integrative Veterinary Medicine (IVM) service at UF; Dr Memon gained knowledge and became an active supporter in this growing area of veterinary medicine. He was instrumental in establishing the IVM service at WSU-Veterinary Teaching Hospital.

Dr Memon has envisioned the need for establishing IVM as part of the veterinary curriculum. He has been a leader in this area, conducting two surveys of the AVMA-accredited colleges to characterize the level of IVM education in veterinary schools. He has published the results along with curriculum recommendations. It is hoped with help from colleagues, Dr Memon will continue promoting IVM as part of the veterinary curricula and support IVM practice worldwide.

Huisheng Xie, DVM, MS, PhD

Dr Xie is Professor Emeritus at University of Florida (UF), and Professor and Founder of Chi University of Traditional Chinese Medicine in Reddick, Florida. He has been teaching and practicing Traditional Chinese Veterinary Medicine (TCVM) since 1983.

Dr Xie received his BS degree of veterinary medicine at the Sichuan College of Animal and Veterinary Sciences in Sichuan, China in 1983. He was a faculty member at the Beijing Agriculture University College of Veterinary Medicine during 1983 to 1987. After receiving his master's in veterinary acupuncture in 1988, he served as an assistant and associate professor in the college until 1994. During this time, he continued his advanced training in human acupuncture at the Beijing College of Traditional Chinese Medicine and the National academy of Traditional Chinese Medicine from 1990 to 1992.

To explore different approaches for studying and advancing TCVM, he moved to the United States in 1994 and began his doctoral training at UF. He investigated using acupuncture as pain control mechanisms in horses and received his PhD in 1999. Believing that TCVM should be available to more veterinarians, Dr Xie founded the Chi Institute of Chinese Medicine in 1998 which has progressed to become Chi University. In addition to offering certifications in various branches of TCVM, Chi University offers MS in TCVM, and MS and doctoral degrees in Integrative Veterinary Medicine.

Dr Xie's academic accomplishments are extensive. He has received numerous achievement awards from Chinese and other international institutions. Dr Xie has been invited to give lectures on veterinary acupuncture for over 100 veterinary organizations or universities of over 20 countries including the WSAVA, AVMA, Western Veterinary Conference, VMX/NAVC, and AAEP etc. He has trained over 10,000 veterinarians from nearly 100 countries. Dr Xie has authored 32 books and over 100 peer-reviewed papers. His textbooks, including *Xie's Veterinary Acupuncture* and *Traditional Chinese Veterinary Medicine – Fundamental Principles*, have been used for TCVM training programs in Asia, Europe, North and South America, Africa, and Australia.

List of Contributors

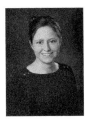

Author – Chapter # 26
Amelia Munsterman, DVM, MS,
MS-TCVM, PhD, Diplomate ACVS-LA,
Diplomate ACVECC, CTCVMP,
CVMMP
Associate Professor, Large Animal Clinical
Sciences, Veterinary Medical Center
Michigan State University, East
Lansing, Michigan, USA

Author – Chapter # 20
Carolina Medina DVM, Diplomate
ACVSMR, CVA, CVPPP
Elanco Animal Health, 2500 Innovation
Way
Greenfield, Indiana, USA

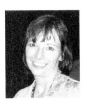

Author – Chapter #23
Cynthia McDowell, DVM, CVA,
MS-TCVM, FAAVA
Cross Point Animal Hospital, LLC
2601 Hopper Road
Cape Girardeau, Missouri, USA

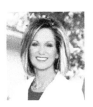

Co-author Chapters # 11, 12
Donna Raditic DVM, ACVIM
(Nutrition)
Nutrition and Integrative Medicine
Consultants
Athens, Georgia, USA

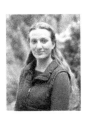

Author – Chapters # 4, 5, 6
Emily Mangan, DVM, CVA, CVCH,
CVFT, CVTP, CVMMP, CCRV
Wisewood Integrative Veterinary
Medicine, LLC
Pleasant Hill, Oregon, USA

**Editor – Section VI: Physical
Rehabilitation
Author/Co-author – Chapters # 13, 14,
15, 16**
Janice Huntingford, DVM, MS-TCVM,
Diplomate ACVSMR, CVA, CVPP
Essex Animal Hospital
355 Talbot St N
Essex, Ontario, N8M2W3, Canada

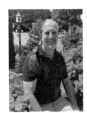

Author – Chapter # 3
John A. Perdrizet, DVM, MS-TCVM,
PhD, Diplomate ACVIM (Large Animal)
The Sanctuary Animal Clinic, 210
Linden Street
Holyoke, Massachusetts, USA

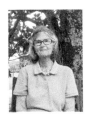

**Editor – Section VIII: Integration of
Complementary Therapies in
Clinical Practice
Author – Chapter # 24**
Judith E. Saik, DVM, PhD, Diplomate
ACVP, CVA, CVCH, CVFT
Winterville Animal Clinic
250 Henry Meyer Rd, Winterville,
Georgia, USA

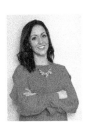

Author – Chapter # 22
Kendra Pope, DVM, Diplomate ACVIM
(Oncology), CVA, CVCH, CVFT, CVTP
Integrative Oncology and Veterinary
Wellness
252 Broad Street, Suite3, Red Bank, New
Jersey, USA

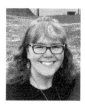

Author – Chapter # 19
Kristina M. Erwin, DVM, CVA, CCRT,
CVPP, CHPV, VHCM
Wholistic Paws Veterinary Services
20600 Gordon Park Sq.
Ashburn, Virginia, USA

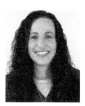

**Editor – Section V: Integrative
Nutrition**
Co-author Chapters # 11, 12
Laura Gaylord, DVM, Diplomate
ACVIM (Nutrition)
Whole Pet Provisions, PLLC
5436 Brushy Meadows Drive
Fuquay Varina, North Carolina, USA

**Editor – Section III: Manual
Therapies**
Author – Chapters # 7, 8
Marilyn Maler, DVM, Diplomate
ACVSMR, CVA, CVCH, CVFT, CVTP,
CVC, EDO
SunSpirit Farm & Veterinary Services, INC
Ocala. Florida, USA

Author – Chapter # 25
Mitchell McKee, DVM, MS-TCVM, CVA,
CVCH, CVFT, CVTP, CTPEP, CTCVMP,
CVMMP
Berry Farms Animal Hospital, Franklin,
Tennessee
Concord Animal Hospital, Brentwood,
Tennessee, USA

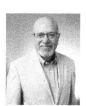

**Co-Editor – Integrative Veterinary
Medicine book**
Editor Sections I, VII
Author – Chapter # 1
Mushtaq A. Memon, BVSc, MSc, PhD,
Diplomate ACT, CVA
Prof Emeritus, Dept of Veterinary
Clinical Sciences
Washington State University
Pullman, Washington, USA

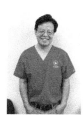

**Co-Editor – Integrative Veterinary
Medicine book**
Editor – Section II: Acupuncture
Huisheng Xie, DVM, PhD
Professor & Founder, Chi University
Reddick, Florida, USA

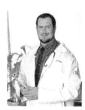

Author – Chapter # 21
Patrick Roynard, DVM, MS, CVA,
Diplomate ACVIM (Neurology), ACVIM
Neurosurgery certificate, CDA
Neurology/Neurosurgery Department
College of Veterinary Medicine
The Ohio State University, Columbus,
Ohio, USA

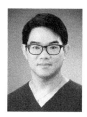

**Author/Co-author – Chapters # 13,
14, 15, 16**
Ronald B. Koh, DVM, MS, Diplomate
ACVSMR, CVA, CCRP, CVMMP, CVCH,
CVFT
Department of Surgical and Radiological
Sciences
School of Veterinary Medicine
University of California, Davis,
California, USA

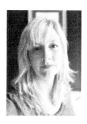

Author – Chapter # 2
Roselle Hartwigsen, BSc, BVSc, MSc, CVA
AnimalQi Wellness Centre
Director, Chi University of TCVM for
South Africa
Rustenburg, South Africa

**Editor – Section IV: Botanical and
Herbal Therapies**
Author – Chapters # 9, 10, 18
Signe Beebe, DVM, CVA, CVCH, CVFT,
CVTP
Instructor, Chi University
Reddick, Florida, USA

Authors – Chapter # 17
Rupali Sodhi, DVM, CVA
Tejinder Sodhi, BVSc & AH (Punjab,
India), CVC
Animal Hospital of Lynnwood
Animal Wellness and Rehab Center
Bellevue and Lynnwood,
Washington, USA

Preface

Integrative Veterinary Medicine (IVM) is a new clinical approach to veterinary medical care that combines conventional (Western) veterinary medicine, as traditionally taught in veterinary schools, with complementary therapies to improve clinical outcomes in patients. The idea for this book stemmed from a publication, co-authored by 26 board-certified veterinarians, which proposed curriculum guidelines for veterinary schools to introduce students to IVM (Open Vet J 6:44–56, 2016). Topics suggested by the publication have been expanded in this book and detailed information is covered in 26 chapters. All chapter authors are talented integrative clinicians with expertise that include one or more AVMA-recognized specializations and/or certification in multiple areas of complementary therapies.

The authors have offered valuable integrative medical approaches in treating patients based upon their long-term experiences in clinical veterinary medicine even though some chapters might challenge a reader's thought processes. Readers are encouraged to have open minds, as well as look for therapies that are evidence-based. One author coaches the reader, "those who dismiss the advantages of integration of therapies, prior to personal exploration, run the risk of stifling scientific method."

The IVM therapies consists of acupuncture, rehabilitation, medical manipulation (chiropractic), physical therapy, nutrition, and botanical medicine etc. Each of these disciplines is inherently individualized; therefore, one cannot expect impressive results from a "one size fits all" approach. Although scientific method is most often linear, the application is circular and follows an authors' insight gathered from years of experience and "learned from patients" based upon outcome of their selected therapies.

The incorporation of IVM approach in your practice can be rewarding for patient outcome, client satisfaction, and professional development. This book contains a compilation of knowledge and wisdom from experienced clinicians to attain that goal. It is your interest and effort that will be the critical factors in the success of your endeavors.

About the Companion Website

This book is accompanied by a companion website:

www.wiley.com/go/memon/veterinary

This website includes

- Integrative Clinical Case Examples
- Clinical Application of Chinese Herbal Medicine
- Videos

Section I

Basic Concepts
(Section Editor – Mushtaq A. Memon)

1

Introduction to Integrative Veterinary Medicine

Mushtaq A. Memon

Introduction

Integrative veterinary medicine (IVM) is defined as combination of complementary therapies with conventional care, which is guided by the best evidence available. With the increasing interest in complementary therapies by human has prompted inquiries and use of these therapies in animals. IVM is preferable term than alternative or holistic medicine. The growing preference for this terminology is exemplified by the renaming the NIH National Center for Complementary and Alternative Medicine's to the National Center for Complementary and Integrative Health. Even though many of the complementary therapies have a long history, such as acupuncture but they have become popular recently in industrialized countries. IVM includes various complementary therapies. Some of the commonly used therapies are acupuncture, rehabilitation, manual and massage therapies, herbal, and integrative nutrition. Veterinary practitioners are frequently asked questions by animal owners about complementary therapies, but the prevalence of integrative medical interventions in veterinary medicine has not been established.

Background

A survey of owners of veterinary oncology patients found that in addition to conventional treatments, the owners often used the therapies regarded as alternative or complementary without the knowledge or supervision of a veterinarian [1]. A survey of one veterinary college's graduates reported that more than two-thirds of these veterinarians encountered clinical situations involving these therapies at least monthly and over 25% experienced them on a weekly or daily basis [2]. Recent publications have emphasized the need for training in this area in veterinary colleges [3]. A survey of the 49 AVMA-accredited colleges revealed that 30.2% offer a formal course in IVM, 33 (76.7%) offered some level of IVM instruction in the curriculum, and 32 (74.4%) provided clinical services in IVM [4]. The most common IVM topics covered in the curriculum were rehabilitation, and acupuncture (Figure 1.1). A retrospective analysis [5] from an IVM service revealed that out of 5,195 patient treatment sessions, 274 patients receiving multiple modalities were most frequently for neurological and orthopedic disease (50.7% versus 49.6% of all presenting complaints, respectively). Older neutered or spayed dogs (mean age = 9 years) and Dachshunds were treated more often than expected based upon general population statistics. Acupuncture, laser therapy, electroacupuncture, and hydrotherapy (Figure 1.2), were frequently administered (>50% patients). In addition to domestic animals, acupuncture is utilized to treat various disorders in zoo and exotic animals [6].

What is in the name: Integrative medicine is defined as combination of complementary and alternative therapies with conventional care, which is guided by the best evidence available [7]. In human medical practice, complementary or alternative are broadly defined which may include acupuncture, nutrition, rehabilitation, laser therapy, hyperbaric oxygen, and other intervention not typically considered mainstream medical practice. However, the term alternative medicine gives impression that certain therapies are a replacement or a mutually exclusive option to conventional care. The critics of complementary medicine term assume that the therapies can and should only be used in tandem, when in some cases a modality may be preferred or exclusive treatment available. Finally, holistic medicine suggests that conventional veterinary practice does not consider the impacts of treatment on the whole animal, an obviously flawed assumption. The growing preference for this terminology is exemplified by the renaming the NIH National Center for Complementary and Alternative Medicine's (NCCAM) to the National Center for Complementary and Integrative Health (NCCIH https://www.nccih.nih.gov).

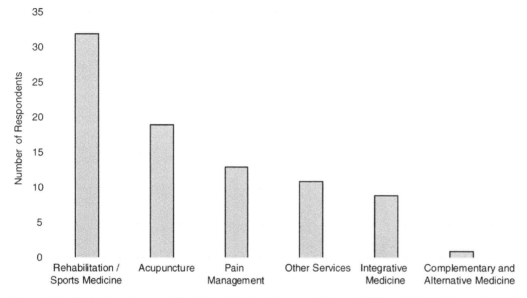

Figure 1.1 Clinical services providing Integrative Veterinary medicine modalities within AVMA-accredited colleges. Memon, Shmalberg and Xie, 2020/University of Toronto Press.

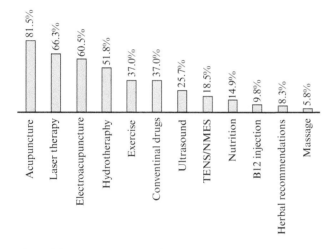

Figure 1.2 The percentage of patients receiving each integrative therapeutic modality at the study site's integrative medicine service. Shmalberg and Memon, 2015 / Hindawi / Licensed under CC BY 4.0.

Veterinary Acupuncture

Veterinary acupuncture, or needle stimulation of various points on the body, generally relies upon an understanding of neuroanatomic and musculoskeletal structures. The proposed physiological effects and possible mechanism of acupuncture are direct neural stimulation, cannabinoid receptor activation, modulation of substance P, release of endogenous opioids, selective activation of nerve fibers, and effect of acetylcholine [8–10]. For additional information on acupuncture, please see Chapters 4, 5, and 6.

Physical Rehabilitation

Physical rehabilitation and sports medicine of horses and dogs has received considerable attention in last about 20 years due to increased participation of these animals in competitive events. This has increased demand for veterinary care for animals injured in an event. The newly approved American College of Veterinary Sports Medicine and Rehabilitation (ACVSMR) has increased academic credibility of this specialty. Some of the commonly utilized rehabilitation modalities include under water treadmill therapy, photobiomodulation or laser therapy, and therapeutic ultrasound. Detailed information on various rehabilitation modalities and their use is discussed in Chapter 13–16 of this book.

Manual Therapies

Manual therapy is broadly defined to include veterinary manipulative therapy, massage, osteopathy, and related techniques. Chapters 7 covers the basic concepts of veterinary manipulative therapy as it related to neurology, biomechanics, and available evidence. Detailed information on massage therapy and myofascial principles are discussed in Chapter 8.

Integrative Nutrition

Nutritional assessment and intervention usually occur in combination with other integrative modalities, such as physical rehabilitation and sports medicine. Animals presented for physical rehabilitation are frequently overweight or obese. Novel trends in nutrition and integrative nutrition in select conditions, such as obesity, performance, and physical rehabilitation are discussed in Chapters 11 and 12.

Herbal Therapies

Botanical and herbal therapies have been utilized for thousands of years. The origins and major systems of herbal therapy with selected evidence-based interventions are described in Chapter 9. Herbal medicine regulation, adverse events and herb-drug interaction, which always is a concern using herbs with Western therapies are discussed in Chapter 10. The clinical application of herbal therapies is discussed with clinical case examples in Chapter 24.

Integrative Therapies – Case Studies

Acute Quadriplegia in Alpaca

A 5-year-old pregnant Huacaya alpaca presented for acute onset of severe weakness and inability to rise (Downer Syndrome). She was found acutely down in the pasture, laterally recumbent and unable to initiate movements (Figure 1.3). Diagnostic tests were performed but no definitive diagnosis was established. Her condition was stabilized using conventional emergency medical procedures. Once stabilized, two weeks after initial presentation, a Traditional Chinese Veterinary Medicine (TCVM) examination was performed. A Global Qi Deficiency pattern was diagnosed based on the presence of quadriparesis

and lethargy. There was Heat in the Upper Burner (Shang Jiao) as evidenced by a red tongue and red oral mucous membranes. False Heat was suspected due to the severe Qi Deficiency causing Yin Deficiency. These deficiencies were most likely a result of her pregnancy, which may have exacerbated a previous underlying Kidney Qi and Yin Deficiency. Quadriparesis may be associated with Deficient Kidney/Spleen Qi causing weakness of the limbs. Seven acupuncture treatments (dry needles, electro-acupuncture, aqua acupuncture) (Figure 1.4) were administered for three months (weekly then every two weeks). Daily physical rehabilitation, including hydrotherapy (Figure 1.5) and walking (Figure 1.6) were provided. By combining acupuncture and physical rehabilitation with conventional treatments and supportive care, the alpaca began walking on her own in approximately 50 days after onset (Figure 1.7) and recovered within three months with a viable fetus. She delivered a normal cria (Figure 1.8) [11].

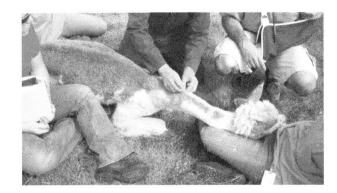

Figure 1.4 Dry needle acupuncture was performed in alpaca with quadriplegia of unknown etiology.

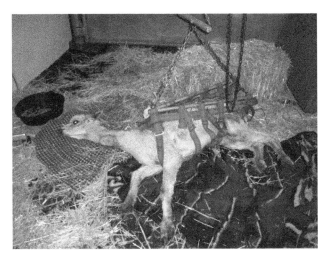

Figure 1.3 A 5-year-old recumbent pregnant alpaca with acute quadriplegia.

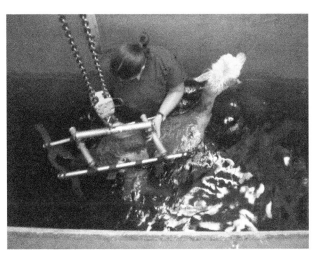

Figure 1.5 Hydrotherapy in a pool was performed in alpaca with quadriplegia of unknown etiology.

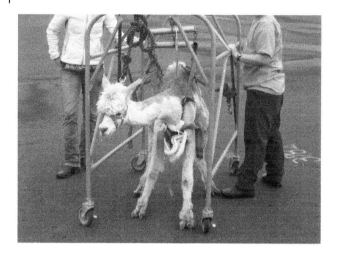

Figure 1.6 Walking with support as a part of rehabilitation was provided to alpaca presented with quadriplegia of unknown etiology.

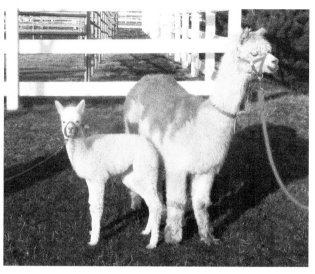

Figure 1.8 A 5-year-old recumbent pregnant alpaca with acute quadriplegia of unknown etiology was treated for six weeks with integrative therapy, including acupuncture. Alpaca delivered a normal cria and shown with the mother 20 days after birth.

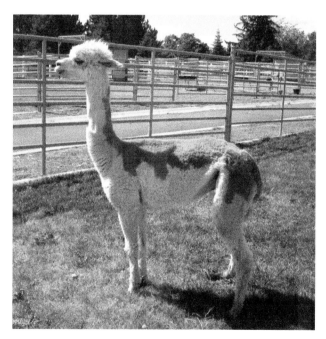

Figure 1.7 By combining acupuncture and physical rehabilitation with conventional treatments and supportive care, the alpaca with quadriplegia began walking on her own in approximately 50 days after onset.

Immune Mediated Hemolytic Anemia (IMHA) in a Dog

A one-year-old spayed female rat terrier dog with IMHA was referred. The referring veterinarian reported that the dog did not respond to treatment with prednisone, azathioprine, and cyclosporine at immunosuppressive doses. She was non-regenerative and had been anorexic and vomiting/regurgitating for about a week. She was transfusion dependent and had been receiving blood roughly every 36 hours.

IMHA causes severe anemia in dogs and is associated with high morbidity and mortality, and mortality as high as 50% of the affected dogs [12]. Treatment relies on nonspecific immune suppression by glucocorticoids to control autoimmune responses targeting red blood cells [13]. Little consensus exists on either the specific drug or combination of drugs to use or their dosages in individual patients [14].

Integrative veterinary medical (IVM) approach was considered in the dog. Traditional Chinese Veterinary Medicine (TCVM) examination of the patient revealed the following. Her nose was cool and dry, the right ear was warmer than the left, warm at Bui-hui and lumbosacral area, the pulse was thready, fast, and superficial. She was depressed (Figure 1.9) but the owner explained her personality which was compatible to Wood. Her sclera of the eyes and mucous membrane of the gums were yellow (Figure 1.10). Her tongue was dry with yellow coating and thicker at the base. Upon diagnostic scan, she was ++ sensitive at BL-22 and BL-23. TCVM pattern diagnosis was Spleen Qi and Blood Qi deficiency with excess heat. A veterinary internist and TCVM practitioner at the hospital worked together and implemented the IVM approach. The conventional therapy included Prednisone 5mg tables (1 tablet by mouth every 12 hours), Cyclosporine 25mg tablets (1 capsule by mouth every 12 hours), Leflunomide 10mg tablets (1 tablet by mouth every 12 hours), Azathioprine 6.5 mg capsules (2 capsules by mouth every 24 hours), Omeprazole 10mg capsules (1 capsule by mouth every 24 hours), and Aspirin 4mg capsules (1 capsule by mouth every 24 hours). TCVM

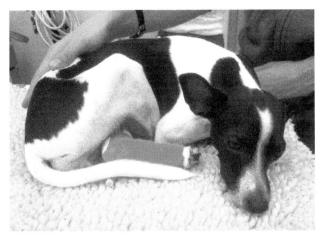

Figure 1.9 One-year-old spayed female rat terrier dog presented depressed with immune mediated hemolytic anemi.

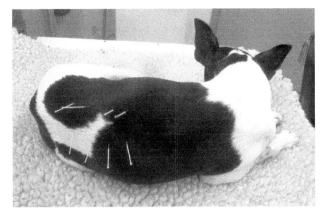

Figure 1.11 Dry needle acupuncture of 1-year-old spayed female rat terrier dog with immune mediated hemolytic anemia.

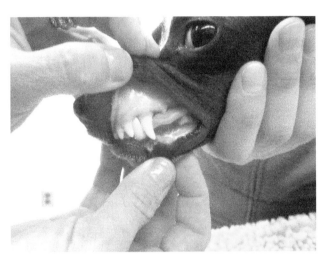

Figure 1.10 One-year-old spayed female rat terrier dog presented with immune mediated hemolytic anemia. Note her yellow sclera of the eye and mucous membranes.

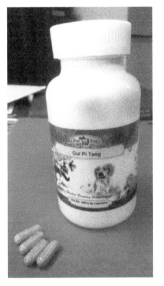

Figure 1.12 Gui Pi Tang was given by mouth twice a day to a 1-year-old spayed female rat terrier dog with immune mediated hemolytic anemia.

treatment included dry needle acupuncture (Figure 1.11) at acupoints BL-18, 20, 21, 22; GV-14, 20; SP-6, 10; ST-36; LI-20; and Gui Pi Tang (Figure 1.12) by mouth every 12 hours.

The patient was examined a day after the acupuncture treatment, and improvement was noticed. The yellowness of the tongue and mucous membranes was decreased (Figure 1.13), the pulse was less thready and fast, ears felt normal, her nose was moist, but she was still sensitive (++) at BL-22, 23. Her PCV (packed cell volume) had improved, therefore less blood transfusion was needed. Acupuncture was repeated and she was discharged from the hospital. After three days, the dog was re-examined; further improvement in the color of her sclera and mucous membrane was noticed. For about three months, the dog was maintained at conventional therapy of only two medications (Azathioprine 6.5 mg and Aspirin 4 mg per day);

and Gui Pi Tang two capsules twice a day. Upon re-examination after about three months of the treatment (Figure 1.14), she showed her Wood personality and didn't allow inserting needles for acupuncture [15].

Chronic Diarrhea in a Cat

A three-and-a-half-year-old spayed female cat (Figure 1.15.) was presented with chronic diarrhea started about four months prior to presentation. Various diagnostic tests (fecal flotation test, CBC, Urine analysis, abdominal ultrasonography) were conducted and the cat was treated with various anthelmintics, including metronidazole, and fenbendazole but no improvement in diarrhea was noticed.

TCVM diagnosis and treatment: The cat was a difficult patient to perform complete TCVM diagnosis. In TCVM,

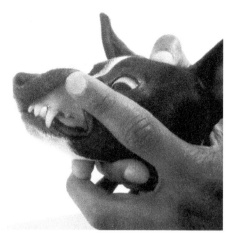

Figure 1.13 The yellowness of the tongue and mucous membranes was decreased after one day of dry needle acupuncture of 1-year-old spayed female rat terrier dog with immune mediated hemolytic anemia.

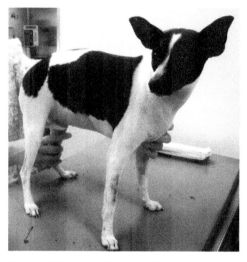

Figure 1.14 About three months after integrative veterinary therapy of a 1-year-old spayed female rat terrier dog with immune mediated hemolytic anemia.

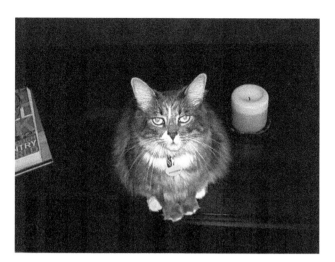

Figure 1.15 A 3.5-year-old spayed female presented with chronic diarrhea recovered with acupuncture therapy.

needles were inserted at GV-1, GV-20, BL-20, BL-21. After one week, aqua acupuncture with diluted B12 was injected at GV-1, 20; BL-20, 21; ST-25, and CV-12. The owner reported decrease in diarrhea. After another week the aqua acupuncture was repeated. The owner was pleasantly surprised to notice that the diarrhea had stopped, and the cat defecated solid stools. The owner couldn't believe her own eyes and got so excited and took a picture of the solid feces and shared with us and with her friends and relatives through social media!

Conclusion

Integrative veterinary medicine is defined as combination of complementary therapies with conventional care, which is guided by the best evidence available. With the increasing interest in complementary therapies by human has prompted inquiries and use of these therapies in animals. IVM is preferable term than alternative or holistic medicine. The growing preference for this terminology is exemplified by the renaming the NIH National Center for Complementary and Alternative Medicine's to the National Center for Complementary and Integrative Health. Some of the commonly used therapies include acupuncture, rehabilitation, manual and massage therapies, herbal and integrative nutrition.

diarrhea is considered stomach cold or cold-damp pattern [16]. It can be caused by stressful environmental changes, sudden change in diet, or unknown etiology. Treatment strategies include warm the middle-*jiao* and eliminate cold; excrete damp and stop diarrhea. The recommended acupuncture points are GV-1, *Bai-hui*, GV-4, ST-36, GB-34, SP-6, SP-9, BL-20, and BL-21. GV-1 is a local point to stop diarrhea, balance water (body fluids), and regulate middle-*jiao*. *Bai-hui* and GV-4 are common points to warm *Yang* to dispel cold-damp. ST-36 and GB-34 are the earth points to strengthen the spleen and stomach. SP-6 and SP-9 strengthen the spleen and eliminate damp. BL-20 and BL-21 are the back-associate points to strengthen the spleen and stomach [16].

As mentioned, the cat was a difficult patient to perform dry needle acupuncture on selected acupoints, therefore a few

References

1 Lana, S.E., Kogan, L.R., Crump, K.A. et al. (2006). The use of complementary and alternative therapies in dogs and cats with cancer. *J Anim Hosp Assoc* 42: 361–365.

2 Memon, M.A. and Sprunger, L.K. (2011). Survey of colleges and schools of veterinary medicine regarding education in complementary and alternative veterinary medicine. *J Am Vet Med Assoc* 239: 619–623.

3 Memon, M.A., Shmalberg, J. et al. (2016). Integrative veterinary medical education and consensus guidelines for an integrative veterinary medicine curriculum within veterinary colleges. *Open Vet J* 6: 41–56. http://www.openveterinaryjournal.com.

4 Memon, M.A., Shmalberg, J., and Xie, H. (2020). Survey of integrative veterinary medicine training in AVMA-accredited veterinary colleges. *J Vet Med Educ* Published Online: March 12, 2020. doi: 10.3138/jvme.2019-0067.

5 Shmalberg, J. and Memon, M.A. (2015). A retrospective analysis of 5,195 treatments in an integrative veterinary medicine service: patient characteristics, presenting complaints, and therapeutic interventions. *Vet Med Int*. doi: 10.1155/2015/983621.

6 Harrison, T.M. and Churgin, S.M. (2022). Acupuncture and traditional Chinese veterinary medicine in zoological and exotic animal medicine: a review and introduction of methods. *Vet Sci* 9: 74. doi: 10.3390/vetsci9020074.

7 Klinger, B., Maizes, V., Schachter, S. et al. (2004). Core competencies in integrative medicine for medical school curricula: a proposal. *Acad Med* 79: 521–531.

8 Ulett, G.A., Han, S., and Han, J. (1998). Electroacupuncture: mechanisms and clinical application. *Biol Psychiatry* 44: 129–138.

9 Cantwell, S.L. (2010). Traditional Chinese veterinary medicine: the mechanism and management of acupuncture for chronic pain. *Top Companion Anim Med* 25: 53–58.

10 Zhang, R., Lao, L., Ren, K., and Berman, B.M. (2014). Mechanism of acupuncture-electroacupuncture on persistent pain. *Anesth* 120: 482–503.

11 Ziegler, J., Bryan, J., Gabrian, K., and Memon, M.A. (2010). Integration of acupuncture, physical therapy and conventional treatments for acute quadriparesis of unknown etiology in an alpaca. *Am J of Traditional Chinese Vet Med* 5: 79–85.

12 Swann, J.W. and Skelly, B.J. (2013). Systematic review of evidence relating to the treatment of immune-mediated hemolytic anemia in dogs. *J Vet Intern Med* 27: 1–9.

13 Swann, J.W. and Skelly, B.J. (2011). Evaluation of immunosuppressive regimens for immune-mediated hemolytic anemia: a retrospective study of 42 dogs. *J Small Anim Pract* 52: 353–358.

14 Swann, J.W., Garden, O.A., Fellman, C.L. et al. (2019). ACVIM consensus statement on the treatment of immune-mediated hemolytic anemia in dogs. *J Vet Intern Med* 33: 1141–1172.

15 Memon, M.A. (2019). Integrative therapy of a dog with immune-mediated hemolytic anemia. In: *TCVM Approach to Veterinary Dermatological and Immune-mediated Diseases. Proc 21st Ann Intn Conf on TCVM*, 99–100.

16 Xie, H. (2007). Acupuncture for internal medicine. In: *Xie's Veterinary Acupuncture*, (ed. Huisheng Xie, Vanessa Preast), 267–308. Ames, IA: Blackwell Publishing Professional. doi:10.1002/9780470344569.

2

Applications of Evidence-based Medicine to IVM and Current Controversies
Roselle Hartwigsen

Understanding Evidence-based Veterinary Medicine and How to Use It

1) The origins of Evidence-based medicine

Evidence-based medicine (EBM) has been practiced for thousands of years with traces being found in ancient Greece and Chinese medicine where testing of medical intervention and data capture were done since the eleventh century [1]. However, it is only in the twentieth century that EBM was formally recognized as a field of study and implemented in the care of patients. EBM is defined as the process of integrating new information and emerging technology into practice [2] and the "contentious, explicit, and judicious use of the current best evidence in making decisions about the care of the individual patients" [3]. EBM evolved as a result of the delay or failure of clinical research to have an impact on patient care and the decision making of the practitioner [3]. Evidence-based veterinary medicine (EBVM) can be understood as a subspeciality of EBM as the implementation is very similar, however, the origin of EVBM is difficult to determine. The first book on EVMB, *Handbook of Evidence-based veterinary medicine* by Crockcroft PD et al. [4], was published in 2003 with very few publications in veterinary literature since then. Crockcroft defined EBVM as "a process of lifelong, self-directed problem based learning" [4]. As veterinarians we continually gain experience from each patient we treat. EVBM uses these "lessons" or experience in a structured and constructive way by combining it with clinical research to result in the best possible outcome for each individual patient. Veterinarians practicing integrative veterinary medicine (IVM) by combining conventional veterinary medicine with complementary medicine (CVM) have been practicing a form of EBVM for years. These practitioners, through experience and literature research, developed treatment strategies on how to successfully use the "new" modalities (CVM) in their patients as these are not taught in veterinary schools. Therefore, the practitioners must rely heavily on literature, which may be of poor quantity and quality, and the knowledge and experience of fellow practitioners that are experts in the fields of CVM.

2) Understanding EBVM

EBVM is combining the clinical experience with the patients' needs and the best available evidence to make treatment decisions with the best possible outcomes for the individual patient.

To be a "good" or successful veterinarian the practitioner needs to use both clinical experience and scientific research in decision making about the individual patient [3]. Neither discipline alone will yield ideal treatment results because research is rapidly revealing new information that must be practically implemented to have any validity. External clinical research can never replace clinical expertise as it is in the expertise that lies the wisdom as to whether the research is applicable to the particular patient [1]. EBVM is not a "cookbook" medicine, and the practitioner should approach each individual case as "new" and work through the EBVM steps to determine the best approach to treat the patient. Practitioners should not fall into a routine of familiar treatments strategies and should constantly educate themselves on new techniques and treatment options available. Humans are often resistant to changes and easily fall into habits and routines; this will cause a stagnation in knowledge and skill development often leading to a decline in good therapeutic outcomes and poor client relations. The EBVM practitioner should be curious and have an open mind to explore and study new modalities, including modalities that have always been seen as "alternative" and use it to treat the patient in an integrative way. This requires the veterinarian to not only be well-read on the

Integrative Veterinary Medicine, First Edition. Edited by Mushtaq A. Memon and Huisheng Xie.
© 2023 John Wiley & Sons, Inc. Published 2023 by John Wiley & Sons, Inc.
Companion Website: www.wiley.com/go/memon/veterinary

latest publications but also have the practical skills and knowledge to apply the new knowledge appropriately to patients. EBVM is often described as a lifelong problem-based learning process [4].

3) How to practice EBVM

The practice of EBVM can be broken into five steps as identified by the Group of Evidence-Based Medicine Resource from McMaster University [1]:

a) Identifying the clinical problem and formulating a specific question
b) Efficient research to find the answer
c) Critically evaluating all research for validity and clinical relevance
d) Integrating knowledge and skills to treat patient
e) Evaluate outcomes.

This process will take effort, time and education and a veterinarian that practice EBVM should take this into account when scheduling appointments or dedicating time to patient treatment.

Step 1:

Identifying the problem and formulating a question. The work of a veterinarian revolves around constant decision-making throughout the day. Decisions on diagnosis, treatments, prognosis, etc. Busy practitioners often do not have the time or resources at hand to research each question and will rely heavily on prioritizing questions and spending time accordingly. To be more efficient and concise when practicing EBVM the question needs to be clear well-structured and answerable. The PICO format can be used to help formulate the question:

P – Patient/Problem. What is the Specie, breed, sex, age, etc., as well as what is diagnosis or problem?
I – Intervention. What treatments are available or needed for treatment?
C – Comparison of intervention. Which modalities i.e., medicine, surgery, complementary, etc., can/should be used and even used together to improve outcome?
O – Outcome. What is the outcome of interventions and how what the success of integrating the interventions?

By using PICO as a starting point, the question can easily be formulated. From here the practitioner can start step two.

Step 2: Efficient research to find the answer.

Good practice based clinical research that are of relevance to the question posed may be challenging to find. Accredited journals from trusted data basis should be consulted first, followed by conference notes/publications and consulting experts within the field. As the practitioner is usually constraint by time and cannot spend eight hours a day reading and evaluating academic papers it is vital to construct a go-to network of trusted resources that can easily be accessed and evaluated quickly. Being familiar with databases such as PubMed and CAB will allow the veterinarian to identify and use keywords more effectively and get relevant results faster. EBVM practitioners should try to connect with one another via social media or within groups to exchange ideas and experiences. Research sources should be valid, relevant, contain all benefits and possible complications as well as be easy to access and useful [1].

Step 3: Critically evaluating all research for validity and clinical relevance.

Not all research is created equally and the peer review system is imperfect and papers in these journals do not necessarily mean that the paper is of useful quality [5]. For this reason, the practitioner needs to be familiar on how to rank articles and journals for usefulness and reliability. In general articles are ranked as follows [6]:

a) Systematic reviews and meta-analysis
b) Randomized clinical trials with conclusive results
c) Randomized clinical trials with inconclusive results
d) Cohort studies
e) Case control studies
f) Cross-sectional surveys
g) Case reports.

Papers can be eliminated from the research effort early on in the process by asking three questions [5]: What was the aim of the study and how was it achieved?

a) What type of study was conducted?
b) Was the study design appropriate?

If all these questions are answered to your satisfaction, you can continue to investigate using a method that you are comfortable and familiar with. One of the acronyms used to evaluate literature is RAAMbo [7]:

R: Represents: What population does this study represent?
A: Allocation: How was the animals allocated in the study groups? Was it randomized etc?
A: Accounted: Did all the animals that started the study complete the study? If not, were the reasons given?
M: Measurements: Was the study evaluated objectively? Were the evaluators blinded to the groups? This is very important especially in observational studies.

The most important outcome of this step is to find and critically evaluate the research available in relation to the relevance of the question posed in Step 1. This should be done in a time saving and efficient manner. The evidence should be ranked and used appropriately in the next step.

Step 4: Integrating knowledge and skills to treat your patient.

Once the practitioner has evaluated the research, a better understanding of the problem as well as the solutions or treatments available, all knowledge is integrated into the treatment plan [1]. CVM should not be overlooked and integrated into the treatment plan should the research show it to be appropriate and successful for the specific problem in question. The more modalities of therapies the practitioner can perform the wider the possibilities of treatment for each patient. Very often combining CVM with conventional therapies in an integrative treatment plan, will have the best possible outcome for the patient.

The treatment plan may change according to the client's ability and preferences. In the age of technology, clients often consult "Dr Google" to self-diagnose their pets and very often tells the veterinarian how they think the condition should be treated. For this reason, veterinarians should be knowledgeable not only on what they are taught in veterinary school but also about alternative therapies suggested on the internet. Veterinarians should be able to easily distinguish between viable alternative or CVM therapies and quackery with no scientific basis and explain this eloquently to their clients. As very little CVM is taught in veterinary schools, practitioners need to search for education in these subjects from reputable universities, institutes and organizations producing research and education. Organizations such as the World Association of Traditional Chinese Veterinary Medicine (WATCVM) or the American Holistic Veterinary Medicine Association (AHVMA) provides useful resources for practitioners and funds a great deal of research into CVM. As the public interest and demand for these therapies are growing, the skills and knowledge of the veterinarians should grow as well [8].

Step 5: Evaluate outcomes.

The outcome of the treatment plan as well as the overall success of the practitioner to perform EBVM should be evaluated [1]. Was the treatment outcome as expected for this specific patient? Did the EBVM applied have the expected results for the patient? If not, why, and how can this be corrected? Were there any changes for the better?

Does the outcome differ significantly from the clinical research? All these questions should be asked, and the outcome critically evaluated.

The practitioner should also do a self-evaluation to gauge the success and efficiency to which EBVM was applied. Was the problem correctly identified? Were the scientific resources used applicable and relevant? Did the practitioner do enough research or spend too much time locating relevant research? Was the evidence correctly integrated and used to treat the patient? Did the practitioner meet the client expectations and work within the preferences subscribed?

Each case should be a learning opportunity for the practitioner and future EBVM practitioners. This will help veterinarians improve their EBVM skills and identify the specific steps where improvement is needed [2]. All veterinary practitioners should aim to document all cases to the highest scientific standard using the correct medical terminology and internationally accepted units. This will help to share knowledge and experience with a wider audience without unfortunate miscommunication and evidence lost in translation. EBVM practitioners should also be encouraged to share their knowledge and experience with other veterinarians at conferences and in peer reviewed journals.

Evidence-based Medicine and Integrative Veterinary Medicine

Lack of understanding has led to confusion surrounding EBVM. Some argue that it is the natural evolution of veterinary science because of the exponential expansion of knowledge and technology available to practitioners. Others suggest that EBVM is a collective effort from corporations and academics to change the traditional way of practicing veterinary medicine by creating "cookie cutter" veterinarians reliant on their research and products. While many are of the opinion that it is merely a new way of looking at the same way of traditional practice [2]. As a profession, veterinarians need to learn how to process a large amount of information and new advances in treatment techniques due to rapid research and development. In the age of information all the latest discoveries are now at our fingertips and available to practitioners even before it is published in a textbook or taught in veterinary schools. Practitioners need an efficient method to weed out what they need and apply the knowledge for a specific patient. EBVM formalizes the process and creates a method to provide a treatment plan with the best possible outcome to patients.

One of the best examples of where EBVM can be successfully implemented is in the use of CVM. Alternative treatment modalities have popped up globally as "cure all" for all sorts of ailments and diseases. Often these therapies have very little or no scientific backing and are practiced by non-veterinary professionals with no or very little education in veterinary science. There are however CVM modalities with excellent clinical research such as herbal medicine and acupuncture, that are taught in certified institutes and universities, all showing excellent treatment results. CVM consists of all therapies and treatments not taught in veterinary school including but not limited to acupuncture, phytomedicine (herbal medicine), food therapy, homeopathy, osteopathy, chiropractic, essential oils, and massage therapy. Clients are aware and enthusiastic about alternative treatment available for their pets, and a growing number of veterinarians are interested in using these therapies to improve the outcomes for their patients. EBVM is an excellent tool to distinguish which of the CVM modalities are valid, proven and indicated for the patient, as well as how to combine different treatments in an integrative tool when using IVM to get the best possible results for the patient and client.

IVM is understood as the use of CVM and conventional medicine together in practice to achieve the best possible outcome for each individual patient as illustrated in figure 2.1. Where conventional veterinary medicine relies heavily on clinical research in decision-making, in CVM clinical published research is somewhat lacking as clinical trials are difficult to standardize and execute. CVM therapies are based on each individual patient and difficult to extrapolate to big research groups. For this reason, CVM practitioners rely heavily on EBVM for practical experience accounts and available clinical research from CVM practitioners in decision-making. The National Centre for Complementary and Integrative health (NCCIH) stresses and supports the development and dissemination of objective evidence-based information on CVM with professional education at its core [9]. The NCCIH has excellent online resource to guide EBVM practitioners in an efficient way to find the most relevant and recent published data on a specific CVM. Other organizations such as the WATCVM has peer reviewed publications available to members that will aid in the decision-making process of EBVM as well as funding of research.

When deciding to use CVM as part of the integrative treatment the veterinarian must satisfy at least one of the following three criteria during step three in the EBVM process: A) There is significant scientific evidence for the efficacy of the therapies. B) There is evidence of the therapy being used in similar population of patients. C) If the therapy has potential to treat a condition for which conventional medicine has failed [8]. Once the veterinarian is satisfied the CVM treatment is appropriate, and will yield good results, an integrated treatment plan is formulated. To integrate CVM successfully into treating a patient the veterinarian should have the necessary training and skill for the specific CVM modality. Currently appropriate training and education in CVM is a challenge due to a lack of accredited teaching institutions. The deficiency of perceived supportive evidence for CVM has created a reluctance to include training in CVM modalities as part of the veterinary curriculum in veterinary schools [10]. Controversies surrounding the validity and efficacy of CVM modalities have been a constant in the academic and clinical setting. Questions about the placebo effect in animals and animal owners or caregivers [11] as well as cyclical regression of chronic diseases are asked when criticizing many of the CVM modalities [8]. The AVMA taskforce on complementary and alternative therapies clearly states that it is the responsibility of the veterinarian to critically evaluate the literature on CVM therapies as the quality of scientific studies varies greatly [12]. Therefore, using the EBVM approach the veterinarian will be able to disseminate quickly between research and therapies applicable and valuable to the patient and those that are poorly designed and has no application for treating the patient.

IVM has been proposed as a model for EVBM courses in veterinary school [8] since it allows students to consider a variety of sources and use critical thinking to tailor make a treatment protocol for a patient. In IVM, the veterinarian must consider conventional treatments as well as available alternatives or complementary therapies. Often a number of different modalities are used to treat the patient for e.g. a dog presenting with chronic atopy will be diagnosed using conventional medicine and lab tests. The treatment may consist of pharmaceuticals, acupuncture, food therapy, and herbal medicine. For each modality, the veterinarian will need to investigate and research the correct application for the specific patient. Often in difficult and chronic cases a multimodal integrative approach delivers the best result.

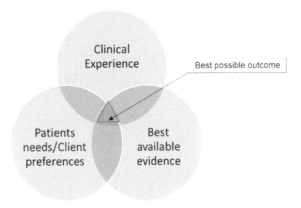

Figure 2.1 Venn diagram explaining Evidence-based veterinary medicine concept.

Conclusion

Veterinarians should familiarize themselves in the practice of EBVM when implementing IVM. By using the five steps structure in research and decision-making a thorough analysis of the problem and solution is made for the patient. The practitioner should be knowledgeable about the strengths and weaknesses of the different CVM modalities appropriate for the patient and how it can be integrated with conventional medicine. Critical thinking and reasoning should be encouraged when doing research on the problem and the veterinarian should be realistic about available skills and experience. A network of peers and experts should be created and cultivated when applying EBVM especially in the use of CVM where published research adhering to the conventional medicine modal is inadequate or lacking. By correctly integrating conventional and complementary medicine in an evidence based model, the outcome will always be to the advantage of the patient and client resulting in the best possible outcomes.

References

1 Masic, I., Miokovic, M., and Muhamedagic, B. (2008). Evidence based medicine–new approaches and challenges. *Acta Inform Med* 16 (4): 219.

2 Schmidt, P.L. (2007). Evidence-based veterinary medicine: evolution, revolution, or repackaging of veterinary practice? *Vet Clin N Am Small Anim Pract* 37 (3): 409–417.

3 Holmes, M.A. and Ramey, D.W. (2007). An introduction to evidence-based veterinary medicine. *Vet Clin North Am Equine Pract* 23 (2): 191–200.

4 Cockcroft, P. and Holmes, M. (2008). *Handbook of Evidence-based Veterinary Medicine*. John Wiley & Sons.

5 Kastelic, J. (2006). Critical evaluation of scientific articles and other sources of information: an introduction to evidence-based veterinary medicine. *Theriogenology* 66 (3): 534–542.

6 Guyatt, G.H. et al. (1995). Users' guides to the medical literature: IX. A method for grading health care recommendations. *Jama* 274 (22): 1800–1804.

7 Jackson, R. (2005). Can we make appraisal simpler? The GATE tool. In: *Conference Report of the 3rd International Conference of Evidence-Based Health Care Teachers & Developers*. Taormina, Sicily.

8 Memon, M.A. et al. (2016). Integrative veterinary medical education and consensus guidelines for an integrative veterinary medicine curriculum within veterinary colleges. *Open Vet J* 6 (1): 44–56.

9 NCCIH (2016). *NCCIH 2016 Strategic Plan*. February 21, 2022; NCCIH 2016 Strategic Plan.

10 Ernst, E. (2011). How much of CAM is based on research evidence? *Evid Based Complement Altern Med Volume 2011(2011)*. doi: 10.1093/ecam/nep044.

11 Conzemius, M.G. and Evans, R.B. (2012). Caregiver placebo effect for dogs with lameness from osteoarthritis. *J Am Vet Med Assoc* 241 (10): 1314–1319.

12 AVMA Alternative and Complementary Therapies Task Force (2001). An insight into the AVMA Guidelines for Complementary and Alternative Veterinary Medicine. *J Am Vet Med Assoc* 218 (11): 1729–1730.

3

Integration of Complementary Therapies with Conventional Therapy: Multimodal Approach

John A. Perdrizet

The Strength of Integrative Medicine: Accepting a New Paradigm for Your Concept of Clinical Practice

Integrative Medicine is a medical paradigm which incorporates the best conventional medicine with the advantageous implementation of complementary/alternative medicine in a coordinated way for the benefit of our patients [1]. The emphasis is on multimodal therapies, and strategies which include two or more components, such as conventional antibiotic therapy with herbal therapy [2, 3], or the use of Traditional Chinese Veterinary Medicine (TCVM) modalities with western medications for the treatment of congestive heart failure [4]. By integrating therapies, the goal is to actuate better clinical outcomes for our patients, and, importantly, to mitigate negative side-effects of those therapies: "*primum non nocere*".

The duality of western vs. alternative medicine should be a celebration of the potential for integration, not a rivalry between insular views and practices. Like the well-known symbol for the dual nature of the universe, the *Tiajitu* (commonly called the Yin-Yang symbol), the combination of these two paradigms can create balance in our goal of optimal patient care. The duality implicit in the Cosmos was observed by ancient healers who incorporated it into their deceptively simple, yet complex web of knowledge that became Traditional Chinese Medicine. Hot and Cold, Internal and External, Excess and Deficiency, Yin and Yang, these dualities guide our diagnostic capabilities, and direct our therapeutic objectives. The practice of western medicine and its materialistic and reductive methods is powerful but does not have a unifying and holistic concept of energy and its profound effects on the body – "the whole is greater than the sum of its parts". This intimate relationship between the organism and energy (Qi, Prana, Vital Force),

is not only acknowledged by alternative medical paradigms but is integral and inseparable in healing, centering, and balancing the patient. This would seem a logical extension of our fundamental western-based science underpinnings; any clinician can still remember the simple and profound equation of the Theory of Special Relativity: $E = MC^2$.

Those who would dismiss Complementary and Alternative Medicine (CAM), prior to personal exploration and open-minded assessment run the risk of stifling the scientific method altogether. These traditions are based on painstaking and detailed observations of the natural world by generations of practitioners transmitted down through the millennia. For example, in the Traditional Chinese Medical Classic *Bencao Gangmu* [5] compiled by Li Shizhen (the equivalent of "Plumbs" pharmacopoeia in 16th century China) there are thirty-two pages devoted to water. Just water. Forty-three different sources of water are described as to their energetics, advantages, indications, and contraindications in the preparation of herbal remedies, as well as applications for specific disharmonies. For example, the energy (Qi) in water can vary as to source – a still pond (calming and centering) versus a rushing stream (moving and dissipating). In contrast to this rich and diverse understanding of water, we in the west just turn on the tap, mix our foods and medicines, and don't give water another thought.

The western medical paradigm is important in our goal of optimal patient care. The inroads attained with imaging modalities, immunological and biochemical therapies, and the advent of DNA diagnostic capabilities are unparalleled and laudable. Yet these are "necessary, but not sufficient" to paraphrase the epidemiologists. With only a three-hundred-year history, modern medicine is decidedly new on the scene [6]. Even with all Western Medicine has to offer, we have all been humbled by difficult cases in which diagnosis and/or successful therapy eludes us. Difficult cases are your

Integrative Veterinary Medicine, First Edition. Edited by Mushtaq A. Memon and Huisheng Xie.
© 2023 John Wiley & Sons, Inc. Published 2023 by John Wiley & Sons, Inc.
Companion Website: www.wiley.com/go/memon/veterinary

opportunity not your failure. These are the moments that understanding an alternative concept to pathogenesis and therapeutics can make all the difference to your patient and their owners: that horse with the undiagnosable lameness? You can make significant progress in diagnosis if you do a TCVM "body scan" [7, 8]. The 16-year-old cat with chronic constipation can have a better life with acupuncture, food therapy, and herbal remedies [9]. With the advantages of multiple options inherent in integration, it is a rare case indeed in which you can look the client in the eye and pronounce that there is nothing more that can be done. With millennia behind the practice of complementary/alternative approaches, it would be foolish not to avail oneself to this diverse and rich body of knowledge. Here is where integration of alternative methods becomes an invaluable addition to your established western veterinary protocols.

Complementary medicine nudges us in the direction of "thinking outside the box", often with welcome success. The author was once confronted with a highly active Labrador retriever that had a chronic indolent lick-granuloma on the dorsum of his paw. The dog was attached by a leash to a frustrated human companion who had tried using a multitude of oral and topical steroids/antibiotics/herbals/etc. to no avail. In taking a thorough history I came upon the fortuitous fact that the owner was an avid runner, yet never took his dog on his three to five-mile daily runs. My treatment plan? Taking the dog on these runs daily- period. One month later the lesion was 90% resolved. The mind-body category of complementary medicine should never be overlooked in our quest for optimal health even in animals.

Preparation: Beginning Your Journey towards Implementing Integrative Medicine

There are many paths to take in improving your patient's health, and client's peace of mind, and it is your task to continually appraise the various methods employed in synthesizing your individualized approach to medicine. The art of medicine is combining clinical experience, scientific evidence, disparate diagnostic and therapeutic modalities, and the values/preferences of our clients for the benefit of our patients. Figure 3.1 shows the information available in assessing the validity of the science used in making medical decisions. Ascending the pyramid, each tier is considered more valid. Although "best evidence" evolves as we ascend the pyramid, we should not ignore information at the base, neither should it be over-emphasized. History has shown us that the greatest medical breakthroughs of the past century include sanitation, antibiotics, vaccines, anesthetics, and the structure and function of DNA. Not one of these breakthroughs involved large scale doubleblind Randomized Controlled Trials or Metanalyses. They involved independent and unconventional scientists often capitalizing on "lab errors" to develop new theories and testable hypothesis (what if Fleming just tossed the mold-contaminated petri dishes from whence penicillin was discovered?). The base of the Evidence Based Medicine (EBM) pyramid remains fertile ground for advances in medicine. We as veterinary clinicians would do well to avoid employing only the top tiers of the EBM pyramid resulting in

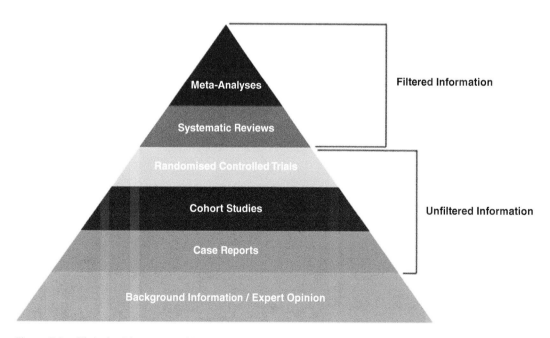

Figure 3.1 Clinical evidence pyramid.

development of lists of protocols, disregarding both the individuality of each patient in a unique environment and the experience and knowledge acquired by the practitioner [10], making the practitioner simply a technician – the antithesis of the integrative approach. Patient-Based rather than Evidence-Based medicine is a more enlightened and productive model. Just because a therapy or protocol cannot be explained, does not preclude its use. As US Surgeon General C. Everett Koop (and others) has said: "*What works is good medicine.*"

The integration of complementary therapies into a clinical practice need not require any major financial burden or alteration of the physical structure of the practice. Primarily, it is your knowledge and novel approach that is most essential. Table 3.1 lists many of the possible modalities available in the pursuit of incorporating complementary medicine into a practice. A holistic view toward practice is important in your quest for integration. To attain this goal, you, the practitioner, must start not with the chosen modality, not with the client, nor with their companion (your patient). Rather, you would be advised to start with yourself. You must accept the concept of universal vital force (or Qi, prana, spirit-energy, or whatever you wish to call it), and you can cultivate it within yourself. Begin to focus (intention) this innate energy on helping your client to heal their companion with you. To obtain accurate information from your client, precise examination findings from your patient, all in the context of a welcoming and supportive environment, you must be your best self! Exercise, nutrition, meditation, mindfulness, Qigong, Tai-Chi, yoga ... the list goes on in the ways available to help you achieve the focused intention and positive vital force necessary to become the empathic, knowledgeable, and successful healer you strive to be [11–13]. Even two minutes of breathing-techniques, or a simple Qigong movement before entering an exam room can make a positive difference.

It is well worth remembering that unlike the western medical paradigm, integrative medicine's success often relies on empowering the client as part of the healing process – acupressure, food-therapy, and *Tui-na* can all be simplified for home use. This gives the owner encouragement, hope, and bonding with their loved one. Do not underestimate the power of the human-animal bond. I have a client who spent every hour of every day for well over a year (living in the barn!) with a severely laminitic overweight Haflinger gelding (metabolic syndrome) doing everything to bring her friend back from an almost predetermined fate. Ten years later, with continued integrative therapies, there is not a trace of hoof malformation, in fact the hoof angle, frog health, and solid convex sole are better than any time before implementing complementary protocols. A client and a case such as this can show you the power of intention, teamwork, and integrative medicine. Intention and expectation are everything [14].

Table 3.1 Complementary/alternative paradigms.

System	Manual	Mind-Body	Bio-electric	Herbal	Miscellaneous
Ayurvedic	Chiropractic	Meditation	Bio-Photons	AromaTherapy	Bacterio-Therapy
Curanderismo	Craniosacral Therapy	Qi Gong	Light Therapy	Ayurvedic	Hydrotherapy
Homeopathy		Reiki	Magnets	Ethno-Botany	Hyper-Barometric O2 Therapy
Iridology	Jin Shin Do	Rolfing	Photo- Bio Modulation	Native American	Nutrition
Naturopathy	Massage	Sufiism	Shockwave	TCVM	Nutraceuticals
Osteopathy	Reflexology	Tai Chi	Ultrasound	Western	Ozone
Shamanism	Shiatsu	"T" Touch			Prolotherapy
Siddha	Tui-na	Yoga			
TCVM					
Tibetan					
Trad. Healer					
Unani					
Witchcraft					

When thinking of beginning or advancing complementary practices into your daily routine it is good to remember Lao Tzu's words from the *Dao De Ching: "A tree as great as a man's embrace springs from a small shoot"* [15]. Start small and keep growing and moving forward. Acupuncture, Chinese food therapy, and Tui-na (Chinese medical massage) are all excellent modalities that can be used throughout the day in a busy practice, without affecting the flow of a traditional western veterinary medical appointment, even before you have mastered the theories and practice behind these modalities – either in a wellness visit, or on a sick patient (from chronic otitis in a Shih Tzu dog to Heaves in an old draft horse). You can pick one acupoint [16] for each patient you examine. Place just one needle (e.g., *Bai hui* – for acceptance/Qi tonification or *Da Feng Men* – for calming and focus, or *GV-14-* to dissipate heat or immune modulation) and leave it in for the duration of the exam. This simple technique will take no more time out of your schedule, will add a new dimension to your practice, will stimulate your interest in furthering your education (remember when you liked medicine), and critically, you will educate your clientele in a whole new way of seeing their companion. As you become familiar with the patient's responses to acupuncture (*de Qi*), you will gain confidence in your technique and your ability to predict patient acceptance of needling. This same approach can be employed on your patient with *Tui-na* or Food Therapy [17, 18]. Learning one or two simple manipulations can have a calming and healing effect on your patient and those observing and performing the techniques. *Tui-na* techniques of *Mo-fa* along the neck, torso, and topline or *Na-fa* along the Yang channel (dorsal mid-line) are easy to learn and teach your staff and clientele. With food therapy, incorporating treats into the client's daily routine for their pet is empowering – try cucumber or melon for that "hot" dog with chronic dermatitis, or a sardine for the chronic renal failure cat; adding mushrooms for immune health and anticarcinogenic effects is universally accepted, and bone broth is a great tonic for older carnivores.

There are many "brick and mortar" in-person locations as well as online/virtual forms/training modules from which to choose when beginning to add a new alternative therapy to your repertoire [19, 20]. Network and seek support from like-minded colleagues, it is amazing how many new perspectives come from multiple opinions gathered on the same presentation. Colleagues with more experience in the field can help you with the nuances of implementing a complementary regime to your practice – a practitioner familiar with acupuncture in your species of interest can save you considerable angst on your first purchase of acupuncture needles. It is best to become familiar and competent in one modality before adding others to your repertoire. This is good for gaining your own confidence and in eliciting a client's favorable impression. As you develop your understanding and expertise in each complementary technique you can begin to set aside time during your weekly schedule in which you can fully immerse yourself in using it on patients. There are often history/clinical examination forms available to download off various websites (e.g., World Association of TCVM has excellent forms for recording TCVM exam findings and check lists to help remember asking pertinent aspects of the patient's history). Develop your own checklists to help fine tune a comprehensive complementary patient evaluation. These aids are critical to prevent "holes" or "lapses" in your records and are important in developing solid data from which to assess progress as the course of therapy unfolds over time. Make sure you schedule enough time to discuss the patient in depth with the client. Success is often the result of clear and open client-doctor communication. Here the art of listening is essential, sometimes this is the key to setting a plan in place which no one before you had considered. Asking pertinent and critical questions to guide the conversation or stimulate the client's memory is also important. This is an opportunity for you to become a teacher for your clients and staff. While I was in my residency, I once asked the late, great Dr. Alexander DeLahunta at Cornell University how he became so knowledgeable in his field (neurology). He gave me his usual intense gaze, smiled, and said (to paraphrase) "when each year you have eighty of the brightest young minds confront you with questions – from that many viewpoints you can't help but become rigorously educated!" If you wish to really know a subject – teach it. Use every opportunity to talk to your clients, staff, and colleagues about what you have learned, to better understand and put it into practice.

With regards to surrounding veterinary practices, it is essential to communicate in a timely manner with veterinarians from which your client may have been referred. This is a suitable time to introduce your newly acquired complementary knowledge to colleagues and begin to network for future referrals. Sending along documentation regarding their patient, and what modalities you have to offer will give them an opportunity to consider referring to you in the future.

There are challenges to the implementation of complementary medicine in today's veterinary practice. The most crucial problem is the incorrect employment of a technique. Every novice surgeon knows the consequences of a poorly tied knot. Recognized sources of information are essential. Secondly, complementary medicine is inherently individualized. You cannot expect impressive results from a "one size fits all" approach. This is where experience, understanding the theory behind a modality, and colleague communication pay off. Thirdly, transparency and discourse are integral to building bridges with clients and colleagues. "Trade secrets" may gain you notoriety but are anathema to the growth and acceptance of integrative medicine. The common good of the profession and community outweigh your individual gain. Fourthly, the most significant obstacle to implementation of complementary modalities is negative attitudes of colleagues who do not believe in integration. Peer-reviewed publications can go a long way toward changing minds – in one survey, 65% of Primary Care clients said they would be more likely to choose a veterinarian who used acupuncture in their clinic [21]. Seek out information to show the financial and reputational advantages to the practice upon implementing a technique.

Examples of Integration: Following the Path of Those before You

There are many examples in the peer-reviewed literature of integrative medicine [22–24]. The use of the herbal *Yunnan Bai Yao* is standard practice in many veterinary hospitals in the prevention and treatment of hemorrhage [25–27]. The use of acupuncture and western pain medications (NSAIDs and Opioids) for the control of pain and improvement of patient outcomes particularly in IVDD surgery is documented [28]. In one study, patients receiving electro-acupuncture alone had better long-term outcomes than those receiving surgical decompression with or without electro-acupuncture [29]. In cases of shock and anesthetic-induced cardiac and respiratory depression, the use of acupoint stimulation at *GV-26* is documented as an adjunct to western therapies [30]. And there are many equine and small animal emergencies for which acupuncture is a useful adjunct to conventional medicine [31–35]. TCVM has become a mainstay of integrative cancer therapy, enhancing radiation and chemotherapeutic protocols, while decreasing their adverse side-effects [36–39]. Epilepsy [40–43], Atopy [44], KCS [45, 46], chronic renal disease [47–49], Heart failure [4, 50], and inappropriate urination [51] are among many of the small animal diseases in which integrative methods are promising. In horses, laminitis [33, 52], sarcoids [53], musculoskeletal diseases [54, 55], and reproductive diseases [56, 57] all have improved outcomes with integrative techniques. The food animal sector has the potential for huge benefits both in reduced costs for medications, and in drug-residue avoidance in our food supply [58, 59]. A benefit the public would assuredly notice.

The power of integration has been proven and published by combining the theory of TCVM immunity with western vaccinology [60]. Simply by inoculating canine patients with distemper vaccine at a classically important immune-stimulating acupoint (GV-*14*) and comparing the humoral immune response (SN titers) to dogs conventionally vaccinated at a non-acupoint location (control), a significant 4-fold increase in titer was measured in the acupoint vaccinated group. Changing the focus from the vaccine to the host, as TCVM theory predicted, led to a promising approach to enhancing vaccine efficacy. Acupuncture points which have been used for immune modulation include *Bai-hui*, GV-1, GV-14, ST-36, LU-1, and LI-4/10/11 [16]. All these acupoints have the potential to enhance the immune response to a given vaccine administered at the acupoint.

A Final Thought on Integration: The Power to Offer Alternatives and Guide Your Client with Difficult Decisions

Finally, the questions of sustainability and costs in the human and animal medical disciplines have significant potential to benefit from CAM in providing alternatives with all aspects of patient care [61]. Not every client can afford the best that western medicine has to offer. Financial constraints can leave a client filled with guilt and angst, and CAM can offer less costly treatment options. This author was recently presented with a four-month-old Male Havanese-cross dog with bilateral tibial fractures. The previous surgical specialty practice offered two alternatives: surgical stabilization for five to seven thousand dollars or euthanasia. The dog was treated with external support, cage rest, NSAIDs, acupuncture, Chinese herbals, *Tui-na*, and food-therapy....and at eight months of age he runs like the wind – for a cost of approximately four-hundred dollars. The incorporation of complementary medicine in your practice can be rewarding for patient outcome, client satisfaction, and professional development. This book contains a compilation of knowledge and wisdom from experienced clinicians to attain that goal. It is your interest and effort that will be the critical factors in the success of your endeavors. Remember Henry Ford's words – "Whether you think you can, or think you can't, you are right" [62].

References

1 Micozzi, M.S. (2019). *Fundamentals of Complementary, Alternative, and Integrative Medicine*, 6e. St. Louis: Elsevier.

2 Bartholomew, M.D. (2017). A controlled *in*-vitro study comparing efficacy of two commercial antibiotic topical compounds and two Chinese herbal medicine topicals against bacteria cultured from 31 canine pyoderma cases. *AJTCVM* 12 (2): 17–28.

3 Hirsch, D.A., Shiau, D.S., and Xie, H. (2017). A randomized and controlled study of the efficacy of *Yin Qiao San* combined with antibiotics compared to antibiotics alone for the treatment of feline upper respiratory disease. *AJTCVM* 12 (2): 39–47.

4 Beebe, S.E. (2009). Treatment of congestive heart failure with conventional pharmaceuticals plus acupuncture, Chinese herbal medicine, and food therapy in a Toy Poodle dog. *AJTCVM* 4 (2): 48–53.

5 Shizhen, L. (2003). The category of waters. In: *Compendium of Materia Medica: Bencao Gangmu*, 1e, vol. 5, (ed. H. Kaimin, and C. Yousheng), 810–844. Beijing: Foreign Languages Press.

6 Thomas, L. (1983). *The Youngest Science*. New York: Penguin Books.

7 Alfaro, A. (2014). Correlation of acupuncture point sensitivity and lesion location in 259 horses. *AJTCVM* 9 (1): 83–87.

8 Le Jeune, S.S. and Jones, J.H. (2014). Prospective study on the correlation of positive acupuncture scans and lameness in 102 performance horses. *AJTCVM* 9 (2): 33–40.

9 Todd, G. (2014). Gastrointestinal, pancreatic, and hepatobiliary disorders. In: *Practical Guide to Traditional Chinese Veterinary Medicine Small Animal Practice* (ed. H. Xie, L. Wedemeyer, C.L. Chrisman et al.), 335–346. Reddick: Chi University Press.

10 Meier, B. and Nietlispach, F. (2019). Fallacies of Evidence-based medicine in cardiovascular medicine. *Am J Cardiol* 125(4): 690–649.

11 Chrisman, C.L. (2008). Experiencing Tao. *AJTCVM* 3 (1): 76.

12 Ferguson, B. (2009). *Qi-gong* for the TCVM practitioner: introduction. *AJTCVM* 4 (1): 84–86.

13 Smith, B. (2008). *Tai Chi* and Traditional Chinese Veterinary Medicine. *AJTCVM* 3 (1): 74–75.

14 Thoresen, A. (2008). Anthropogenic medicine. *AJTCVM* 3 (1): 4–7.

15 Feng, G.-F. and English, J. (1972). *Lao Tzu's Tao De Ching #64*, 1e. New York: Random House.

16 Xie, H. and Preast, V. (2007). *Xie's Veterinary Acupuncture*, 1e. Reddick: Blackwell Publishing.

17 Xie, H., Ferguson, B., and Deng, X. (2008). *Application of Tui Na in Veterinary Medicine*, 2e. Reddick: Chi Institute of Chinese Medicine.

18 Fowler, M. and Xie, H. (eds.) (2020). *Integrative and Traditional Chinese Veterinary Medicine Food Therapy*, 1e. Reddick: Chi University Press.

19 Memon, M. (2015). TCVM around the world and educational opportunities. *AJTCVM* 10 (2): 10–11.

20 Chrisman, C. (2012). Educational opportunities. *AJTCVM* 7 (1): 81.

21 Marks, D. and Schmalberg, J. (2015). Profitability and financial benefits of acupuncture in small animal private practice. *AJTCVM* 10 (1): 43–48.

22 Selmer, M. and Shiau, D.-S. (2019). Therapeutic results of integrative medicine treatments combining traditional Chinese with western medicine: a systematic review and meta-analysis. *AJTCVM* 14 (1): 41–47.

23 Ma, A. (2015). TCVM research around the world from 2005 to 2015. *AJTCVM* 10 (2): 1–9.

24 Dobos, G. and Tao, I. (2011). The model of western integrative medicine: the role of Chinese medicine. *Chin J Integr Med* 17 (1): 11–20.

25 Tang, Z.-L., Wang, X., Yi, B. et al. (2009). Effects of the preoperative administration of *Yunnan Baiyao* capsules on intraoperative blood loss in bimaxillary orthognathic surgery: a prospective, randomized, double-blind, placebo-controlled study. *Int J Oral Maxofacial Surg* 8 (3): 261–266.

26 Adelman, L.B., Olin, S.J., Egger, C.M. et al. (2017). The effect of oral *Yunnan Baiyao* on periprocedural hemorrhage and coagulation parameters in dogs undergoing nasal biopsy: a randomized, controlled, blinded study. *AJTCVM* 12 (2): 29–38.

27 Egger, C., Gibbs, D., Wheeler, J. et al. (2016). The effect of *Yunnan Baiyao* on platelet activation, buccal mucosal bleeding time, prothrombin time, activated partial thromboplastin time, and thromboelastography in healthy dogs: a randomized, controlled, blinded study. *AJTCVM* 11 (2): 27–36.

28 Laim, A., Jaggy, A., and Forterre, F. (2009). Effects of adjunct electroacupuncture on severity of postoperative pain in dogs undergoing hemilaminectomy because of acute thoracolumbar intervertebral disk disease. *JAVMA* 234 (9): 1141–1146.

29 Joaquim, J.G., Luna, S.P., Brondani, J.T. et al. (2010). Comparison of decompressive surgery, electroacupuncture, and decompressive surgery followed by electroacupuncture for the treatment of dogs with intervertebral disk disease with long-standing severe neurologic deficits. *JAVMA* 236 (11): 1225–1229.

30 Hu, X.-Y., Trevelyan, E., Chai, Q.-Y. et al. (2015). Effectiveness and safety of using acupoint Shui Gou (GV 26): a systematic review and meta-analysis of randomized controlled trials. *Acupunct Related Ther* 3(1): 1–10.

31 Magdesian, K.G. (2011). Common acupoints for equine emergencies. *AJTCVM* 6 (2): 36.

32 Xie, H. and Quick, A. (2012). List of TCVM for emergencies. *AJTCVM* 7 (2): 75.

33 Petermann, U. (2011). Comparison of pre- and post-treatment pain scores of twenty-one horses with laminitis treated with acupoint and topical low level impulse laser therapy. *AJTCVM* 6 (1): 13–25.

34 Song, D., Liu, J., Cao, G. et al. (2015). A retrospective study of 67 cases of equine impaction colic treated with the Chinese herbal medicine *Mu Bing Xiao Huang*. *AJTCVM* 10 (1): 49–53.

35 Fowler, M.P., Shiau, D.-S., and Xie, H. (2017). A randomized controlled study comparing *Da Xiang Lian*

Wan to metronidazole in the treatment of stress colitis in shelter/rescued dogs. *AJTCVM* 12 (1): 45–54.

36 Xie, H. and Hershey, B. (2015). Chinese herbal medicine for the treatment of cancer. *AJTCVM* 10 (1): 69–75.

37 Xie, H., Hershey, B., and Ma, A. (2017). Review of evidence-based clinical and experimental research on the use of acupuncture and Chinese herbal medicine for the treatment or adjunct treatment of cancer. *AJTCVM* 12 (1): 69–77.

38 Raditic, D.M. and Bartges, J.W. (2014). Evidence-based integrative medicine in veterinary oncology. *Vet Clin North Am Small Anim Pract* 44 (5): 831–853.

39 Wen, J. and Johnston, K. (2011). Long-term follow-up of canine mammary gland neoplasia in eight dogs treated with surgery and a new Chinese herbal formula. *AJTCVM* 6 (1): 27–31.

40 Chrisman, C.L. (2015). Traditional Chinese veterinary medicine for idiopathic epilepsy in dogs. *AJTCVM* 10 (1): 63–67.

41 Hayashi, A. and Xie, H. (2015). Review of current research on Chinese herbal medicine for epilepsy. *AJTCVM* 10 (1): 31–42.

42 Klide, A.M., Farnbach, G.C., and Gallagher, S.M. (1987). Acupuncture therapy for the treatment of intractable, idiopathic epilepsy in five dogs. *Acupunct Electrother Res* 12 (1): 71–74.

43 Goiz-Marquez, G., Caballero, S., Solis, H. et al. (2009). Electroencephalographic evaluation of gold wire implants inserted in acupuncture points in dogs with epileptic seizures. *Res Vet Sci* 86 (1): 152–161.

44 Xie, H. and Ma, A. (2015). TCVM for the treatment of pruritus and atopy in dogs. *AJTCVM* 10 (2): 75–80.

45 Xie, H. and Shi, D. (2015). TCVM for the treatment of keratoconjunctivitis sicca in dogs. *AJTCVM* 10 (2): 63–68.

46 Jeon, J.H., Shin, M.S., Lee, M.S. et al. (2010). Acupuncture reduces symptoms of dry eye syndrome: a preliminary observational study. *J Altern Complement Med* 16 (12): 1291–1294.

47 Xiong, W., He, F.-F., You, R.-Y. et al. (2018). Acupuncture application in chronic kidney disease and its potential mechanisms. *Am J Chin Med* 46 (6): 1169–1185.

48 Zhong, Y., Menon, M., Deng, Y. et al. (2015). Recent advances in traditional Chinese medicine for kidney disease. *Am J Kidney Dis* 66 (3): 513–522.

49 Donato, L.J. (2010). Acupuncture, Chinese herbal medicine, Tui-Na, and food therapy integrated with other treatments for chronic renal disease of a cat. *AJTCVM* 5 (2): 61–69.

50 Basko, I.J. (1992). Traditional Chinese medical treatment of heart disease. *Probl Vet Med* 4 (1): 132–135.

51 Ferguson, B. (2017). Feline inappropriate elimination and lower urinary tract inflammation: theoretical background and simple management with acupuncture and Chinese herbal medicine. *AJTCVM* 12 (1): 85–88.

52 Sumano Lopez, H., Hoyas Sepulveda, M.L., and Brumbaugh, G.W. (1999). Pharmacologic and alternative therapies for the horse with chronic laminitis. *Vet Clin North Am Equine Pract* 15 (2): 495–516.

53 Thoresen, A.S. (2011). Outcome of horses with sarcoids treated with acupuncture at a single *Ting* point: 18 cases (1995–2009). *AJTCVM* 6 (2): 29–35.

54 Xie, H., Wedemeyer, L., Chrisman, C.L., and Kim, M.S. (eds.) (2015). *Practical Guide to Traditional Chinese Veterinary Medicine Equine Practice*. Reddick: Chi University Press.

55 Haussler, K.K., Hesbach, A.L., Romano, L. et al. (2021). A systematic review of musculoskeletal mobilization and manipulation techniques used in veterinary medicine. *Animals* 11 (10): 2787. doi: 10.3390/ani11102787.

56 Rathgeber, R.A. (2011). Use of acupuncture in equine reproduction. *AAEP Proc* 57: 138–140.

57 Carson, B. (2015). TCVM for equine reproduction. In: *Practical Guide to Traditional Chinese Veterinary Medicine Equine Practice* (ed. H. Xie, L. Wedemeyer, C.L. Chrisman, and M.S. Kim), 219–251. Reddick: Chi University Press.

58 Gao, J., Wang, R., Liu, J. et al. (2022). Effects of novel microecologics combined with traditional Chinese medicine and probiotics on growth performance and health of broilers. *Poult Sci* 101 (2): 101412.

59 Chen, J., Guo, K., and Song, X. et al. (2020). The anti-heat stress effects of Chinese herbal medicine prescriptions and rumen-protected γ-aminobutyric acid on growth performance, apparent nutrient digestibility, and health status in beef cattle. *Anim Sci J* 91 (1): e13361. doi: 10.1111/asj.13361.

60 Perdrizet, J., Shiau, D., and Xie, H. (2019). The effect of acupoint vaccination at GV-14 on the serological response to canine distemper virus vaccine in dogs. *Vaccine* 37 (13): 1889–1896.

61 Lin, J.H., Kaphle, K., Wu, L.S. et al. (2003). Sustainable veterinary medicine for the new era. *Rev Sci Tech* 22 (3): 949–946.

62 "Henry Ford Quotes." BrainyQuote.com BrainyMedia Inc, 2023. https://www.brainyquote.com/quotes/henry_ford_131621

Section II

Acupuncture
(Section Editor – Huisheng Xie)

4

Anatomy and Physiology of Acupuncture
Emily Mangan

Introduction

Traditional Chinese veterinary medicine (TCVM) is a complex and self-referential medical paradigm that relies on the Taoist observation of the known world for explanation of medical phenomenon [1]. TCVM describes the use of four modalities for the treatment of disease: Acupuncture, Chinese herbal medicine, food therapy, and *Tui-na* (a form of medical massage) [1]. Acupuncture has been used to relieve pain and treat disease in veterinary species for more than 2,000 years, and the modality has quickly become the most commonly used TCVM modality in the West [2–9]. This increase in popularity is due to the long history of use, increasing body of scientific evidence to support its safety and efficacy, and its entrance into the public sphere following the NIH Consensus Conference in 1997 and subsequent recognition by the World Health Organization in 1999 [4–7, 9–12]. The rise in popularity of acupuncture in veterinary medicine has closely mirrored the rise of acupuncture popularity in human medicine [4–7].

Acupuncture involves the stimulation of specific anatomical locations on the body, called acupuncture points or acupoints, to produce local and systemic effects [10, 13]. Stimulation of acupuncture points is typically accomplished with thin filiform needles, however, additional methods of stimulation have been described [9, 14]. Acupuncture is minimally invasive, relatively inexpensive, and has few counterindications [9, 15]. Acupuncture has been shown to be effective for a variety of diseases in veterinary species including pain due to injury or post-surgery, anxiety, laminitis, lameness, sarcoidosis, laryngeal hemiplegia, and improving metabolic capacity, as well as a variety of ophthalmological, cardiovascular, respiratory, gastrointestinal, and reproductive disorders [9, 15–26]. As further clinical studies of acupuncture continue to establish efficacy for use, so has the desire of the scientific community to fully elucidate the anatomy and physiologic function of acupuncture and the medical system from which it originates [9, 15, 27]. Scientific studies conducted over the last few decades have elucidated anatomical distinctions of meridians and acupuncture points, as well as physiologic mechanisms for documented effects [27, 28].

Evidence of the Existence of Meridians

Acupuncture relies on the TCVM concept of meridians, which are described as a complex and interconnected network of channels throughout the entire body, connecting the internal organs with each other and the exterior [29]. There are 12 Regular Meridians, each named after their respective TCVM organ, and two extraordinary channels that are commonly discussed in English literature, although there exists a wide variety of named meridians as part of the whole network, which is collectively called *Jing Luo* [29, 30]. Within the TCVM theory, meridians function to carry *Qi* (energy) throughout the body, and acupuncture works to balance this flow of *Qi* within meridians by stimulating acupoints along the meridians [27, 31, 32]. There are 361 transpositional acupuncture points identified on the body, and they are typically found where meridians travel close to the body's surface, and are therefore accessible to manipulation [32, 33].

After the initial studies demonstrating acupuncture efficacy, interest grew in illuminating acupuncture anatomy and mechanisms due to the reasonable and obvious desire to describe the existence of the TCVM meridians. Early studies from the 1980s were performed by injecting technetium-99m as a radiotracer into acupuncture points and found that the radioisotope spread preferentially along meridians, and that injections into non-acupuncture points did not spread in this manner [30, 34, 35].

Integrative Veterinary Medicine, First Edition. Edited by Mushtaq A. Memon and Huisheng Xie.
© 2023 John Wiley & Sons, Inc. Published 2023 by John Wiley & Sons, Inc.
Companion Website: www.wiley.com/go/memon/veterinary

More recent studies providing evidence of the existence of meridians included those that identified propagation of acoustic emission signals from acupoint stimulation along meridians [8, 36], identification that acupoints and meridians had higher electrical conductance and capacitance and lower electrical resistance and impedance compared to surrounding tissues [36–38], and that heat applied to acupoints (but not non-acupoints) would spread along meridians [8, 39]. Yet others have investigated optical [40], magnetic [8], and myoelectrical activities of meridians to differentiate them from surrounding tissues, with positive results [8].

These studies have shown that there exist mechanisms by which to identify meridians from non-meridians, and that allow preferential movement of fluid, electrical current, heat, and light to move within meridians. This is in alignment with proposed meridian functions in accordance with TCVM principles established thousands of years ago, and should encourage further research [30].

Anatomy of Meridians

Although the precise anatomical structure of meridians has yet to be fully elucidated, proposed natures of meridians can be divided into four schools of thought: nerve conduction, interstitial fluid circulation, bioelectrical fields, and connective tissues or fascia [30]. The numerous properties of meridians identified with scientific investigation lends support to these theories, however, of the proposed theories, there is the most scientific evidence available currently in support the neuroanatomical explanation of meridians.

First, studies have shown that meridians correlate with the anatomy of the peripheral nervous system [27]. Second, acupuncture results in a cascade of neurophysiological effects within the spinal cord and brain [27, 41]. Third, studies have shown that the immediate effects of acupuncture are diminished or negated with application of local anesthetic or transection of the peripheral sensory nerve, which indicates that a functional peripheral nervous system is necessary for acupuncture effects [41–43]. It is important to note that while anesthesia or transection of the nerve diminishes the systemic effects of acupuncture, acupuncture stimulation has also been found to stimulate nerve regeneration, and may be helpful for recovery from neurologic injury [44].

When evaluated concurrently, these facts are supportive of a neuroanatomical theory and the alternate proposed structures of fascial, lymphatic, and extracellular fluids, are not as well supported as a single explanation [27]. However, it is likely that acupuncture functions through a variety of mechanisms, and may therefore utilize a variety of anatomical structures for full effect [30]. Because the field of scientific inquiry into TCVM is relatively young, it is likely that additional structures and mechanisms will continue to be proposed and investigated. That being so, currently there is overwhelming evidence from fundamental scientific studies and clinical trials supporting a neuro-anatomic/neurophysiologic basis as a model of meridian structure and function [27].

The advent of advanced diagnostic imaging, such as MRI and high-resolution scintigraphy, have allowed for a more extensive anatomical study of meridians. Classic dissection studies have contributed specific and important foundational information, but frequently small vessels, nerves, and fascia may be accidentally obliterated in the preparation of specimens, even by skilled anatomists. These advanced imaging techniques allow visualization of structures in vivo.

Several striking correlations have been found to support the theory of meridians mirroring peripheral nerves [27]. The Spleen meridian, which courses along the medial aspect of the pelvic limb, directly overlays with the saphenous nerve, and the Lung meridian, which is present on the medial aspect of the thoracic limb, follows the musculocutaneous and lateral antebrachial cutaneous nerves from the upper extremity all the way to the first digit [27, 45]. Similar overlap between meridian and peripheral nerve can be identified with the femoral nerve and distal saphenous sensory nerve branch, as well as every other of the 14 commonly discussed meridians (Table 4.1) [27, 45].

Embryologic studies provide additional evidence for anatomic correlations of meridians [45, 46]. These studies of the development of the nervous system have shown that meridians are well-correlated with the formation of dermatomes in the embryo, which applies both to the development of peripheral nerves in the extremities as well as the trunk [27, 45–47].

Table 4.1 Meridians and associated peripheral nerves.

Meridian	Peripheral Nerve
Large Intestine	Radial
Triple Heater	Radial/posterior interosseous
Small Intestine	Ulnar
Heart	Ulnar
Pericardium	Medial/anterior interosseous
Lung	Musculocutaneous
Liver	Obturator/tibial
Spleen	Femoral (medial branch)
Stomach	Femoral (lateral branch)/deep peroneal
Gallbladder	Sciatic/superficial peroneal/medial plantar
Bladder	Sciatic/tibial/lateral plantar
Kidney	Sciatic/tibial/lateral plantar

Anatomy of Acupuncture Points

Within the theory of TCVM, acupuncture points are locations along meridians near the body surface where *Qi*, or energy, accumulates and are typically depressions that can be externally palpated [48]. Anatomically, the locations of acupuncture points can be characterized into four categories: where peripheral neurovascular bundles bifurcate, penetrate through body fascia, innervate muscles, or innervate tendons [33, 49, 50]. While these characteristics of acupuncture points were first identified in the 1970s, the four categories remain accurate identifiers of acupuncture points in relation to the gross anatomy of the nervous system. These locations of acupuncture points also support the neuroanatomical theory of acupuncture, as they correlate with the structure of peripheral nerves.

In addition to identification of gross anatomy correlations, the characteristics of acupuncture points from a histological perspective have also been investigated [33]. Acupuncture points contain a high density of free nerve endings (specifically Aδ and C nociceptive nerve fibers, as well as non-nociceptive Aβ and Aα nerve fibers,) [32] arterioles and venules, lymphatics, and mast cells, all compared to density in surrounding tissue [48, 51]. Similar studies performed at the meridian level also inform the knowledge base of acupuncture points, mainly that these points have similar characteristics, such as high electrical conductivity and low impudence, as meridians [48]. The electrical properties of acupuncture points and meridians can be partially explained by a high density of gap junctions between cellular components, which facilitate conductance via nitric oxide (NO) [48, 52].

Along the Bladder Channel, there exist acupuncture points (called Back-*shu* acupoints) which are present lateral to the spine bilaterally [33]. In TCVM, treatment of Back-*shu* points influences specific organs and regions in the body. The location of these acupuncture points correlates with spinal nerve roots, and the associated organs said to be affected by stimulating these points have been shown to correlate with the emergence of the spinal nerves that innervate these organs [27, 47]. A recent study utilized MRI contrast to evaluate the TCVM principle of Back-*shu* acupoints [53]. Mice and rats were injected with MRI contrast agents into Back-*shu* acupoints and the migration of the contrast was followed with MRI. The final distribution of the contrast was found to be associated with the internal organ associated with the acupuncture points with TCVM philosophy [53]. This study, while preliminary, is supportive of the TCVM philosophy and invites further research into the topic of anatomical associations of acupoints beyond the well-documented analgesic effects [32, 54, 55].

The Mechanisms of Action of Acupuncture

A variety of theories to describe the effects of acupuncture have been proposed over the last few decades, ranging from fascial to endocrine to neurological [27]. Early studies determined that effects of acupuncture could not be ablated with the application of a proximal tourniquet, which dispelled the theory that effects of acupuncture were solely vascularly mediated [27]. Other early studies found that acupuncture resulted in analgesia, which could be reversed with administration of naloxone, identifying that opioids were an important mechanism [56]. Similar studies also identified that acupuncture was less effective or ineffective when the peripheral nerve was blocked with local anesthetic or transected, which supports the neurophysiological theory [41–43]. While these early studies lacked finesse, they demonstrated that acupuncture requires sensory nerve function as well as inciting centrally-mediated effects [27].

One of the studied acupuncture phenomena is the concept of *De-Qi*, which means the arrival of *Qi*, and defines the moment when acupuncture stimulation is felt or perceived by the patient [13, 57]. *De-Qi* is described as feeling like a heavy, dull, aching pull within the acupuncture point, and can be identified by both the patient and the practitioner placing the needle [13, 57]. Scientifically, *De-Qi* is important for the effect of acupuncture, as it coincides with onset of analgesic effects and correlates with efficacy of acupuncture in that patient [13, 57]. Activation of the thalamus as observed with fMRI is well-correlated with the *De-Qi* sensation during electroacupuncture [27].

Recent technical advancements in biological sciences as well as research methodologies have allowed the formation of an impressive library of high-quality literature on the subject of acupuncture anatomy, mechanisms, and clinical use [27]. There is good evidence now that the mechanisms of acupuncture are neurophysiological in nature and that acupuncture exerts its effects at all levels of the nervous system, which may be characterized as local, segmental (spinal cord), and suprasegmental (brain) effects [10, 27, 47, 48, 58]. Acupuncture for analgesia is a heavily studied topic both in mechanism and in clinical application, with the majority of mechanistic studies focusing on elucidation of analgesic principles [28, 32, 54, 55, 59].

Local Effects of Acupuncture

Local stimulation begins with the insertion of a needle, which functions first as a mechanical irritant. Stimulation of acupuncture points is considered a form of counterirritation, whereby manipulation of the needle results in mechanical and chemical sensory stimulation of local tissues that creates the impetus for a variety of cascades [48]. Stimulation by the needle itself and subsequent deformation of the fascia, induces a local inflammatory response by release of inflammatory mediators including prostaglandins, leukotrienes, bradykinin, and platelet activating factor (Figure 4.1) [48, 51]. Acupoints contain a high concentration of mast cells, which degranulate upon stimulation [60, 61]. Mast cell degranulation is responsible for release of histamine, heparin, kinin protease, and ATP, which results in the clinically evident effect of local hyperemia (visible in non-pigmented skin in hairless regions) and contributes to sensory stimulation [60, 61]. ATP and the metabolite adenosine both serve as neurotransmitters centrally and peripherally, inciting their own cascades [48, 62, 63].

Acupuncture stimulates local nerve fibers mechanically and chemically, including Aδ and C nociceptive nerve fibers and Aβ and Aα non-nociceptive nerve fibers, which are abundantly present in acupuncture points compared to surrounding tissue [48, 51]. Stimulation of sympathetic nerve fibers results in increased release of endogenous opioids (β-endorphins and enkephalins), which mitigate local nociception [48]. Other sources of endogenous opioids include acupuncture-induced release from lymphocytes, macrophages, and granulocytes [58]. Acupuncture also decreases the levels of local inflammatory cytokines, such as tumor necrosis factor-α (TNFα), interleukin 6 (IL-6), and interleukin 1β (IL-1β), which is also proposed to be mediated through endogenous opioids [48, 49].

While the culmination of these effects is complex to parse, the net sum of effect within the tissue is anti-inflammatory and anti-nociceptive. There is a wide variety of local mechanisms that both stimulate and inhibit inflammatory cascades and release endogenous opioids, which interact with a variety of receptors for downstream effect. Local effects are also likely the cause of *De-Qi*, which is important to achieve for acupuncture efficacy. The majority of local mechanisms have clear indications for antinociceptive effects and less clear indications for the other proposed functions of acupuncture. However, the majority of scientific studies have been designed to evaluate the use of acupuncture analgesia specifically, and it is likely there are additional mechanisms that have yet to be elucidated.

Segmental (Spinal Cord) Effects of Acupuncture

Segmental and suprasegmental effects of acupuncture cannot be discussed entirely mutually exclusively from each other, as they are anatomically and physiologically related [48]. However, there are segmental- and suprasegmental-specific actions which are apparent.

Acupuncture stimulation suppresses N-methyl-D-aspartate (NMDA) receptors within the dorsal horn of the spinal cord via endogenous opioids, noradrenaline, and serotonin, which is a well-known anti-nociception mechanism [48, 55]. Acupuncture also suppresses the activities of glial cells within the spinal cord, which results in decreased release of nociceptive-promoting cytokines, including IL-1β, IL-6, TNFα, COX-2, and PGE2 [48, 64, 65].

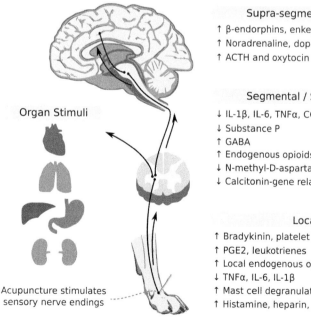

Supra-segmental / Brain
↑ β-endorphins, enkephalins
↑ Noradrenaline, dopamine, serotonin
↑ ACTH and oxytocin

Segmental / Spinal Cord
↓ IL-1β, IL-6, TNFα, COX-2, and PGE2
↓ Substance P
↑ GABA
↑ Endogenous opioids
↓ N-methyl-D-aspartate receptors
↓ Calcitonin-gene related peptide

Local
↑ Bradykinin, platelet activating factor
↑ PGE2, leukotrienes
↑ Local endogenous opioids
↓ TNFα, IL-6, IL-1β
↑ Mast cell degranulation
↑ Histamine, heparin, kinin protease, ATP

Organ Stimuli

Acupuncture stimulates sensory nerve endings

ACTH = adrenocorticotropic hormone, IL-1β = interleukin-1β, IL-6 = interleukin-6, TNFα = tumor necrosis factor-α
COX-2 = cyclooxygenase-2, PGE2 = prostaglandin E2, GABA = γ-amino-butyric acid, ATP = adenosine triphosphate

Figure 4.1 Selected effects of acupuncture at the local, segmental, and suprasegmental levels.

Release of substance P within the spinal cord gray matter is also inhibited by acupuncture stimulation. As substance P typically promotes nociceptive signals and activates glial cells, the inhibition of release of substance P functions to suppress nociception [66]. In addition, acupuncture also deceases calcitonin-gene related peptide (CGRP) release at the synapses between dorsal root ganglion and dorsal horn neurons, as well as increases the release of γ-amino-butyric acid (GABA) at these synapses, which are both inhibitory for nociception [67]. The increase of serotonin within the spinal release previously discussed also functions to accentuate the efficiency of GABA to inhibit nociception signaling [58, 68].

Suprasegmental (Brain) Effects of Acupuncture

With the application of advanced neuroimaging techniques, such as functional magnetic resonance imaging (fMRI), single-photon emission computed tomography (SPECT), and position emission tomography (PET), acupuncture has been shown to activate numerous brain regions in humans, including nucleus raphe magnus in the medulla, locus coeruleus of the pons, hypothalamus, and periaqueductal gray matter of the mesencephalon [10, 41, 48, 54, 55, 59, 69, 70]. These regions are directly or indirectly involved in mitigation of nociception by suppressing neurons of the dorsal horn via β-endorphins, enkephalins, noradrenaline, dopamine, and serotonin [48]. The pituitary gland is also stimulated by acupuncture and releases adrenocorticotropic hormone (ACTH) and oxytocin into the vascular system, which have also been shown to be anti-noticeptive [48].

In another study of acupuncture-induced brain region activation using fMRI, the changes in activity of the thalamus, basal ganglia, and cerebellum due to acupuncture were eliminated with brachial plexus anesthetic block [27, 41].

The majority of research investigating suprasegmental effects has focused on analgesic effects of acupuncture. However, based on the wide variety of brain region activation in response to acupoint stimulation, it is likely that additional, non-analgesic mechanisms are activated by acupuncture that have yet to be investigated.

Summary

Acupuncture has been utilized to treat disease in veterinary species for 2,000 years. In the last few decades, scientific inquiry has demonstrated that acupuncture meridians correlate with anatomical structures, including peripheral nerves, sympathetic ganglion, lymphatic vessels, the vascular system, and fascial planes. A variety of studies into the composition of acupuncture points themselves have found a high density of lymphatics, arterioles and venules, mast cells, and free nerve endings compared to surrounding tissue. Stimulation of acupuncture points results in a cascade of local and central nervous system-mediated effects. Local effects include release of leukotrienes, prostaglandins, bradykinin, and mast cell degranulation, as well as release of local endogenous opioids to culminate in anti-nociceptive and anti-inflammatory effects. Segmental effects include dynorphin and enkephalin release within the central nervous system, which results in neuromodulation within the spinal cord and accounts for various analgesic effects. Suprasegmental effects include activation of various brain regions associated with release of serotonin, endogenous opioids, and other substances which decrease nociception.

The majority of clinical studies have evaluated acupuncture for anti-inflammatory and analgesic properties, although studies investigating uses besides analgesia have shown positive results. While great progress has been made in the last few decades, more research is necessary to fully elucidate acupuncture mechanisms and their clinical applications.

References

1 Gu, S. and Pei, J. (2017). Innovating Chinese herbal medicine: from traditional health practice to scientific drug discovery. *Front Pharmacol* 8: 381.

2 Yu, C. (1995). *Traditional Chinese Veterinary Acupuncture and Moxibustion*. China Agriculture Press.

3 Xie, H. and Chrisman, C. (2009). Equine acupuncture: from ancient art to modern validation. *Am J Trad Chin Vet Med* 4: 1–4.

4 Shmalberg, J. and Memon, M.A. (2015). A retrospective analysis of 5,195 patient treatment sessions in an integrative veterinary medicine service: patient characteristics, presenting complaints, and therapeutic interventions. *Vet Med Int* 2015: 1–11.

5 Memon, M.A. and Sprunger, L.K. (2011). Survey of colleges and schools of veterinary medicine regarding education in complementary and alternative veterinary medicine. *J Am Vet Med Assoc* 239: 619–623.

6 Hunley, S. and Xie, H. (2011). Veterinary acupuncture: current use, trends and opinions. *Am J Tradit Chin Vet Med* 6: 55–62.

7 Xie, H. and Holyoak, G.R. (2021). Evidence-based applications of acupuncture in equine practice. *Am J Tradit Chin Vet Med* 16.

8 Li, J., Wang, Q., Liang, H. et al. (2012). Biophysical characteristics of meridians and acupoints: a systematic review. *Evid Based Complement Alternat Med* 2012: e793841.

9 Xie, H. and Wedemeyer, L. (2012). The validity of acupuncture in veterinary medicine. *Am J Tradit Chin Vet Med* 7: 35–43.

10 Tang, Y., Yin, H.-Y., Rubini, P. et al. (2016). Acupuncture-induced analgesia: a neurobiological basis in purinergic signaling. *Neuroscientist* 22: 563–578.

11 National Institutes of Health (1998). NIH consensus conference: acupuncture. *Jama* 280: 1518–1524.

12 World Health Organization (2020). WHO benchmarks for the practice of acupuncture. Geneva: World Health Organization. https://apps.who.int/iris/handle/10665/340838 (accessed 4 April 2022).

13 Zhang, H., Han, G., and Litscher, G. (2019). Traditional acupuncture meets modern nanotechnology: opportunities and perspectives. *Evid Based Complement Alternat Med* 2019: e2146167.

14 Pellegrini, D.Z., Müller, T.R., Fonteque, J.H. et al. (2020). Equine acupuncture methods and applications: a review. *Equine Vet Educ* 32: 268–277.

15 Xie, H. and Ortiz-Umpierre, C. (2006). What acupuncture can and cannot treat. *J Am Anim Hosp Assoc* 42: 244–248.

16 Xie, H., Colahan, P., and Ott, E.A. (2005). Evaluation of electroacupuncture treatment of horses with signs of chronic thoracolumbar pain. *J Am Vet Med Assoc* 227: 281–286.

17 Faramarzi, B., Lee, D., May, K. et al. (2017). Response to acupuncture treatment in horses with chronic laminitis. *Can Vet J* 58: 823–827.

18 Lee, D., May, K., and Faramarzi, B. (2019). Comparison of first and second acupuncture treatments in horses with chronic laminitis. *Iran J Vet Res* 20: 9.

19 Dunkel, B., Pfau, T., Fiske-Jackson, A. et al. (2017). A pilot study of the effects of acupuncture treatment on objective and subjective gait parameters in horses. *Vet Anaesth Analg* 44: 154–162.

20 Thoresen, A.S. (2011). Outcome of horses with sarcoids treated with acupuncture at a single ting point: 18 cases (1995–2009). *Am J Tradit Chin Vet Med* 6: 29.

21 Kim, M.-S. and Xie, H. (2009). Use of electroacupuncture to treat laryngeal hemiplegia in horses. *Vet Rec* 165: 602–603.

22 Rungsri, P., Trinarong, C., Rojanasthien, S. et al. (2009). The effectiveness of electro-acupuncture on pain threshold in sport horses with back pain. *Am J Tradit Chin Vet Med* 4: 22–26.

23 Bello, C.A.O., Vianna, A.R.C.B., Noqueira, K. et al. (2018). Acupuncture in the restoration of vasomotor tonus of equine athletes with back pain. *J Dairy Vet Anim Res* 7.

24 Ying, W., Bhattacharjee, A., and Wu, S.S. (2019). Effect of laser acupuncture on mitigating anxiety in acute stressed horses: a randomized, controlled study. *Am J Tradit Chin Vet Med* 14: 33–40.

25 Aljobory, A.I., Jaafar, S., and Ahmed, A.S. (2021). Using acupuncture and electroacupuncture in the treatment of laminitis in racing horses: a comparative study. *Iraqi J Vet Sci* 35: 15–21.

26 Angeli, A.L. and Luna, S.P.L. (2008). Aquapuncture improves metabolic capacity in thoroughbred horses. *J Equine Vet Sci* 28: 525–531.

27 Dorsher, P.T. and da Silva, M.A.H. (2022). Acupuncture's neuroanatomic and neurophysiologic basis. *Longhua Chin Med* 5: 8–8.

28 Ma, Y., Dong, M., Zhou, K. et al. (2016). Publication trends in acupuncture research: a 20-year bibliometric analysis based on PubMed. *PLOS ONE* 11: e0168123.

29 Chrisman, C.L. and Xie, H. (2013). The Jing Luo network: an overview of channels and collaterals and their clinical applications. *Am J Tradit Chin Vet Med* 8: 1–13.

30 Chrisman, C.L. and Xie, H. (2011). Research support for the Jing Luo system. *Am J Tradit Chin Vet Med* 6: 1–4.

31 Longhurst, J.C. (2010). Defining meridians: a modern basis of understanding. *J Acupunct Meridian Stud* 3: 67–74.

32 Zhao, Z.-Q. (2008). Neural mechanism underlying acupuncture analgesia. *Prog Neurobiol* 85: 355–375.

33 Xie, H. and Preast, V. (2007). *Xie's Veterinary Acupuncture*. Blackwell Publishing.

34 Kovacs, F.M., Götzens García, V.J., García, A. et al. (1992). Experimental study on radioactive pathways of hypodermically injected technetium-99m. *J Nucl Med* 33 (3): 403–407.

35 Lazorthes, Y., Esquerré, J.-P., Simon, J. et al. (1990). Acupuncture meridians and radiotracers. *Pain* 40: 109–112.

36 Lee, M.S., Jeong, S.-Y., Lee, Y.-H. et al. (2005). Differences in electrical conduction properties between meridians and non-meridians. *Am J Chin Med* 33: 723–728.

37 Falk, C.X., Birch, S., Avants, S.K. et al. (2000). Preliminary results of a new method for locating auricular acupuncture points. *Acupunct Electrother Res* 25: 165–177.

38 Jeong, D.-M., Lee, Y.-H., and Lee, M.S. (2004). Development of the meridian-visualizing system that superimposes a bio-signal upon a body image. *Am J Chin Med* 32: 631–640.

39 Wang, P.Q., Hu, X.L., and Xu, J.S. (2002). The indication of infrared thermal images on … – Google Scholar. *Acupuncture Res* 27: 260.

40 Liu, X., Chen, C., Yu, J. et al. (2010). Light propagation characteristics of meridian and surrounding non-meridian tissue. *Acta Photonica Sin* 39: 29–33.

41 Gu, W., Jiang, W., He, J. et al. (2015). Blockade of the brachial plexus abolishes activation of specific brain regions by electroacupuncture at LI4: a functional MRI study. *Acupunct Med* 33: 457–464.

42 Lu, G.W. (1983). Characteristics of afferent fiber innervation on acupuncture points zusanli. *Am J Physiol-Regul Integr Comp Physiol* 245: R606–R612.

43 Dundee, J.W. and Ghaly, G. (1991). Local anesthesia blocks the antiemetic action of P6 acupuncture. *Clin Pharmacol Ther* 50: 78–80.

44 Wang, H., Cui, J., Zhao, S. et al. (2021). Progress on the experimental research of sciatic nerve injury with acupuncture. *Evid Based Complement Alternat Med* 2021: e1401756.

45 Dorsher, P.T. (2017). Neuroembryology of the acupuncture principal meridians: part 1. The extremities. *Med Acupunct* 29: 10–19.

46 Dorsher, P.T. (2017). Neuroembryology of the acupuncture principal meridians: part 2. The trunk. *Med Acupunct* 29: 77–86.

47 Cheng, K.J. (2011). Neuroanatomical characteristics of acupuncture points: relationship between their anatomical locations and traditional clinical indications. *Acupunct Med* 29: 289–294.

48 Dewey, C.W. and Xie, H. (2021). The scientific basis of acupuncture for veterinary pain management: a review based on relevant literature from the last two decades. *Open Vet J* 11: 203–209.

49 Zhou, W. and Benharash, P. (2014). Effects and mechanisms of acupuncture based on the principle of meridians. *J Acupunct Meridian Stud* 7: 190–193.

50 Maurer, N., Nissel, H., Egerbacher, M. et al. (2019). Anatomical evidence of acupuncture meridians in the human extracellular matrix: results from a macroscopic and microscopic interdisciplinary multicentre study on human corpses. *Evid Based Complement Alternat Med* 2019: 1–8.

51 Zhang, Z.-J., Wang, X.-M., and McAlonan, G.M. (2012). Neural acupuncture unit: a new concept for interpreting effects and mechanisms of acupuncture. *Evid Based Complement Alternat Med* 2012: e429412.

52 Ma, S. (2017). Nitric oxide signaling molecules in acupoints: toward mechanisms of acupuncture. *Chin J Integr Med* 23: 812–815.

53 Kim, J., Bae, K.-H., Hong, K.-S. et al. (2009). Magnetic resonance imaging and acupuncture: a feasibility study on the migration of tracers after injection at acupoints of small animals. *J Acupunct Meridian Stud* 2: 152–158.

54 Wang, S.-M., Kain, Z.N., and White, P. (2008). Acupuncture analgesia: I. The scientific basis. *Anesth Analg* 106: 602.

55 Fry, L.M., Neary, S.M., Sharrock, J. et al. (2014). Acupuncture for analgesia in veterinary medicine. *Top Companion Anim Med* 29: 35–42.

56 Pomeranz, B. and Chiu, D. (1976). Naloxone blockade of acupuncture analgesia: endorphin implicated. *Life Sci* 19: 1757–1762.

57 MacPherson, H. and Asghar, A. (2006). Acupuncture needle sensations associated with De Qi: a classification based on experts' ratings. *J Altern Complement Med* 12: 633–637.

58 Zhang, R., Lao, L., Ren, K. et al. (2014). Mechanisms of acupuncture–electroacupuncture on persistent pain. *Anesthesiology* 120: 482–503.

59 Staud, R. and Price, D.D. (2006). Mechanisms of acupuncture analgesia for clinical and experimental pain. *Expert Rev Neurother* 6: 661–667.

60 Yin, N., Yang, H., Yao, W. et al. (2018). Mast cells and nerve signal conduction in acupuncture. *Evid Based Complement Alternat Med* https://www.hindawi.com/journals/ecam/2018/3524279 (accessed 16 January 2019).

61 Wu, M.-L., Xu, D.-S., Bai, W.-Z. et al. (2015). Local cutaneous nerve terminal and mast cell responses to manual acupuncture in acupoint LI4 area of the rats. *J Chem Neuroanat* 68: 14–21.

62 Takano, T., Chen, X., Luo, F. et al. (2012). Traditional acupuncture triggers a local increase in adenosine in human subjects. *J Pain* 13: 1215–1223.

63 He, J.-R., Yu, S.-G., Tang, Y. et al. (2020). Purinergic signaling as a basis of acupuncture-induced analgesia. *Purinergic Signal* 16: 297–304.

64 Lin, L., Skakavac, N., Lin, X. et al. (2016). Acupuncture-induced analgesia: the role of microglial inhibition. *Cell Transplant* 25: 621–628.

65 Liang, Y., Qiu, Y., Du, J. et al. (2016). Inhibition of spinal microglia and astrocytes contributes to the anti-allodynic effect of electroacupuncture in neuropathic pain induced by spinal nerve ligation. *Acupunct Med* 34: 40–47.

66 McDonald, J.L., Cripps, A.W., and Smith, P.K. (2015). Mediators, receptors, and signaling pathways in the anti-inflammatory and antihyperalgesic effects of acupuncture. *Evid Based Complement Alternat Med* 2015: e975632.

67 Qiao, L., Liu, J., Tan, L. et al. (2017). Effect of electroacupuncture on thermal pain threshold and expression of calcitonin-gene related peptide, substance P and γ-aminobutyric acid in the cervical dorsal root ganglion of rats with incisional neck pain. *Acupunct Med* 35: 276–283.

68 Chen, S., Wang, S., Rong, P. et al. (2014). Acupuncture for visceral pain: neural substrates and potential mechanisms. *Evid Based Complement Alternat Med* 2014: e609594.

69 Lewith, G.T., White, P.J., and Pariente, J. (2005). Investigating acupuncture using brain imaging techniques: the current state of play. *Evid Based Complement Alternat Med* 2: 315–319.

70 Fan, A.Y., Miller, D.W., Bolash, B. et al. (2017). Acupuncture's role in solving the opioid epidemic: evidence, cost-effectiveness, and care availability for acupuncture as a primary, non-pharmacologic method for pain relief and management–white paper 2017. *J Integr Med* 15: 411–425.

5

Traditional Chinese Medical Foundation of Veterinary Acupuncture
Emily Mangan

Brief History of Acupuncture

Traditional Chinese veterinary medicine (TCVM) has been used for the treatment and prevention of disease in veterinary species for 4,000 years, and has utilized acupuncture in horses for the last 2,000 years [1]. Common TCVM modalities include acupuncture, Chinese herbal medicine, *Tui-na*, and food therapy [1]. The oldest surviving text describing a complete and organized system of diagnosis and treatment using acupuncture in humans was *The Yellow Emperor's Classic of Internal Medicine*, dated around 100 BCE [2]. This text described channels within the body in which *Qi*, or vital energy, flowed, as well as the current Taoist philosophies of the time. Later, during the Ming Dynasty (1368–1644), *The Great Compendium of Acupuncture and Moxibustion* was published, which formed the foundation of modern acupuncture [2]. However, there exist records of application of Chinese medicine in horses long before these texts were published.

Some of the earliest records of the application of Chinese medicine in veterinary species describe the practitioner, *Zao Fu*, treating horses with acupuncture during the *Zhou-my-gong* period (947–928 BCE), and the equine veterinary practitioner *Bo Le*, who lived from 659–621 BCE, treating horses and selecting good racehorses from unproven stock (Figure 5.1) [1]. *Bo Le's Canon of Veterinary Acupuncture* is considered the first true and complete veterinary text and included diagrams of equine acupuncture points (Figure 5.2) [1].

The number of veterinary texts available continued to grow over the next millennia, with *Collection of Effective Prescriptions for Equine Diseases* written by *Wang Yu* during the Song dynasty (960–1279 CE), *Treatment of Sick Horses* written by *Bian Guan-gou* during the Yuan dynasty (1279–1368 CE), and *Yuan-Heng's Therapeutic Treatise of Horses* written by *Yu Benyuan* and *Yu Benheng* in 1608 CE [1].

In the 1950s and 1960s, acupuncture had made its way to the West and European veterinarians began investigating its use in horses [1]. However, it wasn't until the 1970s that veterinary acupuncture was introduced to the United States [1]. Despite the long history of use, the scientific method has only been applied to acupuncture within the last 50 years.

Acupuncture does not exist in a vacuum, but rather, is a unique treatment modality in an intricate medical system that has come to be known as traditional Chinese veterinary medicine. The Taoism that formed the foundation of Chinese medicine was based on observation of the natural cycle of the world, including the passing of the seasons, the phases of the moon, and the birth and death of organisms.

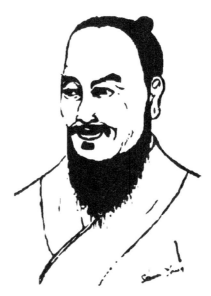

Figure 5.1 Portrait of *Sun Yang (Bo Le)*, an equine veterinary specialist during the *Qing-mu-gong* period (659–621 BCE) [1] From Xie H, Chrisman C. Equine acupuncture: from ancient art to modern validation. Am J Trad Chin Vet Med 2009;4:1–4; with permission.

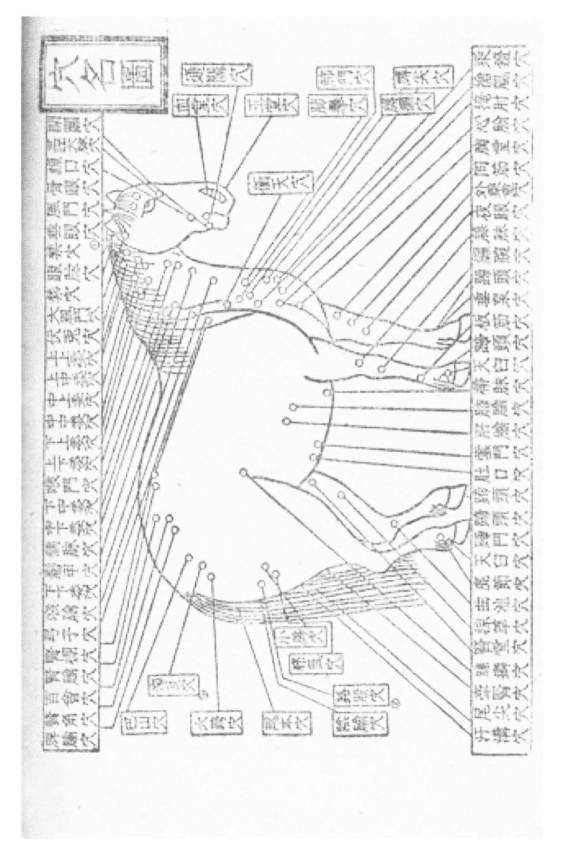

Figure 5.2 Acupoint chart in *Bo Le Zhen Jing* in *Shi Mu An Ji Ji* (published between 618–907 CE) [1] From Xie H, Chrisman C. Equine acupuncture: from ancient art to modern validation. Am J Trad Chin Vet Med 2009;4:1–4; with permission.

The medical philosophy of TCVM relies on several basic theoretical principles derived from these observations, including *Yin/Yang Theory*, the Five Treasures, the Five Element Theory, and the Meridian Theory [3]. These principles are paramount to understanding the philosophy of diagnosis and treatment of disease in TCVM, and from which the practitioner may formulate a *Bian Zheng* (Pattern Diagnosis) which is the basis for selection of TCVM therapy, including acupuncture.

Yin and *Yang* Theory

The concept of *Yin* and *Yang* can be described as the law of opposing forces (Figure 5.3). It is a Taoism principle based on the observation of the dualistic nature of the universe that was first described in the text *Yi Jing (Book of Changes)* around 700 BCE, and applied to medicine sometime between the Spring and Autumn period (722–481 BCE) and the Warring States period (403–221 BCE) [3]. The concept of *Yin* and *Yang* is complex. *Yin* and *Yang* are universal opposites, and everything in the universe can be categorized into *Yin* and *Yang* components [3]. *Yin* refers to the quiet, the dark, and the substantial, and *Yang* refers to the loud, the light, and the insubstantial [4]. Some opposites are intuitive, such as cold (*Yin*) and hot (*Yang*) but others are less intuitive, like fish (*Yin*) and bird (*Yang*), where the fish is more *Yin* than the bird because it is in the cool water and close to the earth, whereas the bird is more *Yang* because it is active and close to the sky [4]. *Yin* or *Yang* designation is dependent on the relative nature of the compared pairs and must always be in balance [4].

Just as *Yin* and *Yang* must remain in balance in the world, so must they remain in balance in the body. The *Yin* governs the structure of the body, the physical nature, tissues, fluids, and cooling, and *Yang* governs the function of the body, the enzymes and nerve impulses, energy, and warming. This balance of the two is homeostasis, and imbalance results in disease. Within TCVM, the concept of *Yin/Yang* is further applied to the internal organs, where they are classified as *Fu* (*Yang*) Organs and *Zang* (*Yin*) Organs [4]. *Yang* organs include Large Intestine, Bladder, Gallbladder, Stomach, Small Intestine, and Triple Heater (Triple Heater is considered an organ in Chinese medicine, and is more spiritual in nature as it does not have an anatomical counterpart) [4]. *Yin* organs include Lung, Kidney, Liver, Spleen, Heart, and Pericardium [4].

In the body, *Yin* provides moisture and cooling, and *Yang* provides warmth and energy. Animals with *Yin* deficiency are not able to adequately cool themselves, and animals with *Yang* deficiency cannot keep warm. Animals with *Yin* Excess have too much cold, and they present with similar temperature preference as those with *Yang* Deficiency, as both conditions result in the feeling of cold. Likewise, *Yang* Excess presents with similar clinical signs to *Yin* Deficiency, in that there is excess Heat in the body, and patients are hot and dry.

Yin/Yang balance must be restored for patient homeostasis. Understanding of these principles is vital for a complete understanding of how imbalances in the body results in disease, and inversely, how these principles may be utilized for therapy.

The Five Treasures (Vital Substances)

Within TCVM, there exists Five Treasures, also known as Vital Substances, consisting of *Jing* (Essence), *Qi* (Energy), *Shen* (Mind), *Xue* (Blood), and *Jin Ye* (Body Fluid) [3, 4]. These substances are necessary for life, and account for the physical properties of TCVM within the body [3, 4]. They impel the function of the body, nourish the body and the mind, and support the function of organs [4]. When the Treasures are depleted or obstructed, disease results [3, 4].

Jing (Essence)

Jing is the essence of an organism. There are two types of *Jing*: prenatal *Jing* and postnatal *Jing*. Prenatal *Jing*, also known as Congenital *Jing*, is the seed of life and is stored in the Kidney. *Jing* is responsible for development of the fetus, for all growth and reproduction, as well as maintaining the life force throughout the organism's life. *Jing* is inherited from one's parents, and *Jing* deficiencies typically result in congenital disorders or sickness in early life. *Jing* is slowly depleted over an individual's lifetime and cannot be replenished. Once *Jing* is exhausted, the animal dies. The conservation of *Jing* is therefore vital to maintain life. Prenatal *Jing* may be supplemented by postnatal *Jing*, which is also known as acquired *Jing*, and is created from

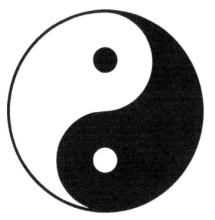

Figure 5.3 The Tai-ji, symbolic of *Yin* (black, right) and *Yang* (white, left).

food. Creating good-quality postnatal *Jing* supplements the continuous depletion of prenatal *Jing* [3, 4].

Qi (Energy)

Qi (energy) is the life force of the world, and where there is *Qi*, there must be life [4]. In TCVM, there are more than 32 types of *Qi* identified, with 8 types being most commonly discussed, each with its own actions, and creation and depletion cycle [3, 4]. The various types of *Qi* each play a specific role in the body: impelling, warming, defending, holding, nourishing, and activity. This chapter will discuss all forms of *Qi* together as a singular concept of life energy [4]. *Qi* may be brought into the body by breathing and by eating, which is then transformed and transported throughout the body in channels, also known as meridians. It is on these channels that acupuncture points are found [3, 4]. Manipulation of acupuncture points has its TCVM physiologic effect on the body by influencing the *Qi* that is flowing within the network of channels within the body [3]. Stagnation of *Qi* within these channels causes stiffness and pain, and deficiency in *Qi* in the body results in weakness and lack of vital functions [3].

Shen (Mind)

Shen is loosely translated as the "mind" or the "spirit" [4]. *Shen* is the outward appearance of all the activities of the body, taking into account personality, mental activity, memory, sleep, and behavior [4]. Shen is what allows clear thought, a focused mind, and inner peace [4]. Shen is stored in the Heart, nourished by *Yin* and Blood, and disturbances in the Heart or in the *Shen* may result in in behavioral abnormalities including anxiety, mania, insomnia, restlessness, hyperactivity, fear, inability to focus, pica, and stereotypies [4].

Xue (Blood)

The TCVM concept of Blood is similar to the Western concept in that Blood contains nutrient *Qi* that circulates throughout the vessels of the body [4]. Blood is formed from food, *Qi*, *Jing*, and Body Fluids, and functions to nourish, moisten, to move *Qi* [4]. Deficiency of Blood may result in anemia, as in Western medicine, but there are other forms of Blood Deficiency in TCVM that do not necessarily result in changes in the hematological profile [4]. Because Blood nourishes tissues and brings moisture, Blood Deficient animals suffer from degeneration of soft tissues and are more prone to soft tissue, tendon, and ligament injury [4]. Blood Stagnation, where the Blood is stagnant within a channel, may result in hematomas, neoplasia, and pain [4].

Jin Ye (Body Fluid)

Jin Ye applies to all the fluids of the body, including intravascular, intraarticular, intraocular, as well as excretions, such as tears, nasal discharge, sweat, urine, gastric and intestinal fluids [4]. *Jin Ye* moistens and nourishes the tissues of the body, and is intimately associated with Blood such that imbalance in one will eventually result in imbalance of the other [4]. The TCVM physiology of water formation, distribution, and excretion is complex and relies on the functions of the Stomach, Spleen, Lung, Small Intestine, Kidney, and Bladder [4]. Disease affecting any of these organs will interrupt the proper flow of *Jin Ye* and result in abnormal fluid homeostasis, leading to effusion, edema, or ascites [4]. Deficiency of *Jin Ye* results in dryness, and obstruction results in edema or Phlegm [4].

Five Element Theory

The cycles of the terrestrial year are featured prominently in the original Taoist observations of the world [4]. In China, there were five distinct seasons identified: spring, summer, late summer, autumn, and winter [4]. Late summer is considered separate from the conventional four seasons because of the heat and humidity of harvest season in China [4]. Each season of the terrestrial year gives rise to an element of the natural world: Wood, Fire, Earth, Metal, and Water (Figure 5.4) [4]. Each season has its own features, bringing

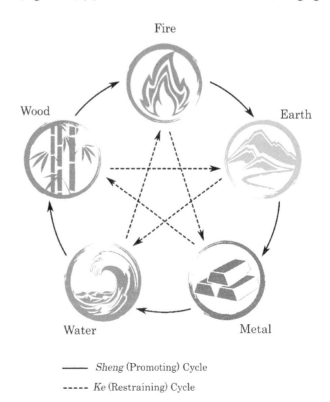

Figure 5.4 Diagram of the Five Element cycle.

new life or disease, and the culmination of these observations developed into the complex system termed the Five Element Theory during the *Zhou* Dynasties (1046 BCE to 221 BCE), which served to explain natural phenomena, including health and disease.

Each element within the theory has its own characteristics and a variety of associated phenomenon, including emotions, tastes, colors, and directions, as well as governing internal organs, body parts, and personality [4]. The Five Elements describe the balance of the forces within the body as well as the relationship of the body to the natural world and the theory may be used within the TCVM framework for diagnosis and treatment of medical conditions [4].

Application to Medicine

Each of the Five Elements is associated with internal organs. In TCVM, the organ is defined not just as the physical organ, but all the functions and associated characteristics and functions of that organ system. The Liver, Heart, Spleen, Lung, and Kidney are representative of their associated elements (Wood, Fire, Earth, Metal, Water, respectively) and all the characteristics governed by those elements. In this way, the concept of an organ in TCVM is expanded from the conventional idea, and when the TCVM organ is intended, it is capitalized ("Kidney") to differentiate it from the typical conventional definition of an organ ("kidney").

The Five Elements follow the cycle of the seasons, with Wood beginning the year in spring, Fire in the summer, Earth in the late summer, Metal in the autumn, and following through to Water in winter, before the cycle begins again. This cycle, the normal progression of the world, is referred to as the *Sheng* Cycle, or Promoting Cycle, and describes the generation and transition of one element to another throughout the course of the year.

The elements are also governed by the *Ke* Cycle, or Restraining Cycle. In contrast to the *Sheng* cycle, the *Ke* cycle describes how each element may be controlled by another. For example, Earth controls Water, which can be seen in the natural world with lakes and river banks containing the water within.

The *Sheng* and *Ke* cycles work together to keep the natural world and the body in balance, promoting and inhibiting in a perpetual circle. An alteration or imbalance of any of the elements and their associated organs has the potential to affect the others, and the imbalance, if not corrected, can propagate, which can transmit the disease process through these cyclic connections to other organ systems.

The application of the Five Element Theory to internal organs, and maintaining balance between the elements, is fundamental to the understanding and practice of TCVM.

Meridians (*Jing Luo*)

Traditional Chinese medicine recognizes meridians, also called channels, which are a complex and interconnected network of channels throughout the entire body that connect the internal organs with each other, as well as to the exterior [5]. This system of channels is called *Jing Luo*, and is categorized into several interlacing networks.

There are 12 Regular Meridians within the body, consisting of 6 *Yin* Meridians, and 6 *Yang* meridians, and each one is associated with a TCVM organ system as defined by the Five Element theory. These meridians exist bilaterally, on the left and right sides of the body, and are paired together in 6 *Yin/Yang* pairs. *Qi* flows through the meridians in a perpetual cycle, traveling from chest to thoracic limb, thoracic limb to head, head to pelvic limb, and pelvic limb to chest, where the cycle begins again.

The 12 Regular Meridians are the Lung, Large Intestine, Stomach, Spleen, Heart, Small Intestine, Bladder, Kidney, Pericardium, Triple Heater, Gallbladder, and Liver. A depiction of meridians is available in Figure 5.5. The two commonly used Extraordinary Meridians are the Governing Vessel and the Conception Vessel. Extraordinary channels are "extraordinary" because they are not associated with a TCVM organ, and they function to assist the Regular Channels. The names of the 12 Regular Meridians and the 2 Extraordinary Meridians are also commonly abbreviated.

Together, the 12 Regular Channels with the Governing Vessel and Conception Vessel, constitute the 14 Regular Channels. These channels are bilateral in the body, except for the Governing Vessel and Conception Vessel, which run along dorsal and ventral midlines, respectively. These 14 channels together serve to transport *Qi* and Blood throughout the body to nourish tissues, coordinate the functioning of the organs, and transmit effects of acupuncture, herbal medicine, and other TCVM treatment modalities [4–6].

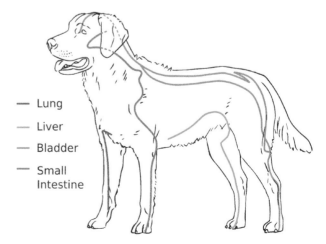

— Lung

— Liver

— Bladder

— Small Intestine

Figure 5.5 A depiction of four meridians within the body.

Transmission of *Qi* by the channels subsequent to acupuncture stimulation is called *De-Qi*, also known as the arrival of *Qi*. This is a feeling experienced by the patient, and may be felt by the practitioner through the needle. The most common descriptions of *De-Qi* include a heavy, pulling, aching feeling, although feelings of pain or tingling may also be reported. In veterinary medicine, practitioners rely on patient response to identify the moment of *De-Qi*, typically a turn of the head, a change in respiratory pattern, muscle twitching, or flinching. The therapeutic effect of acupuncture is correlated with achieving *De-Qi*, meaning the stronger a *De-Qi* response that is obtained, the more potent the treatment [4, 7, 8].

Acupuncture Points

Acupuncture points, or acupoints, are locations on the meridian where *Qi* gathers. They are typically associated with an externally palpable anatomical depression. Each of the 12 Regular Channels and 2 Extraordinary Channels has associated acupuncture points.

Transpositional acupoints, which are points that have been transposed from original use in humans, are characterized by the TCVM organ abbreviation followed by a number, which represents the order of the acupoint on the meridian in the direction of travel. For example, LI-4 represents the 4th acupuncture point along the Large Intestine channel, and KID-27 represents the 27th acupuncture point on the Kidney channel. There are 361 transpositional acupoints identified on the body.

Classical acupoints are another identified type of point, which were originally discovered in the intended species, and are not associated with one of the 14 regular meridians (although there is some overlap with the locations of transpositional acupoints). In the literature, these acupoints are commonly referred to by their Chinese name, although a numbering system has been developed. There are 210 classical acupuncture points described in the horse, and classical acupuncture points in the canine have mostly been adapted from equine and human classical points.

Every acupuncture point has a specific function or indication for use. Acupoints can be stimulated to have a local effect, distal effect, or special effects. Local effects mostly pertain to regional analgesic effect (to treat cervical osteoarthritis, treat acupuncture points located on the neck), distal points for a distant effect (to treat cervical osteoarthritis, select an acupoint on the distal limb on a channel that courses through the area of interest, such as SI-3), or special effect (to treat cervical osteoarthritis, treat an acupuncture point indicated for bone, such as BL-11). Every acupoint has one or many indications, and the selection of which acupoints are necessary to balance the body depends on the patient's Pattern Diagnosis.

Meridian Pathology

Pathology of the meridians results from imbalance in *Yin/Yang*, the Five Elements, or Vital Substances. Imbalance may be Excess or Deficiency, and originates from internal factors (such as congenital abnormality, strong emotions, under- or overfeeding, or activity) or external factors (typically due to invasion of the External Pathogens, but also includes traumatic injury, parasites, poisoning, or iatrogenic factors). The immune system in TCVM is composed of *Wei Qi* (Defensive *Qi*), which controls the opening and closing of skin pores, regulates body temperature, and moistens skin and hair to protect the organs. *Wei Qi* circulates in the superficial regions of the body to defend against invasion of illness.

Excess

In TCVM, there exist six forms of Excessive Pathogenical *Qi*, also called External Pathogens: Wind, Cold, Summer Heat, Dryness, Dampness, Fire. Similar to the Western concept of invading pathogens such as viruses or bacteria, TCVM describes pathogenic factors which invade the body, cause imbalance, and result in disease. These concepts were developed far before germ theory, and were based on generations of observation.

The most commonly encountered form of Excess is Stagnation. Stagnation represents a blockage in a meridian that results in *Qi* or Blood becoming stagnant, which results in pain. Stagnation is seen with all types of pain, including neuropathic pain, pain from injury or surgery, arthritis, or other chronic conditions. The goal of acupuncture treatment for analgesia is to clear the Stagnation.

Deficiency

Deficiency results in weakness or lack of proper function of the body. Deficiency of the Vital Substances may be due to external or internal factors, and is typically identified in older animals and animals with chronic disease. Vital Substances may be depleted by External Pathogens as well as internal causes, such as *Jing* Deficiency or poor diet. The goal of acupuncture therapy is to identify the cause of the deficiency so that it may be tonified to maintain balance.

TCVM Diagnostic System and Methods

Identifying a *Bian Zheng* (Pattern Diagnosis) is the foundation of TCVM diagnosis and treatment. Pattern Diagnoses were developed from the observation that animals with clinical disease (*Zheng*) presented clinical signs (*Bian*) which could be utilized to determine the underlying illness. Over hundreds of years, TCVM practitioners developed the *Si-zhen* (Four Diagnostic Methods) for collecting diagnostic data to be utilized for making diagnosis of disease. The four methods include: Inquiring (*Wen*), Inspection (*Wang*), Smelling/Hearing (*Wen*), and Palpation (*Qie*). Special attention is paid to the characteristics of the tongue and arterial pulses during physical exam.

Inquiring (Wen)

Inquiring is the interrogation of the owner or handler of the animal to obtain information about the patient and the nature and course of disease. When compared to a Western patient history, similar questions are asked (age, duration of illness, clinical signs), with a few additional concepts to aid in the ultimate goal of identifying a Pattern Diagnosis, such as the time of day that clinical signs occur or are most prominent, temperature preferences, questions to better understand the patient's constitution, and a detailed dietary history.

Inspection (Wang)

Inspection of a patient begins at the earliest possible moment, ideally before the patient has noticed the practitioner, to allow for the best and unaltered observation of the patient's *Shen*, constitution, and obvious clinical signs. Inspection takes into account everything about an animal – the behavior and mental state, posture, gait, appetite, thirst, and appearance of the tongue, ears, eyes, nose, lips, skin, and excretions.

Shen

Shen is a patient's mental state, spirit, or way of going. The *Shen* is responsible for how well the body functions and how the animal behaves and reacts to the world around them. Inspection of the *Shen* occur at the earliest moment during the exam. Good *Shen* is characterized by a patient with bright eyes and a strong will to live. They are happy, balanced, responsive to their environment, and move their ears and eyes to watch and listen. Patients with decreased or poor *Shen* may show signs of exhaustion, weariness, with dull eyes and droopy or still ears. The head may be low, and the patient may have dulled responses to their environment. Sick patients with good *Shen* have a more favorable prognosis than sick patients with poor *Shen*.

Shen Disturbance is defined as an unbalanced Shen, resulting in mania, confusion, aggression, fear, and other abnormal behaviors. *Shen* Disturbance is usually readily observable or easily identifiable from inquiring.

Tongue Diagnosis

Evaluation of the tongue is paramount to successful pattern diagnosis, as the tongue reflects the internal workings of the body. The tongue is evaluated for color, shape, size,

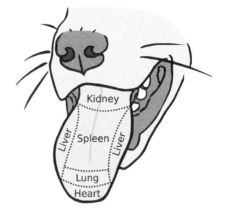

Figure 5.6 The regions of the tongue and the associated TCVM organs.

coating, and moisture level. Each region of the tongue corresponds to a different TCVM organ (Figure 5.6). The tip of the tongue represents the Heart, the mid tip (just caudal to the tip of the tongue) represents the Lung, the center of the tongue represents the Spleen, the caudal aspect of the tongue represents the Kidney, and the sides of the tongue represent the Liver. Changes in the color, coating, size, and shape in these regions of the tongue indicate imbalances in the associated organ system (Figure 5.7 and Table 5.1).

Smelling/Hearing (Wen)

The use of smelling and hearing in TCVM is arguably much more important than in Western medicine. While it is common to auscultate the heart, lungs, or gastrointestinal system, or smell for ketones or otic yeast, TCVM also pays attention to subtle changes in the sound of the breath, the quality of the voice, the sound of chewing, or the specific scent of the skin and mouth.

Palpating (Qie)

Palpation of the characteristics of the arterial pulse can reveal pathological conditions in the body. Along with tongue diagnosis, the pulse is one of the pillars of the Pattern Diagnosis, as it reflects changes and imbalances in the organs, *Qi*, and Blood. In small to moderately sized animals, including cats, dogs, pigs, and goats, the pulse is taken on the femoral artery. In the horse, the pulse is taken on the carotid artery low in the jugular groove, and in the cow, the pulse can be taken on the median caudal artery of the tail.

The pulse is felt at three levels, superficial, middle, and deep, and evaluated for strength and character. The pulse is also felt at three positions on both the right and left sides of the body, typically simultaneously with the practitioner's ring, middle, and index fingers. Each position on the artery is representative of a TCVM organ system. The left pulse from proximal to distal in a small animal (or cranial to caudal in a horse) indicates Heart, Liver, and Kidney

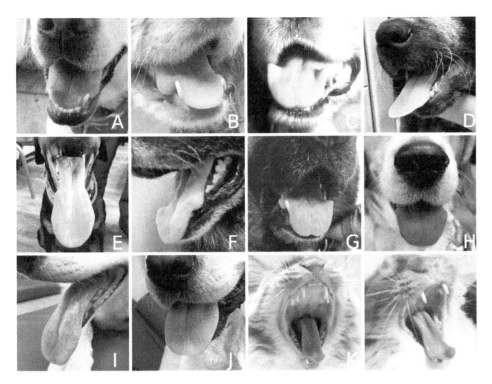

Figure 5.7 Examples of different tongue colors. A – Normal tongue. B – Pale dry tongue. C – Pale wet tongue. D – Pale tongue, especially pale in the region of the Heart. This puppy had multiple cardiac defects. E – Pale tongue in the Kidney and Spleen regions. F – Pale tongue in the Kidney and Spleen regions with redness in the Liver region. G – Redness in the Heart region. H – Deep red tongue. I – Pale and gray tongue with Phlegm. J – Purple tongue in the Spleen and Kidney regions. K – Red tongue, especially in the Heart and Spleen regions. L – Normal tongue. This is the same cat seen in K after treatment with acupuncture.

Table 5.1 Characteristics of the tongue interpreted with Traditional Chinese Medicine.

CHARACTER	CHARACTERISTIC	INTERPRETATION
COLOR	Peach-flower pink	Normal
	Pale	*Qi* or Blood Deficiency
	Red	Heat or *Yin* Deficiency
	Deep red	Heat *Yin* Deficiency
	Purple	Stagnation or Cold
	Yellow	Dampness
COATING	Thin	Normal
	White	Exterior Pattern or Cold Pattern Damp, Phlegm
	Yellow	Heat Pattern
	Grey-black	Heat, Cold-Damp, or Deficiency Cold
	Dry	*Yin* or Blood Deficiency
	Wet	*Qi* or *Yang* Deficiency Damp-Cold
	Sticky	Phlegm, Camp
SHAPE	Swollen	*Qi* Deficiency, Kidney *Yang* Deficiency
	Small, soft	*Jing* Deficiency
	Flat, wide	Blood Deficiency

Yin, and the right pulse in the same positions indicates Lung, Spleen, and Kidney *Yang*. The pulse may also be attributed to the *Yang* organs. In general, the left pulse provides information about the *Yin* and Blood within the body, and the right pulse about the *Qi* and *Yang* (Figure 5.8 and Table 5.2).

Equine Acupuncture Point Scan

The acupuncture point scan (APS) examination is performed by gentle stimulation of acupuncture points along the horse's body with a blunt instrument, such as a finger, needle cap, or acupuncture guide tube. This technique reveals areas of hypersensitivity, known as "*A-shi*" acupoints. Studies of APS in equids has shown an 82.4% sensitivity and 78.4% specificity in diagnosing the anatomic location of naturally occurring lameness [9]. Beyond diagnostic capabilities for musculoskeletal aberrations, APS can also be used to diagnose internal medicine conditions or as a form of confirmatory lameness diagnostic. For example, in a horse that is lame in the forefoot, PC-1 and LI-18 are commonly sore and function as diagnostic points. When the lame foot receives acupuncture treatment, the APS positivity at PC-1 and LI-18 resolves, indicating the APS sensitivity was indeed due to the forefoot lameness.

Table 5.2 Pulse palpation descriptions and their significance.

Pulse	Description	Significance
Floating	Easily palpated with light pressure, and cannot feel with deep pressure	Early phases of invasion of External Pathogen
Deep	Cannot be felt with light pressure, and can only be felt with deep pressure	Interior pattern
Rapid	Pulse rate is faster than expected	Heat, *Yin* Deficiency
Slow	Pulse rate is slower than expected	Cold, *Yang* deficiency
Full	Forceful in all three levels	Excess, Stagnation
Thin	Soft and weak, but clearly defined	*Yin* and/or Blood Deficiency
Weak	Soft and weak at all levels	*Qi* Deficiency
Slippery	Rounded and rolling, smooth	Phlegm, Heat
Choppy	Irregular and rough	Stagnation, *Yin* Deficiency
Soft	Easily felt with superficial pressure, not well defined with deep pressure. May be thready or forceless.	Spleen *Qi* Deficiency, Damp
Wiry	Firm and straight like a guitar string	Stagnation, Liver imbalance, Wind

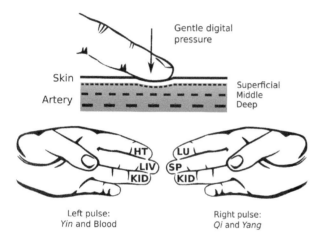

Figure 5.8 Palpation at three depths (superficial, middle, and deep), and at the three levels (index finger, middle finger, ring finger).

Pattern Diagnosis (*Bian Zheng*)

The strategy of constructing a Pattern Diagnosis typically involves collecting clinical information with the *Si-zhen* (Four Diagnostic Methods), categorizing the clinical signs, and then synthesizing the information.

Most Pattern Diagnoses are formulaic in their nomenclature such that a single diagnosis expresses (1) Which organ is affected, (2) What Vital Substance is affected, and (3) How the Vital Substance has been affected. Examples of this formula include Liver *Qi* Stagnation, Kidney *Jing* Deficiency, and Liver *Yang* Rising. Many Pattern Diagnoses do not fit this formulaic naming pattern, such as Phlegm Misting Mind or Bladder Damp Heat, but these Patterns are still descriptive of the clinical condition.

Pattern Diagnosis is important because selection of acupuncture points, based on the actions of the specific acupoint, is determined based on the underlying Pattern. In general, the selected acupoints should have indications to restore balance. Every acupuncture point has nuances of use, so careful reading of an acupuncture atlas for formulation of an acupuncture treatment is recommended for best results.

Conclusion

Traditional Chinese veterinary medicine has been used for the treatment and prevention of disease in veterinary species for thousands of years. TCVM philosophy is based in the Taoist observation of the universe, including terrestrial cycles, life, death, and disease. The theory of *Yin-Yang*, the Five Elements, Meridians, and the Five Treasures are the basic principles that form the foundation of traditional Chinese veterinary medical philosophy. Understanding of these principles allows practitioners to form a *Bian Zheng* (Pattern Diagnosis), which allows prescription of modalities, including acupuncture and herbal medicine, for the treatment and prevention of disease in veterinary patients.

References

1 Xie, H. and Chrisman, C. (2009). Equine acupuncture: from ancient art to modern validation. *Am J Trad Chin Vet Med* 4: 1–4.
2 White, A. and Ernst, E. (2004). A brief history of acupuncture. *Rheumatology* 43: 662–663.

3 Chrisman, C.L. and Xie, H. (2010). The paradigm shift to Bian Zheng for conventionally trained veterinarians. *Am J Tradit Chin Vet Med* 5: 1–7.

4 Xie, H. and Preast, V. (2013). *Traditional Chinese Veterinary Medicine: Fundamental Principles*, 2e. Chi Institute Press.

5 Chrisman, C.L. and Xie, H. (2013). The Jing Luo network: an overview of channels and collaterals and their clinical applications. *Am J Tradit Chin Vet Med* 8: 1–13.

6 Xie, H. and Preast, V. (2007). *Xie's Veterinary Acupuncture*. Blackwell Publishing.

7 Kuo, T.-C., Chen, Z.-S., Chen, C.-H. et al. (2004). The physiological effect of DE *QI* during acupuncture. *J Health Sci* 50: 336–342.

8 MacPherson, H. and Asghar, A. (2006). Acupuncture needle sensations associated with De *Qi*: a classification based on experts' ratings. *J Altern Complement Med* 12: 633–637.

9 Le Jeune, S.S. and Jones, J.H. (2014). Prospective study on the correlation of positive acupuncture scans and lameness in 102 performance horses. *Am J Tradit Chin Vet Med* 9: 33.

6

Integrative Acupuncture: Clinical Approaches and Current Scientific Literature

Emily Mangan

Introduction

Acupuncture exists within the philosophical framework of traditional Chinese veterinary medicine (TCVM) with over 2,000-year history of use in veterinary species [1]. Acupuncture is the stimulation of acupuncture points (acupoints) which are externally palpable depressions present on the body surface that are associated with peripheral nerve bifurcation, transition through facial planes, and innervation of muscle and tendon [2–5]. Acupuncture points have been characterized histologically by a high density of free nerve endings, arterioles, venules, lymphatics, and mast cells compared to surrounding tissues [2, 3, 6, 7]. Acupuncture points are most commonly found on meridians, which is a TCVM concept that describes a complicated network of channels throughout the body that interconnect internal organs with each other and the body surface to facilitate the transmission of energy and nourishment [8, 9]. Scientifically, meridians align with the peripheral nervous system and the current, best supported hypothesis for acupuncture function lies in the neuroanatomic and neurophysiologic mechanisms described in the literature [2, 10].

Meridians and acupuncture points have been found to have specific properties that define them from surrounding tissue, including higher electrical conductance and capacitance [11–13], lower electrical resistance and impedance [11–13], propagation of heat along meridians [14, 15], and preferential transmission of fluids along meridian lines [8, 16, 17]. Acupuncture meridians have also been defined optically [18], magnetically [14], with acoustic signals [11, 14] and by the myoelectrical activities [14].

This data strongly supports neuroanatomical and neurophysiologic mechanisms of acupuncture. While there is a near-exponential growing body of evidence for the use of acupuncture in veterinary medicine developed over the last 50 years, it is still a young field and there remain swaths of clinical conditions that still require exploration and validation via blinded, controlled clinical trials.

Evidence-based Studies

In the West, the most frequent applications of acupuncture in standard clinical practice include analgesia for postoperative, geriatric, and sports medicine applications [19], nausea [20, 21], neurological disorders including intervertebral disc disease, and epilepsy, and has been shown to have cardiovascular, gastrointestinal motility, and respiratory effects [19, 22–33]. Beyond these categories which have the support of high-quality clinical studies, acupuncture may be applied in a great many situations for treatment of a wide variety of conditions, although there is need for randomized blinded, placebo-controlled studies, as the majority of information available on additional clinical conditions has been taken directly from TCVM philosophy or experience of practitioners.

Analgesia

Acupuncture stimulation has potent analgesic properties, which remain the best studied of all the clinical applications [7, 34, 35]. There is great interest in both human and veterinary medicine for analgesic uses, as acupuncture is

Integrative Veterinary Medicine, First Edition. Edited by Mushtaq A. Memon and Huisheng Xie.
© 2023 John Wiley & Sons, Inc. Published 2023 by John Wiley & Sons, Inc.
Companion Website: www.wiley.com/go/memon/veterinary

non-pharmaceutical, does not interact with medications, is safe when used appropriately, and is efficacious.

Analgesic effects of acupuncture, which have been rigorously explored scientifically, have been determined to be due to a cascade of effects, beginning with needle stimulation within an acupoint [7, 34, 35]. Stimulation creates local counterirritation within the acupoint characterized by release of local inflammatory mediators and endogenous opioids, and stimulates Aα, Aβ, Aδ, and C nerve fibers [2, 6]. Stimulation progresses segmental effects by release of endogenous opioids and cytokines within the spinal cord [2, 36, 37], and culminates in suprasegmental effects, characterized by specific and consistent brain region activation and release of β-endorphins, enkephalins, noradrenaline, dopamine, and serotonin [2, 10, 38].

Acupuncture for post-surgical analgesia has been explored in the literature with encouraging results. In a study evaluating post-surgical analgesia in dogs undergoing routine ovariohysterectomy, acupuncture, and pharmacopuncture (1/10th the standard dose) with morphine and carprofen were just as effective as standard doses of parenteral morphine or carprofen [39]. Another study investigated acupuncture analgesia for soft tissue surgery in dogs undergoing mastectomy and the finding suggest that high-frequency electroacupuncture may be more effective in this clinical setting at managing post-operative pain than the standard dose of morphine [40]. Electroacupuncture (EAP) for post-operative pain management after hemilaminectomy for thoracolumbar intervertebral disc disease in dogs resulted in significantly lower total dose of fentanyl in the first 12 hours post operatively in dogs that received EAP, as well as significantly lower pain scores in the first 36 hours after surgery, compared to dogs receiving conventional pain management alone [41].

Clinical studies also support the use of acupuncture for pain associated musculoskeletal conditions. Acupuncture was found to be more effective for thoracolumbar pain in horses compared to phenylbutazone, and in a study of lameness in dogs, acupuncture improved quality of life, comfort, and mobility compared to conventional treatments alone [23, 42, 43].

While acupuncture has powerful analgesic properties, it should never be relied upon as a sole method of analgesia for procedures, and is best utilized as part of a comprehensive multimodal analgesic plan.

Neurologic Disorders

Studies investigating the efficacy of acupuncture for the treatment and management of neurologic conditions has shown it is effective for epilepsy, cervical spondylomyelopathy, and intervertebral disc disease [44–49]. Gold bead implantation into acupuncture points decreased seizure

frequency with reduced doses of anticonvulsant mediations, acupuncture treatment resulted in return to function in 85% of dogs with cervical spondylomyelopathy compared to 20% in the conventional treatment group, and the application of acupuncture for animals suffering from intervertebral disc disease (IVDD) is one of the best-studied neurologic applications [44, 45]. Dogs suffering ambulatory paraparesis have a significantly shorter time to recovery of ambulation proprioception when treated with electroacupuncture compared to corticosteroids, and a greater percentage of recovery compared to surgery or corticosteroids alone [46–48].

Cardiovascular

Acupuncture is effective for lowering high blood pressure, normalizing heart rate, and reducing heart rate variability [50]. The mechanisms of cardiovascular effect are still under-researched, but the current hypothesis includes sympathetic and parasympathetic regulation. Stimulation at the acupoint GV-26 increased cardiac output, stroke volume, heart rate, mean arterial pressure, and pulse pressure, and decreased total peripheral resistance [51]. The acupoints PC-6 and BL-15 were found to significantly increase heart rate in animals with induced xylazine-induced bradycardia, and these same points also significantly decreased heart rate in animals with glycopyrrolate-induced tachycardia. [52, 53] This is an example of dual-direction regulation: a physiologic response to stimulation of acupuncture points facilitates homeostasis [19]. These last two studies, where the same two acupoints either increased or decreased heart rate, is an excellent example of this principle [19].

Respiratory

Acupuncture is known to produce a parasympathomimetic-like effects as well as modulate the balance between the sympathetic and parasympathetic nervous systems [50]. While the mechanisms of respiratory effect are not fully elucidated, there is data showing that acupuncture has clinical indications for the management of respiratory conditions. Needling of GV-26 was found to cause a faster return to spontaneous ventilation in anesthetized turtles compared to epinephrine, as well as faster time to movement, and faster time to complete recovery [54]. In a cross-over study of tracheal collapse in small breed dogs, acupuncture treatment resulted in improved heart rate variably, reduced coughing, and reductions in oxidative stress after exercise compared to no treatment [50].

Gastrointestinal

Acupuncture has a homeostatic effect on the parasympathetic and sympathetic nervous systems, which is apparent in its effect on the cardiovascular and respiratory regulation. These same principles also influence gastric and intestinal motility. Acupuncture stimulation at ST-36 and BL-27 have been shown to increase intestinal motility, and stimulation at PC-6 and ST-36 were found to slow gastric emptying time [55, 56]. These studies also demonstrate the principle of dual-direction regulation.

Acupuncture also has antiemetic properties. Dogs with vasopressin-, hydromorphone-, or morphine-induced vomiting showed reduction of vomiting/retching episodes after acupuncture stimulation [57–59].

While more clinical studies are indicated, these studies demonstrate that acupuncture influences gastrointestinal motility, gastric emptying time, nausea, and vomiting.

Sedation

When comparing sedation after injection of dexmedetomidine administered either intramuscularly in gluteal muscles versus into GV-20, dogs that received injection into GV-20 had significantly increased sedation and analgesia, with longer duration of action. [60] Stimulation of GV-20 was also found to reduce EEG spectral edge frequency and achieve acceptable levels of sedation [61].

Immunostimulation

A study by Perdrizet *et al.* investigated immunostimulation properties of acupuncture by way of injection of the canine distemper vaccine into GV-14 versus control in 100 healthy dogs. There was a significant increase in canine distemper virus serum neutralization titers following injection at GV-14 compared to control [62].

Evidence-based Acupuncture Summary

Acupuncture has been found to be effective for the treatment of a variety of clinical applications and to influence the sympathetic and parasympathetic nervous system. While more research is required to further elucidate mechanisms and quantify effects, these studies demonstrate clinical efficacy of acupuncture mechanisms in veterinary species.

Acupuncture Methods

There is a wide variety of modalities available to stimulate acupuncture points, each with their own indication and efficacy. While dry needling is the traditional method of stimulation, other methods, such as electroacupuncture or laser therapy, are growing in popularity in the veterinary field. Selection of a specific acupoint stimulation modality depends on diagnosis and patient goals, patient

preferences, and tolerances, availability for follow up, and practitioner comfort.

Dry Needling

Dry needling is the insertion of a thin needle into the acupuncture point and may include various manipulations of the tissue including pricking, lifting, spinning, or fanning (Figure 6.1) [63]. The proposed mechanism of dry needling is direct disruption of tissue, resulting in stimulation of nerve fibers and mast cell degranulation, as well as additional stimulation from fascial interactions due to needle manipulation, and all resulting cascades previously discussed.

Dry needle acupuncture is less potent than some other methods, and typically requires frequent initial treatments (1–2x weekly for several weeks) followed by a period of elongation of interval between treatments, for clinical resolution or stable management of disease.

Electroacupuncture

Electroacupuncture (EAP) is the use of low-amplitude electrical current to stimulate acupuncture points and meridians (Figure 6.1). Electrical leads from an electrostimulation device that generates electrical current are connected to a set of acupuncture needles, which completes the circuit within the body [35, 63]. The amplitude of the wave is adjusted to patient tolerance [63]. Compared to dry needling alone, EAP provides more stimulation, which provides a longer lasting and more potent effect [32]. The electrical frequency utilized for treatment has been shown to influence the neurochemical mediators released [2]. Low-frequency stimulation (2–10 Hz) preferentially releases enkephalins, endorphins, noradrenaline, and acetylcholine, and has been shown to be effective for analgesia for chronic conditions. Moderate frequency (50–100 Hz) stimulation has been shown to preferentially release dynorphins and be muscarinic and GABAergic, and high frequency (200 Hz) has been shown to release serotonin [2]. High-frequency acupuncture has a short duration of action, but is potent and may be effective for acute or surgical pain [63].

Aqua-acupuncture

Aqua-acupuncture or aquapuncture is the injection of a variety of substances subcutaneously or intramuscularly into acupuncture points, depending on the described depth of the acupoint itself [63]. Commonly injected fluids include saline, Vitamin B_{12}, autologous blood, and pharmaceuticals [63]. Injection of fluid into an acupuncture point provides local distention of the area and prolonged stimulation of the tissue, thereby providing a longer lasting treatment than dry needling alone.

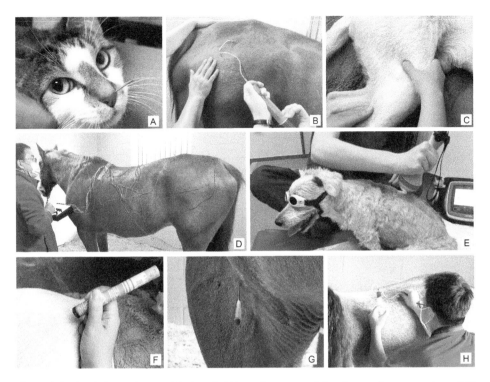

Figure 6.1 A – A domestic cat with chronic kidney disease receiving dry needle acupuncture at *Shan-gen* to stimulate appetite. B – Administration of pneumo-acupuncture at BL-54 for treatment of muscle atrophy secondary to equine protozoal myeloencephalitis (EPM). C – Figure 6.7 A yellow Labrador Retriever receiving acupressure at GB-33. D – Electroacupuncture is administered to an equine patient with sacroiliac osteoarthritis. E – Photobiomodulation (cold laser) therapy at *Hua-tuo-jia-ji* along the site of a hemilaminectomy for treatment of intervertebral disc disease (IVDD). F – A yellow Labrador Retriever receiving moxibustion at *Bai-hui*. G – Hemoacupuncture at *Xiong-tang* resulting in a drop of dark stagnant blood. H – Aqua-acupuncture with vitamin B_{12} is administered via a winged infusion set along the Bladder Meridian in an equine patient with back pain.

Pharmacopuncture

Pharmacopuncture is a form of aquapuncture, and is defined by the injection of small amounts (1/10th the standard parenteral dose) of medications into acupuncture points [60, 64–66]. Pharmacopuncture with analgesics and sedatives have been shown to be efficacious in veterinary species in achieving sedation and decreasing requirements of additional analgesic after surgical procedures [39, 64–66].

Hemo-acupuncture

Hemoacupuncture or hemopuncture is the treatment of an acupuncture point with the specific intent to cause bleeding from the acupoint (Figure 6.1). In Chinese medicine, this is considered a release of Excess and Heat, and is useful for conditions of high fever, severe stagnation, or severe inflammation, such as laminitis [3, 63].

Pneumoacupuncture

Pneumoacupuncture is the injection of air into the subcutaneous space for treatment of regional muscle atrophy or to release fascial adhesions (Figure 6.1) [67]. Historically,

pneumoacupuncture was performed by cutting a small hole in the skin and then lifting the skin manually to create negative pressure and facilitate influx of air. With the advent of medical instruments, air can simply be injected with a hypodermic needle and syringe, which also allows direct quantification of the injected air.

The principles of pneumoacupuncture for treatment of muscle atrophy have been hypothesized to cause a release of fascial tension which allows unrestricted blood and lymphatic flow and increased nutrient availability to tissues.

Implantation

Occasionally, acupuncture points may be sterilely implanted with a bead or wire made of surgical stainless steel, gold, or titanium [63, 68]. The goal of implantation acupuncture is to provide prolonged stimulation of acupoints that have been shown to relieve symptoms in the patient [68].

Moxibustion

Moxa is a dried herb, typically *Artemisia sinesis* (mugwort), that is frequently processed into a roll and lit on one end until it is smoking, and then held above the acupuncture point or needle to provide a warming stimulation (Figure 6.1) [63]. Moxibustion is particularly useful in patients that feel cold due to suffering from the Cold pathogen or *Yang* deficiency, patients who are elderly, or those who live in cold climates.

Acupressure

In patients aversive to more invasive techniques, or for owners looking to safely provide stimulation at home, acupressure may be of clinical use. Acupressure is the application of pressure over an acupuncture point either with digits or wooden or plastic massage stick to provide stimulation (Figure 6.1) [63]. Typically, the acupoint is stimulated by pushing, rubbing, or pinching for 1–3 minutes before moving on to the next acupoint.

Photobiomodulation (Cold Laser)

Utilizing infrared photobiomodulation (frequently referred to as cold laser) for stimulation of acupuncture points (Figure 6.1) has shown to be efficacious for a variety of conditions, especially analgesia, when compared to therapy of sham-acupuncture points [10, 69]. Efficacy has been shown between 630–904 nm at 5–500 mW [63]. The current data shows that photobiomodulation produces ATP locally, similar to mast cell degranulation, which can then activate cascades directly or via its metabolite adenosine, as well as directly depolarize axons [10, 63, 69].

Designing an Integrative Treatment Plan

Acupuncture has been shown to be an effective therapy for many veterinary complaints. Despite its efficacy, acupuncture works best as part of an integrative treatment plan. Acupuncture has few contraindications, does not interfere with medications, and can be performed in a kennel or run, during anesthesia or recovery from anesthesia, and is known for its anti-nausea, analgesic, and appetite stimulating properties, which makes it a great addition to any critical care, oncological, or pain management case. While the best efficacy of acupuncture is seen when the patient is being treated based on TCVM examination and pattern diagnosis, acupuncture may still be effective when performed based on Western diagnosis.

Acupuncture Point Selection

Every acupoint has an indication for use. Many acupoints share indications but differ in their nuances, and some work best when used with other acupoints. The selection of the correct acupoint prescription is a major component

of what determines the efficacy of treatment. The traditional Chinese veterinary medical philosophy, from within which acupuncture was developed, informs the selection of acupoints. There are many methods by which to select an acupoint for treatment of any given diagnosis, including local, meridian, Five Element, and *A-shi*.

Local acupoints are defined as acupoints that are located anatomically near the area of pathology [3]. For example, acupoints surrounding the stifle can be used for the treatment of stifle pain, or paravertebral acupoints for spinal pain [63].

If the meridian affected by pathological changes can be identified, then acupoints treating the unbalanced meridian can be treated. One may treat the Bladder and Kidney meridian for pathology of the urogenital system or the Liver meridian for hepatic disease. Meridian acupoint selection can also be utilized for treatment of a distant area that the meridian courses through. For example, treatment of acupoints on the Small Intestine meridian on the distal thoracic limb are beneficial for cervical pain, as the Small Intestine meridian travels over the area of pathology.

The Five Element Theory associates the traditional Chinese veterinary medicine organs with one of the Five Elements: Wood, Fire, Earth, Metal, Water [3]. This theory describes both the *Sheng* and *Ke* cycles, as well as pathological changes within the cycles. These principles may be utilized for the selection of therapeutic acupoints based on their elemental associations.

Myofascial trigger points are identified as *A-shi* points in TCVM [3]. These points are local areas of pain, typically involving pathology of muscle and connective tissue, which may be identified with palpation.

Duration and Frequency of Treatment

The suggested duration of acupuncture therapy in veterinary species typically ranges from 15–30 minutes, with special, severe cases benefitting from >60 minutes of treatment time [70]. The required frequency of treatment depends on the patient being treated, the disease process, and the type of stimulation used, although is typically one session every 1 to 8 weeks [70]. An elderly patient with a chronic condition will need more frequent treatments than a young animal with acute illness. Typically, patients are initially treated once to twice per week for 3–4 visits, then once weekly, then once every other week, continuing to taper to a monthly or as-needed basis [71]. Several acupuncture treatments may be needed to identify if the patient will respond well to acupuncture treatment.

Acupuncture Cautions and Contraindications

Acupuncture should be avoided in areas of the skin with dermatitis or other infectious skin infections, as needling may introduce pathogens from the exterior of the body. In animals that are visibly dirty, such as horses or other livestock animals, the skin should be cleansed first before needling.

Acupuncture needles should not be inserted into open wounds or neoplastic lesions. Acupuncture may be safely utilized away from the edges of the wound or neoplasia to provide local effect without disruption of abnormal tissue, a technique which is commonly called "Circle the Dragon." [63] Acupuncture should be used with caution in pregnant animals, as many acupuncture points may have an ecbolic effect and result in abortion or preterm labor. While acupuncture has been shown to be an effective adjunct management modality for seizures, electropuncture specifically should be avoided in these patients. Electroacupuncture leads also should not cross the heart or the brain, and should not be used in animals with cardiac pacemakers. While there are no documented ill effects of crossing the heart or the brain with electroacupuncture, it is unnecessary to do so.

Practitioners should use caution when needling acupuncture points over the abdomen or thorax as to not induce a peritonitis or pneumothorax. Thorough understanding of anatomy is necessary to safely needle these acupoints, and frequently a non-invasive method, such as acupressure, laser, or moxibustion, is recommended. Likewise, practitioners should be mindful of acupoints located over articular spaces, and if these acupoints are chosen for treatment, sterile preparation of the skin is recommended.

Occasionally, with strong *De-Qi* response, animals may attempt to bite or remove acupuncture needles with their mouths. Animals should be monitored closely, especially with acupuncture treatment of the face and forelimbs, to prevent accidental ingestion of acupuncture needles.

Clinical Applications

Acupuncture is minimally invasive and relatively inexpensive, although like any modality, acupuncture has appropriate uses, indications, and contraindications [19, 22]. There are some clinical presentations where acupuncture alone may be enough for management or resolution of clinical signs, however, acupuncture is typically best utilized as an integrative component of a comprehensive treatment plan. While acupuncture exists within a medical philosophy of Traditional Chinese Veterinary medicine (TCVM), which can aid in the diagnosis and treatment of clinical disease with acupuncture, acupuncture may still be effectively utilized when applied from a Western approach.

Post-surgical Pain

Acupoints: LI-4, ST-36, SI-9, BL-20, BL-23, LIV-3, GV-20, GV-14, *Shen-shu*, *Bai-hui*

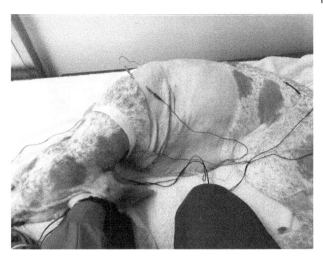

Figure 6.2 A six-year-old female spayed Bracco Italiano undergoing acupuncture therapy after left forelimb amputation.

Case example: An 8-year-old female spayed Bracco Italiano underwent amputation of the left thoracic limb due to pathological fracture secondary to osteosarcoma (Figure 6.2). After surgery, she appeared painful, requiring a high dose of fentanyl CRI and frequent lidocaine infusion through the soaker catheter embedded at the surgical site. Two days after surgery, she had yet to attempt to rise, and was inapparent. She received a mixture of dry needle and EAP at GV-20, GV-14, SI-9, BL-20, BL-21, BL-54, LIV-3, LI-4, *Bai-hui*, and *Shen-shu* for 30 minutes. She appeared more comfortable at the end of her first treatment and within 10 minutes, she attempted to stand for the first time since surgery. Shortly afterward, she ate for the first time since hospital admittance. She received repeat acupuncture therapy while hospitalized for the next four days, and once discharged, continued acupuncture and rehabilitation twice weekly for the next four weeks until she was able to ambulate well on her own.

Cervical Pain

Acupoints: LI-4, LI-16, SI-3, SI-16, BL-10, BL-11, TH-16, GB-20, GB-21, *Jing-jia-ji*

Case example: A six-year-old female spayed Beagle presented with a three-month history of cervical pain with stereotypical head carriage and pain on cervical lateral and vertical flexion (Figure 6.3). MRI did not reveal a compressive lesion and no myelopathy was present. The patient had trialed gabapentin, methocarbamol, and TENS with little improvement. She received electroacupuncture (20 Hz for 30 minutes) at bilateral cervical *Jing-jia-ji*, SI-3, BL-10, GV-14, GB-21, and *Bai-hui*. Immediately after her first treatment, she was able to shake her body (as if drying herself) pain free, and maintain a more normal head carriage. She was seen once weekly for two more weeks, and

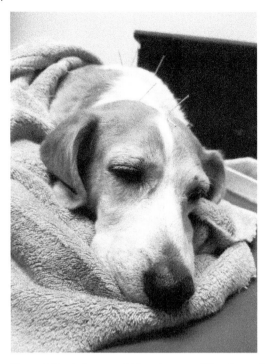

Figure 6.3 A six-year-old female spayed Beagle receiving acupuncture for cervical pain.

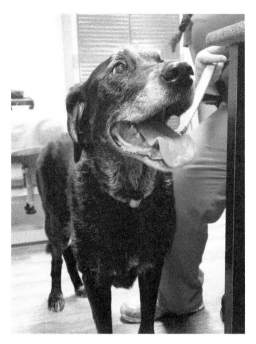

Figure 6.4 A 10-year-old female spayed Labrador Retriever who received acupuncture once every two weeks for maintenance of degenerative joint disease.

then once every other week for four weeks. By the end of her treatment (total of seven sessions), she no longer displayed clinical signs of cervical pain.

Degenerative Joint Disease

Acupoints: LI-10, ST-36, BL-11, BL-23, BL-60, KID-3, GB-34, GB-39, *Bai-hui*, *Shen-shu*

For hip, add: BL-54, GB-29, GB-30, *Jian-jiao*

For stifle, add: ST-35a/b, ST-34, SP-9, BL-54, BL-40, GB-32, GB-33, LIV-8

For tarsus, add: ST-41, SP-6, BL-54, BL-62, KID-3, KID-7

For shoulder, add: LI-14/LI-15, ST-10, SI-9, SI-10, TH-14, GB-21

For elbow, add: LU-5, LI-11, HT-3, SI-8, PC-3, TH-10, *Zhou-shu*

For carpus, add: LI-4, LU-7, LU-9, SI-4, HT-5, HT-7, PC-6, TH-4

Case example: A 10-year-old female spayed Labrador Retriever presented for slowing down and inability to climb the stairs to the front porch (Figure 6.4). Her body condition score was 7/9 and her muscle condition score of her hind limbs was 1/3. During the exam, she had difficulty with postural transitions, and suffered from bilateral carpal hyperextension. Based on physical exam and radiographs, she was diagnosed with moderate to severe bilateral osteoarthritis of the coxofemoral joints, with mild to moderate bony changes of the stifles, elbows, and carpi. She had already been prescribed carprofen, gabapentin, and fish oil supplement. She received dry needle and electroacupuncture at GV-20, BL-23, BL-54, GB-29, GB-30, GB-34,

KID-3, ST-36, GV-14, *Bai-hui*, *Jian-jiao*, and *Shen-shu*. She slept through her treatment, which was uneventful. The following day, she was slightly worse at home and slept most of the day, but 48 hours after treatment, her owner called to say she had more energy than she'd had in the last several years and was spending more time out in the yard. She received weekly acupuncture for the next four weeks, and was maintained with one session every two weeks.

Intervertebral Disc Disease (IVDD)

Acupoints: LI-10, ST-36, BL-23, BL-11, BL-40, KID-1, GV-14, *Bai-hui*, *Shen-shu*, *Liu-feng*

Case example: A six-year-old male neutered Pug mix presented for acute onset of paraplegia following a jump down from the couch (Figure 6.5). He was deep-pain negative upon arrival to the hospital. A compressive disc extrusion was identified at T13/L1 on MRI and he immediately underwent a right-sided hemilaminectomy. He received electroacupuncture (80/120 Hz for 30 minutes) at KID-1, GV-14, Bai-hui, LI-4, *Liu-feng*, *Shen-shu*, GV-20, ST-36 after recovery from anesthesia. He received daily inpatient therapy. By the following day, he had recovered deep-pain sensation of his hind limbs. By the third day of daily treatment, he had slight motor visualized at his hip flexors. By seven days after surgical decompression and initial acupuncture therapy, he was paraparetic and was discharged. He continued to receive acupuncture treatment once weekly for eight weeks, and eventually regained his ability to ambulate enough to have a good quality of life, although he continued to display proprioceptive ataxia.

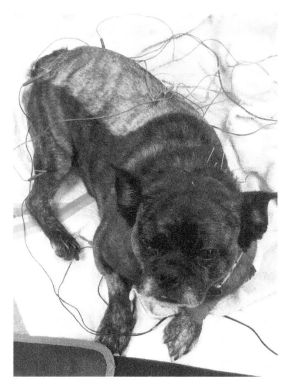

Figure 6.5 A six-year-old male neutered Pug mix receiving acupuncture for acute-onset paraplegia following episode of compressive disc extrusion and hemilaminectomy.

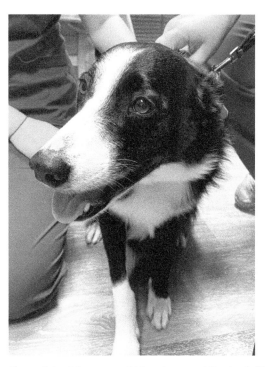

Figure 6.6 A four-year-old female spayed Border Collie who received weekly acupuncture treatments for management of epilepsy.

Seizures

Acupoints: SP-10, BL-17, BL-18, GB-20, LIV-3, GV-1, GV-20, GV-21, *Nao-shu*

Case example: A four-year-old female spayed Border Collie presented with acute onset of high-frequency, long-duration generalized seizures (Figure 6.6). Routine evaluation, including MRI, toxin panel, and evaluation of spinal fluid, revealed no significant findings. She was diagnosed with cryptogenic epilepsy, and prescribed daily levetiracetam with diazepam as needed. While the frequency of seizures decreased, she was still having multiple seizures per week, and was started on phenobarbital, after which, she was still having one to two seizures per week. She received dry-needle acupuncture at bilateral *Nao-shu*, *Da-feng-men*, GV-20, GB-20, BL-17, SP-10, and LIV-3, and aqua-acupuncture with Vitamin B_{12} in bilateral *An-shen*. She received treatment once weekly for one month, and only suffered two seizures during this time. She continued weekly acupuncture for an additional four weeks, where she only had one seizure. Based on her excellent response, she received acupuncture weekly. She never underwent dose reduction of anticonvulsants based on owner preference.

Diarrhea

Acupoints: ST-36, SP-6, BL-20, BL-21, GB-34, GV-1
  Chronic diarrhea, add: LI-10, BL-25, SP-9

  Acute or diarrhea with blood/mucus, add: ST-37, GV-14, *Wei-jian*

Case example: A six-year-old female spayed Beagle presented for a several-month history of chronic watery diarrhea (Figure 6.7). She had been adopted from a shelter and had never had normal stool. She was minimally responsive to dietary fiber. She was under the care of an internal medicine specialist upon referral. She received dry needle acupuncture at GV-20, electroacupuncture at BL-20, BL-21, ST-36, LI-10, GV-14, *Bai-hui*, *Shen-shu*, and aqua-acupuncture at GV-1. About an hour after her acupuncture treatment, her owner called: the dog had had her first normal bowel movement since adoption four months ago. She continued to receive acupuncture every other week for several weeks, before tapering to once monthly for maintenance. She never relapsed.

Constipation and Megacolon

Acupoints: ST-25, ST-37, SP-6, BL-20, BL-21, BL-25, TH-6, GV-1, CV-12

Case example: A 14-year-old male neutered cat presented with increasing straining to defecate, vomiting, and anorexia, and was diagnosed with megacolon (Figure 6.8). He underwent manual deobstipation several times before referral for acupuncture. He received dry needle acupuncture at BL-20, BL-21, ST-37, GV-1, and *Bai-hui*. He had little improvement following his first treatment. He was treated

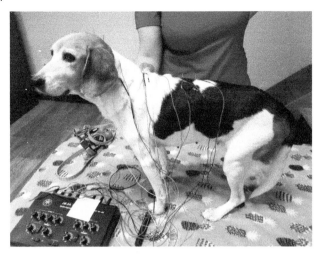

Figure 6.7 A six-year-old female spayed Beagle receiving acupuncture for chronic diarrhea.

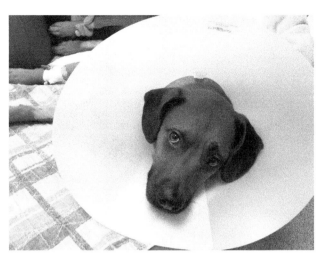

Figure 6.9 A three-year-old female intact Rhodesian Ridgeback who received acupuncture to resolve vomiting.

At this point in her clinical presentation, she was dehydrated, and her vomitus consisted of saliva and bile or nonproductive retching. She received aqua-acupuncture with Vitamin B_{12} at PC-6, CV-23, CV-12, which resolved her vomiting within 10 minutes.

Appetite Stimulation

Acupoints: ST-36, ST-37, BL-21, PC-6, GB-34, CV-12, *Jian-wei*, *Shan-gen*

Case example: A four-month-old female intact cat was surrendered to the shelter with history of severe upper respiratory infection (Figure 6.10). She suffered from oral and ocular ulceration and produced copious nasal and ocular discharges. She had a body condition score of 3/9 and was completely anorexic since admission. She was receiving IV fluids, doxycycline, saline nebulization, and many other conventional treatments. Acupuncture consisted of dry-needling of PC-6, BL-21, GV-14, and *Bai-hui* with needling of *Shan-gen* after 10 minutes, for a total treatment time of 20 minutes. The needles were removed, and a fresh plate consisting of a buffet of five different warmed wet cat foods, and a small plate of dry cat foods, were offered. She ate half of the offered foods, which was her first interest in food at all since admission.

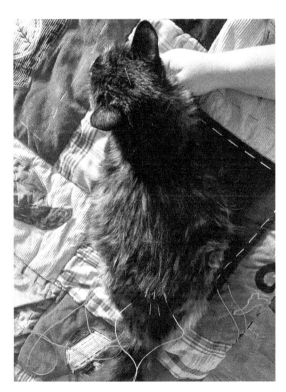

Figure 6.8 A 14-year-old male neutered cat receiving electroacupuncture for treatment of megacolon.

weekly for three weeks, when his owner noted he was straining less in the litterbox. After six weeks of weekly treatments, he was able to defecate normally. He was maintained on acupuncture every other week, as well as his conventional therapies, for maintenance of his quality of life.

Antiemesis

Acupoints: PC-6, GB-34, CV-12 CV-22, CV-23

Case example: A three-year-old female intact Rhodesian Ridgeback presented with acute gastroenteritis (Figure 6.9).

Congestive Heart Failure

Acupoints: LI-10, ST-36, BL-14, BL-15, HT-7, CV-14, CV-17, *An-shen*

Case example: A 13-year-old male neutered Terrier mix presented after diagnosis of congestive heart failure three months prior (Figure 6.11). He recovered from the initial episodes and was maintained on conventional medications, but had started to show more exercise intolerance and coughing at night. He received electroacupuncture at LI-10, ST-36, BL-14, BL-15, *Bai-hui*, and GV-14, and

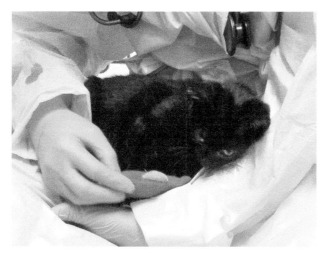

Figure 6.10 A four-month-old female intact Domestic Short Hair who received acupuncture for appetite stimulation.

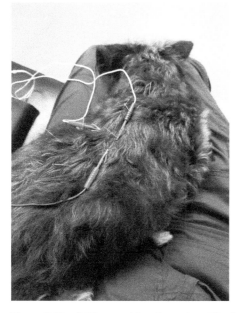

Figure 6.11 A 13-year-old male neutered Terrier mix receiving acupuncture for congestive heart failure.

aqua-acupuncture with Vitamin B_{12} at HT-7 and CV-14. After his first visit, he slept through the night without coughing. The next week, he was more active outside. He continued once weekly acupuncture for two more weeks, and then received every other week acupuncture to maintain his quality of life until he suddenly decompensated 18 months after his first acupuncture treatment and was euthanized.

Chronic Renal Disease

Acupoints: ST-36, BL-20, BL-21, BL-23, BL-24, KID-3, *Shan-gen*

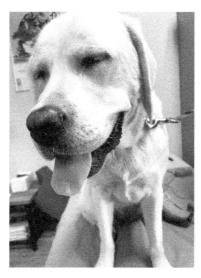

Figure 6.12 A one-year-old female intact yellow Labrador Retriever who received frequent acupuncture for management of renal dysplasia.

Case example: A one-year-old female intact yellow Labrador Retriever presented with a history of diagnosis of renal dysplasia a few months previous, as well as urinary incontinence (Figure 6.12). She was receiving subcutaneous fluids at her local veterinary clinic twice weekly and was fed a prescription renal diet. On presentation, her blood urea nitrogen was 35 mg/dL, her creatinine was 3.0 mg/dL, and her SDMA was 30ug/dL. She received dry-needle acupuncture at BL-20, BL-21, BL-23, BL-24, GV-20, GV-14, *Shen-shu*, and *Bai-hui*, and aqua-acupuncture with Vitamin B_{12} at BL-39. After her first treatment, her appetite improved. She received acupuncture every 2–4 weeks for several months, at which time her creatinine had decreased to 2.6mg/dL, she had a good appetite, and her urinary incontinence had resolved.

Summary

Acupuncture requires additional education to be used effectively by practitioners, but it is safe, inexpensive, and necessitates little special equipment. It is well-tolerated by most patients, and has been utilized in dogs, cats, horses, cows, birds, rabbits, and reptiles as well as other exotic and zoo species. Acupuncture is effective for analgesia due to injury or post-surgery, anxiety, nausea, vomiting, laryngeal hemiplegia, intervertebral disc disease, and management of many orthopedic and internal medicine conditions and is also an effective adjunct therapy for cardiovascular, respiratory, gastrointestinal, and renal diseases. As acupuncture has only been rigorously studied for less than 50 years in western countries, frequent exploration of current available literature is recommended as the field is progressing rapidly.

References

1 Xie, H. and Chrisman, C. (2009). Equine acupuncture: from ancient art to modern validation. *Am J Trad Chin Vet Med* 4: 1–4.

2 Dewey, C.W. and Xie, H. (2021). The scientific basis of acupuncture for veterinary pain management: a review based on relevant literature from the last two decades. *Open Vet J* 11: 203–209.

3 Xie, H. and Preast, V. (2007). *Xie's Veterinary Acupuncture*. Blackwell Publishing.

4 Zhou, W. and Benharash, P. (2014). Effects and mechanisms of acupuncture based on the principle of meridians. *J Acupunct Meridian Stud* 7: 190–193.

5 Maurer, N., Nissel, H., Egerbacher, M. et al. (2019). Anatomical evidence of acupuncture meridians in the human extracellular matrix: results from a macroscopic and microscopic interdisciplinary multicentre study on human corpses. *Evid Based Complement Alternat Med* 2019: 1–8.

6 Zhang, Z.-J., Wang, X.-M., and McAlonan, G.M. (2012). Neural acupuncture unit: a new concept for interpreting effects and mechanisms of acupuncture. *Evid Based Complement Alternat Med* 2012: e429412.

7 Zhao, Z.-Q. (2008). Neural mechanism underlying acupuncture analgesia. *Prog Neurobiol* 85: 355–375.

8 Chrisman, C.L. and Xie, H. (2011). Research support for the Jing Luo System. *Am J Tradit Chin Vet Med* 6: 1–4.

9 Chrisman, C.L. and Xie, H. (2013). The Jing Luo network: an overview of channels and collaterals and their clinical applications. *Am J Tradit Chin Vet Med* 8: 1–13.

10 Dorsher, P.T. and da Silva, M.A.H. (2022). Acupuncture's neuroanatomic and neurophysiologic basis. *Longhua Chin Med* 5: 8–8.

11 Lee, M.S., Jeong, S.-Y., Lee, Y.-H. et al. (2005). Differences in electrical conduction properties between meridians and non-meridians. *Am J Chin Med* 33: 723–728.

12 Falk, C.X., Birch, S., Avants, S.K. et al. (2000). Preliminary results of a new method for locating auricular acupuncture points. *Acupunct Electrother Res* 25: 165–177.

13 Jeong, D.-M., Lee, Y.-H., and Lee, M.S. (2004). Development of the meridian-visualizing system that superimposes a bio-signal upon a body image. *Am J Chin Med* 32: 631–640.

14 Li, J., Wang, Q., Liang, H. et al. (2012). Biophysical characteristics of meridians and acupoints: a systematic review. *Evid Based Complement Alternat Med* 2012: e793841.

15 Wang, P.Q., Hu, X.L., and Xu, J.S. (2002). The indication of infrared thermal images on body surface along 14 meridian lines. *Acupuncture Res* 27: 260.

16 Kovacs, F.M., Götzens García, V.J., García, A. et al. (1992). Experimental study on radioactive pathways of

17 hypodermically injected technetium-99m. *J Nucl Med* 33 (3): 403–407.

17 Lazorthes, Y., Esquerré, J.-P., Simon, J. et al. (1990). Acupuncture meridians and radiotracers. *Pain* 40: 109–112.

18 Liu, X., Chen, C., Yu, J. et al. (2010). Light propagation characteristics of meridian and surrounding non-meridian tissue. *Acta Photonica Sinica* 39: 29–33.

19 Xie, H. and Ortiz-Umpierre, C. (2006). What acupuncture can and cannot treat. *J Am Anim Hosp Assoc* 42: 244–248.

20 Kotani, N., Hashimoto, H., Sato, Y. et al. (2001). Preoperative intradermal acupuncture reduces postoperative pain, nausea and vomiting, analgesic requirement, and sympathoadrenal responses. *Anesthesiol J Am Soc Anesthesiol* 95: 349–356.

21 Dundee, J.W. and Ghaly, G. (1991). Local anesthesia blocks the antiemetic action of P6 acupuncture. *Clin Pharmacol Ther* 50: 78–80.

22 Xie, H. and Wedemeyer, L. (2012). The validity of acupuncture in veterinary medicine. *Am J Tradit Chin Vet Med* 7: 35–43.

23 Xie, H., Colahan, P., and Ott, E.A. (2005). Evaluation of electroacupuncture treatment of horses with signs of chronic thoracolumbar pain. *J Am Vet Med Assoc* 227: 281–286.

24 Faramarzi, B., Lee, D., May, K. et al. (2017). Response to acupuncture treatment in horses with chronic laminitis. *Can Vet J* 58: 823–827.

25 Lee, D., May, K., and Faramarzi, B. (2019). Comparison of first and second acupuncture treatments in horses with chronic laminitis. *Iran J Vet Res* 20: 9.

26 Dunkel, B., Pfau, T., Fiske-Jackson, A. et al. (2017). A pilot study of the effects of acupuncture treatment on objective and subjective gait parameters in horses. *Vet Anaesth Analg* 44: 154–162.

27 Thoresen, A.S. (2011). Outcome of horses with sarcoids treated with acupuncture at a single ting point: 18 cases (1995–2009). *Am J Tradit Chin Vet Med* 6: 29.

28 Kim M.-S. and Xie H. (2009). Use of electroacupuncture to treat laryngeal hemiplegia in horses. *Vet Rec* 165: 602–603.

29 Rungsri, P., Trinarong, C., Rojanasthien, S. et al. (2009). The effectiveness of electro-acupuncture on pain threshold in sport horses with back pain. *Am J Tradit Chin Vet Med* 4: 22–26.

30 Bello, C.A.O., Vianna, A.R.C.B., Noqueira, K. et al. (2018). Acupuncture in the restoration of vasomotor tonus of equine athletes with back pain. *J Dairy Vet Anim Res* 7.

31 Ying, W., Bhattacharjee, A., and Wu, S.S. (2019). Effect of laser acupuncture on mitigating anxiety in acute stressed horses: a randomized, controlled study. *Am J Tradit Chin Vet Med* 14: 33–40.

32 Aljobory, A.I., Jaafar, S., and Ahmed, A.S. (2021). Using acupuncture and electroacupuncture in the treatment of laminitis in racing horses: a comparative study. *Iraqi J Vet Sci* 35: 15–21.

33 Angeli, A.L. and Luna, S.P.L. (2008). Aquapuncture improves metabolic capacity in thoroughbred horses. *J Equine Vet Sci* 28: 525–531.

34 Wang, S.-M., Kain, Z.N., and White, P. (2008). Acupuncture analgesia: I. The scientific basis. *Anesth Analg* 106: 602.

35 Fry, L.M., Neary, S.M., Sharrock, J. et al. (2014). Acupuncture for analgesia in veterinary medicine. *Top Companion Anim Med* 29: 35–42.

36 Lin, L., Skakavac, N., Lin, X. et al. (2016). Acupuncture-induced analgesia: the role of microglial inhibition. *Cell Transplant* 25: 621–628.

37 Liang, Y., Qiu, Y., Du, J. et al. (2016). Inhibition of spinal microglia and astrocytes contributes to the anti-allodynic effect of electroacupuncture in neuropathic pain induced by spinal nerve ligation. *Acupunct Med* 34: 40–47.

38 Gu, W., Jiang, W., He, J. et al. (2015). Blockade of the brachial plexus abolishes activation of specific brain regions by electroacupuncture at LI4: a functional MRI study. *Acupunct Med* 33: 457–464.

39 Luna, S.P.L., Martino, I.D., Lorena, S.E.R.D.S., et al. (2015). Acupuncture and pharmacopuncture are as effective as morphine or carprofen for postoperative analgesia in bitches undergoing ovariohysterectomy. *Acta Cirúrgica Bras* 30: 831–837.

40 Gakiya, H.H., Silva, D.A., Gomes, J. et al. (2011). Electroacupuncture versus morphine for the postoperative control pain in dogs. *Acta Cir Bras* 26: 346–351.

41 Laim, A., Jaggy, A., Forterre, F. et al. (2009). Effects of adjunct electroacupuncture on severity of postoperative pain in dogs undergoing hemilaminectomy because of acute thoracolumbar intervertebral disk disease. *J Am Vet Med Assoc* 234: 1141–1146.

42 Lane, D.M. and Hill, S.A. (2016). Effectiveness of combined acupuncture and manual therapy relative to no treatment for canine musculoskeletal pain. *Can Vet J* 57: 407–414.

43 Silva, N.E.O.F., Luna, S.P.L., Joaquim, J.G.F. et al. (2017). Effect of acupuncture on pain and quality of life in canine neurological and musculoskeletal diseases. *Can Vet J* 58: 941–951.

44 Klide, A.M., Farnbach, G.C., and Gallagher, S.M. (1987). Acupuncture therapy for the treatment of intractable, idiopathic epilepsy in five dogs. *Acupunct Electrother Res* 12: 71–74.

45 Sumano, H., Bermudez, E., and Obregon, K. (2000). Treatment of wobbler syndrome in dogs with electroacupuncture. *Dtsch Tierarztl Wochenschr* 107: 231–235.

46 Yang, J.W., Jeong, S.M., Seo, K.M. et al. (2019). Effects of corticosteroid and electroacupuncture on experimental spinal cord injury in dogs. *J Vet Sci* 4: 97–101.

47 Hayashi, A.M., Matera, J.M., and Pinto, A.C.B.D.C.F. (2007). Evaluation of electroacupuncture treatment for thoracolumbar intervertebral disk disease in dogs. *J Am Vet Med Assoc* 231: 913–918.

48 Han, H.-J., Yoon, H.-Y., Kim, J.-Y. et al. (2010). Clinical effect of additional electroacupuncture on thoracolumbar intervertebral disc herniation in 80 paraplegic dogs. *Am J Chin Med* 38: 1015–1025.

49 Joaquim, J.G.F., Luna, S.P.L., Brondani, J.T. et al. (2010). Comparison of decompressive surgery, electroacupuncture, and decompressive surgery followed by electroacupuncture for the treatment of dogs with intervertebral disk disease with long-standing severe neurologic deficits. *J Am Vet Med Assoc* 236: 1225–1229.

50 Chueainta, P., Punyapornwithaya, V., Tangjitjaroen, W. et al. (2022). Acupuncture improves heart rate variability, oxidative stress level, exercise tolerance, and quality of life in tracheal collapse dogs. *Vet Sci* 9: 88.

51 Clifford, D.H., Lee, D.C., and Lee, M.O. (1983). Effects of dimethyl sulfoxide and acupuncture on the cardiovascular system of dogs. *Ann N Y Acad Sci* 411: 84–93.

52 Lee, H.-H., Oh, H.-W., Han, J.-W. et al. (2007). The efficacy of needle-acupuncture at Nei Guan (PC06) and Xin Shu (BL15) on bradycardia in dogs. *J Vet Clin* 24: 345–349.

53 Cho, Y.-H., Jun, H.-K., Kim, N.-J. et al. (2008). The efficacy of needle-acupuncture at Nei Guan (PC06) and Xin Shu (BL15) on canine tachycardia. *J Vet Clin* 25: 359–362.

54 Davies, A., Janse, J., and Reynolds, G.W. (1984). Acupuncture in the relief of respiratory arrest. *N Z Vet J* 32: 109–110.

55 Chae, M., Jung, J., Seo, M. et al. (2019). Ultrasonographic observation of intestinal mobility of dogs after acupunctural stimulation on acupoints ST-36 and BL-27. *J Vet Sci* 2: 221–226.

56 Radkey, D.I., Writt, V.E., Snyder, L.B.C. et al. (2019). Gastrointestinal effects following acupuncture at Pericardium-6 and Stomach-36 in healthy dogs: a pilot study. *J Small Anim Pract* 60: 38–43.

57 Tatewaki, M., Strickland, C., Fukuda, H. et al. (2005). Effects of acupuncture on vasopressin-induced emesis in conscious dogs. *Am J Physiol-Regul Integr Comp Physiol* 288: R401–R408.

58 Koh, R.B., Isaza, N., Xie, H. et al. (2014). Effects of maropitant, acepromazine, and electroacupuncture on vomiting associated with administration of morphine in dogs. *J Am Vet Med Assoc* 244: 820–829.

59 Scallan, E.M. and Simon, B.T. (2016). The effects of acupuncture point Pericardium 6 on hydromorphone-induced nausea and vomiting in healthy dogs. *Vet Anaesth Analg* 43: 495–501.

60 Pons, A., Canfrán, S., Benito, J. et al. (2017). Effects of dexmedetomidine administered at acupuncture point GV20 compared to intramuscular route in dogs. *J Small Anim Pract* 58: 23–28.

61 Kim, M.-S. and Nam, T.-C. (2006). Electroencephalography (EEG) spectral edge frequency for assessing the sedative effect of acupuncture in dogs. *J Vet Med Sci* 68: 409–411.

62 Perdrizet, J.A., Shiau, D.-S., and Xie H. (2019). The serological response in dogs inoculated with canine distemper virus vaccine at the acupuncture point Governing Vessel-14: a randomized controlled trial. *Vaccine* 37: 1889–1896.

63 Pellegrini, D.Z., Müller, T.R., Fonteque, J.H. et al. (2020). Equine acupuncture methods and applications: a review. *Equine Vet Educ* 32: 268–277.

64 Reginato, G.M., Xavier, N.V., Alonso, B.B. et al. (2020). Pharmacopuncture analgesia using flunixin meglumine injection into the acupoint GV1 (Ho Hai) after elective castration in horses. *J Equine Vet Sci* 87: 102911.

65 Scallan, E.M., Eckman, S.L., Coursey, C.D. et al. (2021). The analgesic and sedative effects of GV20 pharmacopuncture with low-dose hydromorphone in healthy dogs undergoing ovariohysterectomy. *Can Vet J* 62: 1104–1110.

66 Santos Godoi, T.L.O., Villas-Boas, J.D., Almeida, N.A.D.S. et al. (2014). Pharmacopuncture versus acepromazine in stress responses of horses during road transport. *J Equine Vet Sci* 34: 294–301.

67 Xie, H., Asquith, R.L., and Kivipelto, J. (1996). A review of the use of acupuncture for treatment of equine back pain. *J Equine Vet Sci* 16: 285–290.

68 Jaeger, G.T., Larsen, S., Soli, N. et al. (2006). Double-blind, placebo-controlled trial of the pain-relieving effects of the implantation of gold beads into dogs with hip dysplasia. *Vet Rec* 158: 722–726.

69 Law, D., McDonough, S., Bleakley, C. et al. (2015). Laser acupuncture for treating musculoskeletal pain: a systematic review with meta-analysis. *J Acupunct Meridian Stud* 8: 2–16.

70 Xie, H. and Holyoak, G.R. (2018). Tips to improve acupuncture results for lameness in horses. In: *Proceedings of the 64th Annual Convention of the American Association of Equine Practitioners*, 330–336. San Francisco, California: American Association of Equine Practitioners.

71 le Jeune, S., Henneman, K., and May, K. (2016). Acupuncture and equine rehabilitation. *Vet Clin North Am Equine Pract* 32: 73–85.

Section III

Manual Therapies
(Section Editor – Marilyn Maler)

7

Veterinary Manipulative Therapy: Neurology, Biomechanics, and Available Evidence

Marilyn Maler

Introduction

Manipulative therapy of animals as a standardized modality is a fairly recent development compared to manipulative therapy of humans. While Danial David Palmar established the first chiropractic school in 1897, it would be nearly a century later before a recognized program of animal chiropractic arose. Sharon Willoughby Blake DVM, DC is considered the founder of modern animal chiropractic. While practicing as a veterinarian, Dr. Willoughby witnessed the positive effects of chiropractic therapy on both herself and her canine patients. She subsequently earned a Doctorate of Chiropractic and then sought to educate her colleagues on animal chiropractic. She founded the American Veterinary Chiropractic Association and the first postgraduate animal chiropractic training program which was the main training program from 1989 to 2001. The development of the manipulative modality of animal osteopathy took a similar path, but instead it arose in Europe initially. Despite originating in the United States, osteopathy of humans became more popular in Europe, followed by osteopathy practice on animals.

It should be noted that while modern animal manipulative therapy education in the United States was developed from established human chiropractic techniques, the widely used term "chiropractic" in reference to manipulative therapy on animals has been legally challenged as a term that is strictly in reference to humans. Thus, the terms "spinal manipulation" or simply "manipulation" are now used to describe the modality instead.

Manipulation in Practice

While the terms mobilization and manipulation are often used interchangeably, they are different manual techniques in practice. Mobilization techniques use repetitive graded passive movements and can be applied to musculoskeletal soft tissue or joints. The unique biomechanical characteristic of manipulation is the application of a nonrepetitive, high velocity, low amplitude (HVLA) thrust directed to an articular or axial joint. There is low to moderate evidence to support manipulation as a therapy to reduce local pain, address muscle hypertonicity, and increase joint range of motion (ROM) [1]. As the HVLA thrust cannot be resisted by the patient, manipulations are thought to be less safe than mobilizations. A thorough knowledge of anatomy and biomechanics, good palpation skills, and well developed "feel" of joint motion is essential to perform manipulations safely and effectively [2, 3].

While manipulations are typically associated with the chiropractic and osteopathic practice, physiotherapists sometimes also use manipulations as part of their therapy. Osteopathic treatment may also consist of cranial therapy and visceral mobilization. In the United States, the legalities of which practitioners are allowed to perform manipulations on animals and the education requirements are covered in each state's veterinary practice act.

Joint Mechanics of Manipulative Therapy

Manipulation aims to correct a subluxation, a term which has caused confusion among medical practitioners. In manipulative therapy, subluxation refers to a hypomobility of a joint within the normal physiologic ROM. The term subluxation should not be confused with a luxation or dislocation which is characterized by hypermobility [4].

There are three zones of joint motion as described starting from the neutral position: physiologic, paraphysiologic,

Integrative Veterinary Medicine, First Edition. Edited by Mushtaq A. Memon and Huisheng Xie.
© 2023 John Wiley & Sons, Inc. Published 2023 by John Wiley & Sons, Inc.
Companion Website: www.wiley.com/go/memon/veterinary

and pathologic. The physiologic zone is where mobilization occurs and includes the active ROM and passive ROM. In the active ROM, the patient can actively move the joint themselves. The passive ROM is outside the active ROM and requires an outside force to move into and within. The paraphysiologic zone is where the HVLA thrust of manipulation occurs. In between the physiologic and paraphysiologic zones is the elastic barrier and is where joint end-feel is evaluated. In the pathological zone, anatomical limits of the joint are exceeded, and injury occurs [2, 3]. (Figure 7.1)

To determine if any subluxation is present and before any HVLA is applied, the joint should be evaluated for ROM and end-feel in all potential directions. (Figure 7.2) The normal ROM of joints will vary between species, within species and even within a spinal region on an individual. Joint end-feel is palpated at the elastic barrier. It will start as soft and resilient and will become firmer and restrictive as end of motion is reached. An abnormally restrictive end-feel will occur earlier within the ROM or will have a more abrupt and hard feeling [2, 3].

Theoretical Mechanism of Subluxation Effects

Numerous theories have been put forth to explain how a subluxation can cause deleterious effects on the body. The theories can be broadly grouped into three mechanism-oriented classifications and are not mutually exclusive. The first classification is encroachment of the intervertebral canal or spinal canal. Structures such as hypertrophied facet joint capsules, bulging disks, or enlarged intra-foraminal ligaments may encroach on the pressure sensitive nervous and vascular tissues of the intervertebral foramen or spinal canal and compromise their function. The second classification is based on the subluxation

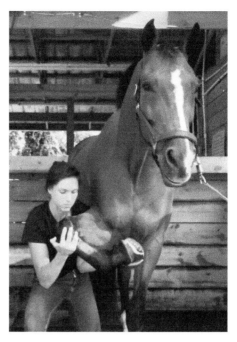

Figure 7.2 Joint motion in all directions should be evaluated before manipulation. An example of mobilization within the passive range of motion. To the untrained eye, the amount of mobility seen in this picture may appear excessive, but it is in fact normal. (Courtesy of Ashley Reid).

causing altered afferent input to the central nervous system which in turn alters function. In this theory, spinal manipulation corrects the biomechanics of the spine which then restores normal afferent input to the central nervous system. The third classification is founded on theories that during subluxation or misalignment, dentate ligaments may put abnormal traction on the spinal cord, causing cord distortion and consequently dysfunction. Each of these mechanisms has some supporting research, but deficiencies in studies are also noted, thus no conclusions are made currently [4].

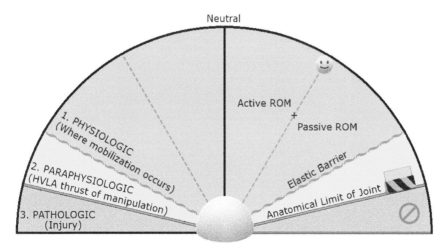

Three Zones of Joint Motion

Figure 7.1 The three zones of joint motion. (Courtesy of Ashley Reid).

Neurology of Pain Relief

While spinal manipulative therapy is commonly used to treat back and neck pain in human and veterinary integrated medicine, the mechanism of action for pain relief is not yet fully understood. Studies have reported potential pain-relieving effects from peripheral nervous system changes, spinal cord mechanisms, and supraspinal processes [5, 6]. There is support for the segmental/spinal cord mechanisms as the main contributor of pain relief [7].

Peripheral Mechanisms

It has been proposed that manipulative therapy provides pain inhibition through release of the hormone cortisol, which is known to have an anti-inflammatory effect on the periphery [8]. However, studies of blood and plasma cortisol levels showed inconsistent results after spinal manipulation [8, 9]. The conflicting results prevent drawing any conclusions about the role of cortisol as a method of pain inhibition at the present and more research is needed to make any determination of cortisol's role in spinal manipulation pain relief.

Another proposed peripheral mechanism of spinal manipulation pain relief is through an effect on sensitization of nociceptive fibers by reactive oxygen species. This is supported by animal studies that show spinal manipulation may provide pain relief by preventing an increase in the reactive oxygen species [10] or increasing serum antioxidant enzymes in humans [11]. While these studies are promising, more research is needed to determine if these mechanisms contribute specifically to pain relief through spinal manipulation.

A third potential peripheral mechanism of pain relief is through a reduction of pro-inflammatory and pro-nociceptive mediators (chemokines, TNF-α, and IL-1β) that are elevated during spine pain. These mediators are involved in peripheral sensitization of nociceptors. Research has suggested that spinal manipulation may decrease these pro-inflammatory responses, and this may in turn provide pain relief by altering peripheral inflammation and sensitization of nociceptors [10, 12]. A recent review determined that more well-controlled research with consistent results is needed before drawing conclusions about this proposed mechanism of pain relief [8].

Segmental/Spinal Cord Mechanisms

There is significant support that manipulation affects mechanoreceptors such as Golgi tendon organs and muscle spindle cells [13] to induce reflex muscle relaxation and pain inhibition [14]. The segmental effects of spinal manipulation on pain threshold and sensitivity are supported by systematic reviews and meta-analysis of related literature [15–17]. Several studies have shown an increased pain pressure threshold (decreased pain sensitivity) either local to the spinal manipulation application site or in the related dermatome [18–20]. Similar effects have been reported in myofascial tissue related to the treated spinal segment, indicating an effect on the myotome also [21–23]. The duration of these segmental effects has yet to be clarified, but appears to be short-lived, lasting only about ten minutes [24]. Although the studies are few, the effects of pain pressure sensitivity of manipulation compared to mobilization appear to be similar [18, 25–27]. Despite the large volume of support for the segmental effects of spinal manipulation, there are two recent studies showing conflicting results [28, 29].

Attenuation of temporal summation of afferent nociceptive fibers is also proposed as a segmental mechanism of pain relief. Repeated or constant stimulation of afferent nociceptive fibers will result in temporal summation, causing increased action potential firing and enhanced pain. There are numerous behavioral studies that support attenuation of temporal summation as a method of pain relief from spinal manipulation [30–36]. It is suggested that specifically C-fibers are modulated but there are no studies confirming this from a neurophysiological basis [7]. C-fibers may also play a role in spinal manipulation induced pain relief through central sensitization. This occurs when repeated stimulation of C-fibers induce synaptic plasticity in the spinal cord. Central sensitization is associated with chronic pain syndromes and can result in secondary hyperalgesia and allodynia. There is supportive but scarce research on central sensitization modification as a mechanism of pain relief from spinal manipulation [7, 37].

Supraspinal Mechanisms

The widespread hypoalgesia attributed to spinal manipulation has been attributed to supraspinal mechanisms but this assumption is debated as there is difficulty creating control groups, negating the placebo effect, and eliminating the interference of other causes of hypoalgesia associated with spinal manipulation [7, 27, 30, 38]. A recent review pointed out the shortcomings of research supporting supraspinal mechanisms and indicated that altered ascending information (spinal) was a likely the cause of the brain changes reported [39].

Evidence in Veterinary Medicine

Early equine chiropractic received much skepticism, partially due to the dubious ability for a practitioner to induce significant motion in the spine of such a large patient. This argument has been refuted by research on chiropractic effects on equine spinal kinematics [40]. Further, several studies using pressure algometry have demonstrated spinal manipulation's effect of increasing the spinal pain nociceptive threshold (decreased sensitivity) in horses [41, 42].

Other effects attributed to manipulation include an improvement in trunk and pelvic reflexes [43], enhancement of symmetry of the range of motion of the carpus and tarsus [44], less thoracic spine extension, reduced inclination of the pelvis, and improved pelvic motion symmetry [45]. More research is needed to confirm these findings and assess clinical relevance. A 2021 review of mobilization and manipulation techniques used in veterinary medicine concluded that there is a growing body of supporting evidence for equine spinal manipulation, but clinical trials of spinal manipulation of canines are severely lacking [1].

Summary

Despite initial skepticism of its effectives by a large portion of veterinarians, manipulation as a modality on animals has grown steadily since its inception and is now a generally accepted addition to integreted treamtment plans. This growth is primarily attributed to client and practitioner observations of its effectiveness on pain management and performance enhancement as while research is generally supportive, large scale clinical trials are lacking.

References

1 Haussler, K.K., Hesbach, A.L., Romano, L. et al. (2021 October). A systematic review of musculoskeletal mobilization and manipulation techniques used in veterinary medicine. *Animals* 11 (10): 2787.

2 Haussler, K.K. (April 1, 2016). Joint mobilization and manipulation for the equine athlete. *Vet Clin Equine Pract* 32 (1): 87–101.

3 Haussler, K.K. (December 1, 2009). Review of manual therapy techniques in equine practice. *J Equine Vet Sci* 29 (12): 849–869.

4 Henderson, C.N. (October 1, 2012). The basis for spinal manipulation: chiropractic perspective of indications and theory. *J Electromyogr Kinesiol* 22 (5): 632–642.

5 Bialosky, J.E., Bishop, M.D., Price, D.D. et al. (October 1, 2009). The mechanisms of manual therapy in the treatment of musculoskeletal pain: a comprehensive model. *Man Ther* 14 (5): 531–538.

6 Gyer, G., Michael, J., Inklebarger, J., and Tedla, J.S. (September 1, 2019). Spinal manipulation therapy: is it all about the brain? A current review of the neurophysiological effects of manipulation. *J Integr Med* 17 (5): 328–337.

7 Gevers-Montoro, C., Provencher, B., Descarreaux, M. et al. (2021 August). Neurophysiological mechanisms of chiropractic spinal manipulation for spine pain. *Eur J Pain* 25 (7): 1429–1448.

8 Kovanur-Sampath, K., Mani, R., Cotter, J. et al. (June 1, 2017). Changes in biochemical markers following spinal manipulation-a systematic review and meta-analysis. *Musculoskelet Sci Pract* 29: 120–131.

9 Valera-Calero, A., Gallego-Izquierdo, T., Malfliet, A., and Pecos-Martín, D. (January 8, 2019). Endocrine response after cervical manipulation and mobilization in people with chronic mechanical neck pain: a randomized controlled trial. *Eur J Phys Rehabil Med* 55 (6): 792–805.

10 Duarte, F.C., Kolberg, C., Riffel, A.P. et al. (July 1, 2019). Spinal manipulation therapy improves tactile allodynia and peripheral nerve functionality and modulates blood oxidative stress markers in rats exposed to knee-joint immobilization. *J Manipulative Physiol Ther* 42 (6): 385–398.

11 Kolberg, C., Horst, A., Moraes, M.S. et al. (February 1, 2015). Peripheral oxidative stress blood markers in patients with chronic back or neck pain treated with high-velocity, low-amplitude manipulation. *J Manipulative Physiol Ther* 38 (2): 119–129.

12 Roy, R.A., Boucher, J.P., and Comtois, A.S. (September 1, 2010). Inflammatory response following a short-term course of chiropractic treatment in subjects with and without chronic low back pain. *J Chiropr Med* 9 (3): 107–114.

13 Bolton, P.S. and Budgell, B.S. (January 1, 2006). Spinal manipulation and spinal mobilization influence different axial sensory beds. *Med Hypotheses* 66 (2): 258–262.

14 Pickar, J.G. (September 1, 2002). Neurophysiological effects of spinal manipulation. *Spine J* 2 (5): 357–371.

15 Coronado, R.A., Gay, C.W., Bialosky, J.E. et al. (October 1, 2012). Changes in pain sensitivity following spinal manipulation: a systematic review and meta-analysis. *J Electromyogr Kinesiol* 22 (5): 752–767.

16 Honoré, M., Leboeuf-Yde, C., and Gagey, O. (2018 December). The regional effect of spinal manipulation on the pressure pain threshold in asymptomatic subjects: a systematic literature review. *Chiropr Man Ther* 26 (1): 1–8.

17 Millan, M., Leboeuf-Yde, C., Budgell, B., and Amorim, M.A. (2012 December). The effect of spinal manipulative therapy on experimentally induced pain: a systematic literature review. *Chiropr Man Ther* 20 (1): 1–22.

18 Alonso-Perez, J.L., Lopez-Lopez, A., La Touche, R. et al. (October 1, 2017). Hypoalgesic effects of three different manual therapy techniques on cervical spine and psychological interaction: a randomized clinical trial. *J Bodyw Mov Ther* 21 (4): 798–803.

19 Fernández-De-Las-Peñas, C., Pérez-De-Heredia, M., Brea-Rivero, M. and Miangolarra-Page, J.C. (2007 June).

Immediate effects on pressure pain threshold following a single cervical spine manipulation in healthy subjects. *J Orthop Sports Physiol Ther* 37 (6): 325–329.

20 Fernández-Carnero, J., Fernández-de-las-Peñas, C., and Cleland, J.A. (November 1, 2008). Immediate hypoalgesic and motor effects after a sinle cervical spine manipulation in subjects with lateral epicondylalgia. *J Manipulative Physiol Ther* 31 (9): 675–681.

21 de Camargo, V.M., Alburquerque-Sendín, F., Bérzin, F. et al. (May 1, 2011). Immediate effects on electromyographic activity and pressure pain thresholds after a cervical manipulation in mechanical neck pain: a randomized controlled trial. *J Manipulative Physiol Ther* 34 (4): 211–220.

22 Dorron, S.L., Losco, B.E., Drummond, P.D., and Walker, B.F. (2016 December). Effect of lumbar spinal manipulation on local and remote pressure pain threshold and pinprick sensitivity in asymptomatic individuals: a randomised trial. *Chiropr Man Ther* 24 (1): 1–9.

23 Laframboise, M.A., Vernon, H., and Srbely, J. (2016 June). Effect of two consecutive spinal manipulations in a single session on myofascial pain pressure sensitivity: a randomized controlled trial. *J Can Chiropr Assoc* 60 (2): 137.

24 Honoré, M., Leboeuf-Yde, C., Gagey, O., and Wedderkopp, N. (2019 December). How big is the effect of spinal manipulation on the pressure pain threshold and for how long does it last?–secondary analysis of data from a systematic review. *Chiropr Man Ther* 27 (1): 1–2.

25 Fryer, G., Carub, J., and McIver, S. (April 1, 2004). The effect of manipulation and mobilisation on pressure pain thresholds in the thoracic spine. *J Osteopath Med* 7 (1): 8–14.

26 Thomson, O., Haig, L., and Mansfield, H. (June 1, 2009). The effects of high-velocity low-amplitude thrust manipulation and mobilisation techniques on pressure pain threshold in the lumbar spine. *Int J Osteopath Med* 12 (2): 56–62.

27 Salom-Moreno, J., Ortega-Santiago, R., Cleland, J.A. et al. (June 1, 2014). Immediate changes in neck pain intensity and widespread pressure pain sensitivity in patients with bilateral chronic mechanical neck pain: a randomized controlled trial of thoracic thrust manipulation vs non–thrust mobilization. *J Manipulative Physiol Ther* 37 (5): 312–319.

28 Aspinall, S.L., Jacques, A., Leboeuf-Yde, C. et al. (October 1, 2019). No difference in pressure pain threshold and temporal summation after lumbar spinal manipulation compared to sham: a randomised controlled trial in adults with low back pain. *Musculoskelet Sci Pract* 43: 18–25.

29 Honoré, M., Picchiottino, M., Wedderkopp, N. et al. (2020 December). What is the effect of spinal manipulation on the pressure pain threshold in young, asymptomatic subjects? A randomized placebo-controlled trial, with a cross-over design. *Chiropr Man Ther* 28 (1): 1–0.

30 Aspinall, S.L., Leboeuf-Yde, C., Etherington, S.J., and Walker, B.F. (2019 December). Manipulation-induced hypoalgesia in musculoskeletal pain populations: a systematic critical review and meta-analysis. *Chiropr Man Ther* 27 (1): 1–9.

31 Bialosky, J.E., Bishop, M.D., Robinson, M.E. et al. (2008 December). The influence of expectation on spinal manipulation induced hypoalgesia: an experimental study in normal subjects. *BMC Musculoskelet Disord* 9 (1): 1–9.

32 Bialosky, J.E., George, S.Z., Horn, M.E. et al. (February 1, 2014). Spinal manipulative therapy–specific changes in pain sensitivity in individuals with low back pain (NCT01168999). *J Pain* 15 (2): 136–148.

33 Bialosky, J.E., Bishop, M.D., Robinson, M.E. et al. (December 1, 2009). Spinal manipulative therapy has an immediate effect on thermal pain sensitivity in people with low back pain: a randomized controlled trial. *Phys Ther* 89 (12): 1292–1303.

34 Bishop, M.D., Beneciuk, J.M., and George, S.Z. (May 1, 2011). Immediate reduction in temporal sensory summation after thoracic spinal manipulation. *Spine J* 11 (5): 440–446.

35 George, S.Z., Bishop, M.D., Bialosky, J.E. et al. (2006 December). Immediate effects of spinal manipulation on thermal pain sensitivity: an experimental study. *BMC Musculoskelet Disord* 7 (1): 1–0.

36 Randoll, C., Gagnon-Normandin, V., Tessier, J. et al. (May 4, 2017). The mechanism of back pain relief by spinal manipulation relies on decreased temporal summation of pain. *Neuroscience* 349: 220–228.

37 Song, X.J., Huang, Z.J., Song, W.B. et al. (January 1, 2016). Attenuation effect of spinal manipulation on neuropathic and postoperative pain through activating endogenous anti-inflammatory cytokine interleukin 10 in rat spinal cord. *J Manipulative Physiol Ther* 39 (1): 42–53.

38 Martínez-Segura, R., De-La-Llave-Rincón, A.I., Ortega-Santiago, R. et al. (2012 September). Immediate changes in widespread pressure pain sensitivity, neck pain, and cervical range of motion after cervical or thoracic thrust manipulation in patients with bilateral chronic mechanical neck pain: a randomized clinical trial. *J Orthop Sports Physiol Ther* 42 (9): 806–814.

39 Meyer, A.L., Amorim, M.A., Schubert, M. et al. (2019 December). Unravelling functional neurology: does spinal manipulation have an effect on the brain?-A systematic literature review. *Chiropr Man Ther* 27 (1): 1–30.

40 Haussler, K.K., Bertram, J.E., and Gellman, K. (1999). In-vivo segmental kinematics of the thoracolumbar spinal region in horses and effects of chiropractic manipulations. *Proc Am Ass Equine Practnrs* 45: 327–329.

41 Haussler, K.K. and Erb, H.N. (November 21, 2003). Pressure algometry: objective assessment of back pain

and effects of chiropractic treatment. *Proc Am Ass Equine Practnrs* 49: 66–70.

42 Sullivan, K.A., Hill, A.E., and Haussler, K.K. (2008 January). The effects of chiropractic, massage and phenylbutazone on spinal mechanical nociceptive thresholds in horses without clinical signs. *Equine Vet J* 40 (1): 14–20.

43 Haussler, K.K., Manchon, P.T., Donnell, J.R., and Frisbie, D.D. (March 1, 2020). Effects of low-level laser therapy

and chiropractic care on back pain in Quarter Horses. *J Equine Vet Sci* 86: 102891.

44 Guest, J. and Cunliffe, C. (2014 June). The effects of chiropractic treatment on the range of motion of the carpus and tarsus of horses. *Equine Vet J* 46: 40–41.

45 Alvarez, C.G., L'ami, J.J., Moffatt, D. et al. (2008 March). Effect of chiropractic manipulations on the kinematics of back and limbs in horses with clinically diagnosed back problems. *Equine Vet J* 40 (2): 153–159.

8

Massage Therapy and Myofascial Principles

Marilyn Maler

Introduction

Massage therapy is the manipulation of the skin, muscle, or superficial soft tissues either manually or with an instrument or mechanical device for therapeutic purposes. It has been developed over thousands of years and across the world as a method to promote and restore health. There are over 80 different forms of massage, ranging from soft and pleasurable to deep and uncomfortable. This discussion will be limited to some of the most commonly used forms of therapeutic massage. With the more recent boom of research on myofascia and its relationship to whole body function, the importance of many forms of massage as myofascial therapeutic treatments is recognized.

Massage Therapy

Massage differs from other forms of manual therapy such as stretching and mobilization techniques in that massage typically does not involve changes in joint position as part of the prescribed treatment. The techniques used vary widely in the force, depth, speed, and tissues that are targeted. There is obvious overlap in massage therapy and myofascial treatment as it is impossible to employ massage without affecting the fascia enveloping the musculoskeletal system. Thus, discussion in the next section on myofascial principles will be partially applicable to massage therapy as well.

Development of Massage Therapy

Defined by Hippocrates as "the art of rubbing," massage has an extensive history. References of massage date back to 2500 BC, making it one of the first treatment modalities ever documented. Although first described in China,

ancient Greeks and Indians also implemented massage, but it was the Roman empire that notably embraced massage therapy for sport and war injuries [1, 2].

Like other forms of manual therapy, massage therapy was originally applied to humans and subsequently to domesticated animals. Early animal massage therapists were initially trained as human massage therapists that adapted their training to animals. Numerous animal massage schools and certification programs arose in the 1980s–1990s, but there is still no universally accepted standard of education or certification for animal massage therapists as there is for human massage therapists. In the United States, the legal requirements for animal massage therapy are determined by each state's veterinary board. It was shown that the training and experience of the therapist is an important factor in the effectiveness of massage [3].

Massage is generally considered safe and has a low risk of adverse effects. Contraindications to massage are not absolute rules based on empirical data, but rather guidelines grounded on common sense. Potential contraindications include acute inflammation, skin infection, nonconsolidated fracture, burns, active cancer tumor, deep vein thrombosis, and rhabdomyolysis [4–6].

Massage as Therapy for Musculoskeletal Pain and Dysfunction in Humans

The force, speed, depth, and pressure used in different forms of massage therapy to mobilize the tissues is highly varied, a factor that makes comparing research on massage therapy difficult. A 2014 review of massage therapy research indicates that moderate pressure massage is more effective than light pressure massage for improving chronic pain conditions; where moderate pressure massage involves moving the skin and light pressure massage involves lightly stroking

Integrative Veterinary Medicine, First Edition. Edited by Mushtaq A. Memon and Huisheng Xie.
© 2023 John Wiley & Sons, Inc. Published 2023 by John Wiley & Sons, Inc.
Companion Website: www.wiley.com/go/memon/veterinary

but not moving the skin [7]. It is theorized that the need for moderate pressure versus light pressure massage indicates involvement in stimulation of pressure receptors which in turn can activate the vagus nerve. The stimulation of the vagus nerve is theorized as the mechanism for massage therapy's effects on gastric function, heart rate, blood pressure, and cortisol levels [7]. A massage research review of years 2013–2016 covered approximately 20 randomized controlled trials conducted on pain syndromes. Results suggest massage is effective in reducing pain, increasing range of motion and/or improving function in several types of musculoskeletal pain/dysfunction categories, including back and neck pain, knee and upper limb arthritis, and muscle pain [8].

Despite research that claims widespread benefits of massage for pain, there are recent reviews that question the validity of such claims. Recent reviews found no studies of moderate to high strength to support claims of pain relief [9, 10]. This finding is consistent with an earlier review of sports massage that concluded there were only equivocal results on blood flow, blood lactate removal, and delayed onset of muscle soreness, with blood lactate removal following exercise more efficiently removed through active recovery strategies rather than through massage [11]. It is noted that applying scientific principles to the study of massage and other forms of manual therapy presents methodological challenges for researchers

In addition to other design challenges, the skill and experience of the therapist is a variable which is not easily reproduced across studies.

Research in Animals

In 2002 the Jack Meagher Institute published a small but pivotal equine study showing the positive effects of increased range of motion demonstrated as increased stride length on horses massaged for 20 minutes using direct pressure, cross-fiber friction, and compression. In this small, controlled study, horses underwent treadmill locomotion evaluation to record stride lengths before and after massage. The specific muscles targeted with massage therapy were major muscles involved in the planned work: the supraspinatus, triceps brachii, biceps femoris, and superficial gluteal muscles. After massage, the stride length at the walk increased by 3.6% (4.8 inches) and the stride length at the trot increased by 1.2% (1.7 inches). Due to increased range of motion, a decreased stride frequency was documented [12]. Although these findings imply a positive effect of sports massage on athletic performance in the horse, the findings are not considered clinically significant due to the small sample size. These findings were consistent with larger studies involving human athletes which demonstrated that therapeutic massage induced improvements in flexibility

and range of motion [13, 14]. Similarly, a subsequent comparative crossover design study demonstrated that massage to the caudal muscles of the equine hind limb, that is the superficial gluteal, semitendinosus, biceps femoris, and semimembranosus muscles, significantly increased both passive and active hind limb protraction. This study measured active hind limb protraction as increased stride length, a result supportive of the previous Jack Meagher study [15]. Other studies showed massage therapy in horses resulted in lowered mechanical nociceptive thresholds within the thoracolumbar region as measured by pressure algometry [16] and a reduction in stress-related behavior [17].

Despite these few promising equine studies, there is still not ample controlled research to support longstanding claims that massage can increase blood flow, promote relaxation, reduce muscle hypertonicity, increase tissue extensibility, reduce pain, and promote return to normal function [11, 12, 18]. Despite of a lack of clear evidence of massage therapy benefits in horses, its use and acceptance by animal owners and veterinarians has grown. A recent international survey of veterinary groups on rehabilitation modalities used in horse treatments revealed that massage was used by 69% of the respondents [19].

Research and literature covering the use of massage in small animals is minimal. Techniques originally described for humans are being used on small animals and the indications and purported benefits extrapolated from human and equine research [2]. Massage use in dogs and cats includes indications outside the common musculoskeletal/athletic massage therapy in horses and also includes: control of postoperative swelling and edema, support to intensive care patients, osteoarthritis and orthopedic rehabilitation, chronic pain and palliative care of geriatric and cancer patients [2].

Massage Techniques

Depending on the patient, diagnosis, and desired outcome, different techniques are employed by therapists. While there are some preferred techniques for specific issues, the final choice is usually based on practitioner's experience and opinion of the superiority of certain techniques for desired outcomes. Independent of the techniques chosen, the therapist should evaluate the tissue and take note of the tissue's tone, temperature, moisture content (hydration), pliability, elasticity, and contour [20]. Massage may be performed using the fingers, palms, knuckles, elbows and even shoulders. Mechanical devices are becoming more common and mostly provide vibration or percussion to the tissues. Mechanical devices do not provide the evaluation of tissues and the feedback changes in tissue that is only possible through the therapist's hands, so it is not advised to rely solely on mechanical devises for treatments.

Massage may be divided broadly as medical or therapeutic massage in which there is a specific injury or physiological goal being addressed or sports massage in which improved athletic outcomes/injury prevention is the goal. Common Therapeutic massage techniques performed in equine and small animal rehabilitation include effleurage, petrissage, tapotage, friction, and skin rolling [2, 6, 20]. To treat equine back pain, massage sessions of 20 to 30 minutes are recommended with the addition of passive mobilization likely improving results [6, 20].

Sports massage is performed either before or after competition. The rationale behind pre-exercise or pre-competition massage is that it prepares muscles for the upcoming activity. Post exercise or post competition massage is chosen based on the claim of enhanced removal of metabolic waste. Neither claim is fully supported by research. Sport massage techniques are numerous and most often focuses on various "point therapies" such as stress point therapy and trigger point therapy, and use techniques such as compression, direct pressure, friction, effleurage, and myofascial release [6].

Description of Techniques

Effleurage or stroking: This technique is commonly used at the beginning and at the end of massage sessions and as a transition between other techniques. It is a technique that prepares the patient and the superficial tissues for deeper work and is used to promote venous and lymphatic fluid return. Effleurage uses long and slow rhythmic strokes with pressure being applied as the therapist's hands are moving away from their own body and preferably in the direction of venous return of the patient [20].

Petrissage or kneading: This is a technique that is firmer and deeper than effleurage and involves a large portion of muscle while using the hands in a down, around, and up motion in an attempt to recreate the compression and relaxation cycle of a working muscle. On the large muscles of horses, the therapist would use a loosely clenched fist with alternating hands in which one hand is pushing down while the other is coming up. The benefits of kneading are enhanced circulatory and lymph flow, decreased muscle tension, and mobilization of scar tissue including adhesions following a hematoma [6, 20].

Skin rolling: The skin is picked up between the fingers and thumb rolled over the underlying tissues in a continuous manner. Skin rolling, although seemingly superficial, is mobilizing the subcutaneous fascia which is contiguous with the fascia throughout the whole body and thus may have much further reaching physiological effects. It is also used to improve circulatory flow through the dermis [6, 20].

Friction: The technique is chosen when specific local work is required. This technique is unique in that the direction of pressure is cross fiber meaning that the force direction is in a transverse manner across the directional flow of the underlying tissue fibers. In this technique it is important that the practitioner's index finger is supported by a second finger so that the pressure is deep and firm to ensure the skin and underlying tissue move as one in order to be effective and to prevent blister formation. Friction is used for the mobilization and breakdown of scar tissue and adhesions [6, 20] and muscular contractures, trigger point elimination, myofascial release, and to promote pain relief [2].

Tapotage: This is a percussion-based technique in which cupped hands, the edge of the hand or tips of the fingers are used to induce tissue vibration, activation of the cutaneous reflex, and consequent vasodilation. Tapotage variations include beating (hitting lightly with closed fist), slapping (hitting lightly with fingers), hacking (hitting with edge of the hand), tapping (using fingertips), and cupping (hitting with hands formed into a cup shape), which makes a characteristic sound when applied. Tapotage is frequently used in respiratory physiotherapy to help loosen and eliminate accumulated lower airway secretions. It is also utilized to increase blood flow prior to exercise and to promote muscle recovery and relaxation after exercise [6].

Vibration and shaking: This type of massage produces coarse and energetic vibration of tissue. This technique is used in therapeutic and sports massage. It is employed with tapotage to disperse mucus from the lower respiratory tract and improve respiratory function. Benefit claims are reduced edema in tissues and muscle relaxation [1]. Vibration is the technique that many modern mechanical devices replicate.

Compression: Compression technique utilizes rhythmic pressure in a pumping motion to repeatedly compresses a muscle against the underlying bone, which has the effect of flattening and separating the muscle fascicles [6].

Direct pressure: Direct pressure technique is commonly used for "point therapies" such as trigger point therapy. It is a form of compression that involves applying and holding pressure to create a temporary ischemia of the area, after which extracellular fluid and blood are redistributed and the area becomes more pliable when palpated [6].

Myofascial release therapy: This therapy has become an area of increased interest recently, coinciding with the boom in fascial research in the early 2000s. Myofascial release therapy is not technically single technique, but a combination of several massage techniques. Myofascial release therapy is intended to affect the three-dimensional subcutaneous fascial web surrounding the muscles, tendons and ligaments. By releasing myofascial restrictions, greater freedom of movement may be achieved [6].

Lymphatic drainage: Manual lymphatic drainage encompasses a set of specific techniques based on gentle, superficial gliding movements, such as effleurage, to promote lymph flow. It is used for post-operative swelling and lymphedema. Lymphatic drainage purpose is to move accumulated fluids and lymph from the interstitial areas and back into circulation [1, 2].

Myofascial Principles

A Contemporary View of Fascia

Fascia is a fast-growing area of research, both for its own sake and as a potential explanation as a mechanism of action for several therapies including acupuncture, massage, and osteopathic and chiropractic medicine. The first International Fascia Research Congress originated in 2007 and has been held every 2–3 years thereafter. The volume of peer-reviewed research papers on this topic has grown steadily, particularly since 2005.

Fascia was historically regarded as a simple packing material covering the more important tissues such as muscles, organs, vessels, and nerves. The importance of fascia's own functions and its integration into other body systems has recently come to light. It is no longer regarded as an inert tissue as it has been shown to not only have adaptable mechanical properties, but also immune, proprioceptive and nociceptive functions.

The Fascia Nomenclature Committee (2014) was formed from the Fascia Research Society founded in 2007 and proclaimed a widely accepted modern description of fascia as follows. "The fascial system consists of the three-dimensional continuum of soft, collagen-containing, loose and dense fibrous connective tissues that permeate the body. It incorporates elements such as adipose tissue, adventitia, and neurovascular sheaths, aponeuroses, deep and superficial fasciae, epineurium, joint capsules, ligaments, membranes, meninges, myofascial expansions, periosteum, retinacula, septa, tendons, visceral fasciae, and all the intramuscular and intermuscular connective tissues including endo-/peri-/epimysium. The fascial system interpenetrates and surrounds all organs, muscles, bones and nerve fibers, endowing the body with a functional structure, and providing an environment that enables all body systems to operate in an integrated manner." [21]

Myofascia is fascia associated with skeletal muscle and is anatomically divided into the epimysium, perimysium, and endomysium. Current understanding of the expansiveness and interconnectedness of all fascia brings new light to myofascial therapies. Therapy on the myofascia may affect the entire fascial system and thus the entire body. Conversely, factors outside the fascial system (pH, sympathetic tone, toxins, etc.,) may affect the fascia in a way that requires fascial therapy to be expanded beyond the direct work on the fascial tissue itself.

Mechanical Properties of Fascia

The mechanical properties of fascia are pivotal to its structural and musculoskeletal function, as alterations in fascial stiffness or compliance have been shown to alter intermuscular force transmission and thus likely muscle mechanics [22–25]. The mechanical properties of fascia are not static and can be altered by many internal and external factors [25].

Fascia can alter its stiffness (the resistance to external deformation) through two mechanisms: cellular contraction (usually myofibroblasts) and the modification of the fluid characteristics [26]. The presence of intrafascial myofibroblasts is well documented in normal fascia, the active contraction of which may augment fascial stiffness [27, 28]. In the short term, the force derived from cellular contraction is not considered sufficient to have a significant impact on mechanical joint stability or normal biomechanics but is considered to effect motoneuronal coordination when viewed over the longer term of several minutes. Over days to months, cellular contraction forces can induce long-term and severe tissue contractures [27, 29] and excessive long-term myofibroblast activity has been documented in fibrosis and several types of pathological fibrotic contractures [28].

This cellular contractility seems independent from a direct synaptic signal transmission from the central nervous system such as with skeletal muscle contractions. Instead, this fascial cellular contractility is influenced via the expression of various cytokines within the ground substance of the fascia. One of these cytokines, Transforming Growth Factor β1 (TGF-β1) is positively influenced by the sympathetic nervous system [28]. Chronic shifts in the autonomic nervous system toward a more sympathetic status may therefore increase fascial stiffness, and thus affect the development, prevention and treatment of musculoskeletal pain conditions [26, 28]. Cellular contraction may also be altered by the pH level in the ground substance, with a more acidic level leading to increased fascial stiffness. The importance of this information, if verified, is that therapeutic strategies to modify the acidity of the ground substance, such as via moderate exercise and nutritional modifications, might help relieve conditions associated with enhanced fascial stiffness [28].

A second method of altering fascial stiffness is modification of the fluids water and hyaluronic acid (HA) and is likely the method of short-term fascial stiffness changes; while long-term stiffness is likely driven by cell contraction as discussed previously. Water bound in the tissue will substantially affect the mechanical stiffness of fascia [30]. HA acts as a gliding lubricant between the fibrous fascial layers and between the fascia and underlying muscle. While HA facilitates movement at physiological levels, it may cause restrictions at higher levels [31]. Increased fascial stiffness may also occur due to the thixotropic qualities of HA in which HA will become more viscous in the absence of mechanical loading, such as occurs with immobilization or physical inactivity [26].

In addition to cellular contraction and fluid modifications, fascial stiffness is also increased by aging, fibrous cross-linking of fascia, extracellular matrix deposition and neuromuscular diseases. Fascial stiffness is decreased by corticosteroids and stretch induced tissue elongation. Factors that show ambiguous effects include tissue hydration, HA, estrogen, and genetic makeup [25].

Myofascial Force Transmission

The previously described ability of fascia to change its tensional state is of great significance when considering body wide myofascial continuity in movement, therapy and training. The "insertion moves toward origin" explanation for musculoskeletal movement has been challenged with the deeper understanding of myofascia. The simplified concept of a motion occurring by a muscle contraction solely transmitting forces through myotendinous junctions onto osseous insertions is outdated. Force transmission through intermuscular and extra muscular fascial tissues has been documented in animals, but the amount of contribution of these non-myotendinous fascial tissues is disputed [32]. Altered stiffness or compliance outside the normal range has been shown to change the amount of intermuscular force transmission shared by the myofascial tissue and may have a significant effect on muscular movement mechanics [22–24].

Myofascial Chains

Contradictory to historical descriptions of skeletal muscles working as independent units, recent research suggests that skeletal muscles work in a synchronous manner along anatomical chains commonly termed myofascial chains. The existence of myofascial chains is becoming more accepted as fact as evidence accumulates and the capability of force transmission via myofascial chains is a topic of recent increased interest [33]. Though there are several proposed models of muscle chains and muscle slings, the model of Anatomy Trains by Thomas Myers is one of the most widely accepted and referenced myofascial chain explanations [33]. In this scheme, there are 12 sets of lines through the outer layer of myofascia. With regards to location, these lines have some commonality to the meridians of acupuncture. A systematic review covering six of the twelve myofascial lines proposed by Myers concluded that there is strong empirical support for three of the six lines

studied, ambiguous results for two lines and poor evidence for one line [34]. Similar myofascial lines have been proposed for dogs and horses [35].

Trigger Points and Myofascial Therapy

A trigger point (TrP) is a point from which symptoms, primarily referred pain, are originated. TrPs may be either active or latent. Active TrPs are painful at rest or during normal physiological movement while latent TrPs are not spontaneously painful and only become painful when provoked by pressure. A TrP in the muscle is termed a myofascial trigger point (mTrP). TrPs may also be found in ligament, tendon, periosteum, etc., and are named as TrPs for the respective tissue [36].

Myofascial trigger points (mTrP) are frequently a cause of musculoskeletal pain and while they have been a target of manual therapists for several centuries, they have only become a focus of myofascial scientific research in the last several decades and are now a well-researched phenomenon. A mTrP is defined as "a hyperirritable spot in skeletal muscle that is associated with a hypersensitive palpable nodule in a taut band." [37] The sarcomeres in a mTrP are contracted and thus shortened, causing the adjacent sarcomeres to become elongated. (Figure 8.1) Therapy on mTrP's is primarily directed at releasing the contraction knot of the shortened sarcomeres of the mTrP which will then allow the elongated adjacent sarcomeres to return to normal length.

Characteristic findings of a mTrP are localized hypoxia causing an energy crisis as the center of pathological changes, altered EMG potential which is interpreted as motor endplate malfunction, and changes in biochemistry including a decreased pH and increased inflammatory mediators which in turn lead to peripheral sensitization of nociception. Ischemia and hypoxia lead to pain, connective tissue shortening and pathological crosslinks in the collagenic tissue of the myofascia. Pathological crosslinks in myofascia will then cause associated muscle dysfunction [36]. Chronic mTrPs exhibit rigor complexes as a result of the energy crisis from hypoxia, and connective tissue shortening and adhesions from the local inflammatory processes [36]. While muscle release techniques (e.g., dry needling, shockwave) may treat the rigor complexes, they may not address the connective tissue pathology effectively. Manual techniques have been described that propose to address both the rigor complexes and connective tissue changes through myofascial trigger point therapy IMTT®. Other manual methods of myofascial therapy that also have varying degrees of proof of efficacy include Rolfing, Myofascial Induction Therapy, Connective Tissue Manipulation, and Fascial Manipulation® [37].

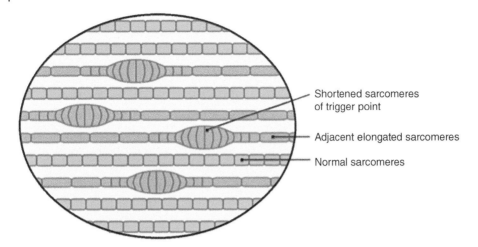

Figure 8.1 Myofascial trigger points within a taunt band of muscle.

Summary

While manual therapists have long touted the benefits of massage and myofascial therapy on whole body health and healing, these claims have often been met with skepticism. It is only in the last few decades that clinical research on fascia has been able to explain not only the importance of myofascia as a major player in musculoskeletal system function, but also explore fascia's role in immunity, proprioception, and nociception. It is expected that with this expansion of knowledge, that fascial therapy as an accepted and prescribed treatment will also expand.

References

1 Goats, G.C. (September 1, 1994). Massage–the scientific basis of an ancient art: part 1. The techniques. *Br J Sports Med* 28 (3): 149–152.

2 Formenton, M.R., Pereira, M.A., and Fantoni, D.T. (December 1, 2017). Small animal massage therapy: a brief review and relevant observations. *Top Comp Anim Med* 32 (4): 139–145.

3 Moraska, A. (January 1, 2007). Therapist education impacts the massage effect on postrace muscle recovery. *Med Sci Sports Exerc* 39 (1): 34–37.

4 Vickers, A. and Zollman, C. (September 9, 2000). ABC of complementary medicine: massage therapies. *Br Med J* 321 (7261): 1254–1257.

5 Hernandez-Reif, M., Field, T., Krasnegor, J., and Theakston, H. (January 1, 2001). Lower back pain is reduced and range of motion increased after massage therapy. *Int J Neurosci* 106 (3–4): 131–145.

6 Bromiley, M. (March 27, 2013). *Equine Injury, Therapy and Rehabilitation*, 3e. Oxford, UK: John Wiley & Sons, 76–129.

7 Field, T. (November 1, 2014). Massage therapy research review. *Complement Ther Clin Pract* 20 (4): 224–229.

8 Field, T. (August 1, 2016). Massage therapy research review. *Complement Ther Clin Pract* 24: 19–31.

9 Miake-Lye, I., Lee, J., Lugar, T. et al. Massage for pain: an evidence map [Internet].

10 Miake-Lye, I.M., Mak, S., Lee, J. et al. (May 1, 2019). Massage for pain: an evidence map. *J Altern Complement Med* 25 (5): 475–502.

11 Hemmings, B.J. (November 1, 2001). Physiological, psychological and performance effects of massage therapy in sport: a review of the literature. *Phys Ther Sport* 2 (4): 165–170.

12 Scott, M. and Swenson, L.A. (September 1, 2009). Evaluating the benefits of equine massage therapy: a review of the evidence and current practices. *J Equine Vet Sci* 29 (9): 687–697.

13 Kokkonen, J. and Allred, J. (May 1, 2002). The effects of chronic sports massage on strength and flexibility. *Med Sci Sports Exerc* 34 (5): 47.

14 Coles, M.G., Jones-Harvey, V.N., Greer, F.A., and Gilbert, W.D. (May 1, 2005). Effect of sports massage on range of motion, peak torque, and time to peak torque: 1351: board# 206: 2: 00 PM-3: 30 PM. *Med Sci Sports Exerc* 37 (5): S264.

15 Hill, C. and Crook, T. (2010 November). The relationship between massage to the equine caudal hindlimb muscles and hindlimb protraction. *Equine Vet J* 42: 683–687.

16 Sullivan, K.A., Hill, A.E., and Haussler, K.K. (2008 January). The effects of chiropractic, massage and phenylbutazone on spinal mechanical nociceptive thresholds in horses without clinical signs. *Equine Vet J* 40 (1): 14–20.

17 McBride, S.D., Hemmings, A., and Robinson, K. (2004). A preliminary study on the effect of massage to reduce stress in the horse. *J Equine Vet Sci* 2 (24): 76–81.

18 Ramey, D.W. and Tiidus, P.M. (2002 May). Massage therapy in horses: assessing its effectiveness from empirical data in humans and animals. *Compendium* 24 (5): 418–423.

19 Wilson, J.M., McKenzie, E., and Duesterdieck-Zellmer, K. (June 11, 2018). International survey regarding the use of rehabilitation modalities in horses. *Front Vet Sci* 5: 120.

20 Bromiley, M.W. (1999). Physical therapy for the equine back. *Vet Clin North Am Equine Pract* 15 (1): 223–246.

21 Bordoni, B., Mahabadi, N., and Varacallo, M. (2022 January). Anatomy, fascia. [Updated 2021 July 22]. In: *StatPearls* [Internet]. Treasure Island, FL: StatPearls Publishing. https://www.ncbi.nlm.nih.gov/books/NBK493232.

22 Smeulders, M.J. and Kreulen, M. (December 1, 2007). Myofascial force transmission and tendon transfer for patients suffering from spastic paresis: a review and some new observations. *J Electromyogr Kinesiol* 17 (6): 644–656.

23 Yucesoy, C.A. and Huijing, P.A. (December 1, 2007). Substantial effects of epimuscular myofascial force transmission on muscular mechanics have major implications on spastic muscle and remedial surgery. *J Electromyogr Kinesiol* 17 (6): 664–679.

24 Huijing, P.A., Voermans, N.C., Baan, G.C. et al. (2010 October). Muscle characteristics and altered myofascial force transmission in tenascin-X-deficient mice, a mouse model of Ehlers-Danlos syndrome. *J Appl Physiol* 109 (4): 986–995.

25 Zügel, M., Maganaris, C.N., Wilke, J. et al. (December 1, 2018). Fascial tissue research in sports medicine: from molecules to tissue adaptation, injury and diagnostics: consensus statement. *Br J Sports Med* 52 (23): 1497.

26 Wilke, J., Schleip, R., Yucesoy, C.A., and Banzer, W. (January 1, 2018). Not merely a protective packing organ? A review of fascia and its force transmission capacity. *J Appl Physiol* 124 (1): 234–244.

27 Schleip, R., Gabbiani, G., Wilke, J. et al. (April 2, 2019). Fascia is able to actively contract and may thereby influence musculoskeletal dynamics: a histochemical and mechanographic investigation. *Front Physiol* 10: 33.

28 Schleip, R. and Klingler, W. (2019 October). Active contractile properties of fascia. *Clin Anat* 32 (7): 891–895.

29 Castella, L.F., Buscemi, L., Godbout, C. et al. (May 15, 2010). A new lock-step mechanism of matrix remodelling based on subcellular contractile events. *J Cell Sci* 123 (10): 1751–1760.

30 Haut, T.L. and Haut, R.C. (January 1, 1997). The state of tissue hydration determines the strain-rate-sensitive stiffness of human patellar tendon. *J Biomech* 30 (1): 79–81.

31 Pavan, P.G., Stecco, A., Stern, R., and Stecco, C. (2014 August). Painful connections: densification versus fibrosis of fascia. *Curr Pain Headache Rep* 18 (8): 1–8.

32 Maas, H. and Sandercock, T.G. (2010 October). Force transmission between synergistic skeletal muscles through connective tissue linkages. *J Biomed Biotechnol* 2010.

33 Krause, F., Wilke, J., Vogt, L., and Banzer, W. (2016 June). Intermuscular force transmission along myofascial chains: a systematic review. *J Anat* 228 (6): 910–918.

34 Wilke, J., Krause, F., Vogt, L., and Banzer, W. (March 1, 2016). What is evidence-based about myofascial chains: a systematic review. *Arch Phys Med Rehabil* 97 (3): 454–461.

35 Ahmed, W., Kulikowska, M., Ahlmann, T. et al. (2019 December). A comparative multi-site and whole-body assessment of fascia in the horse and dog: a detailed histological investigation. *J Anat* 235 (6): 1065–1077.

36 Gautschi, R. (2012). Trigger points as a fascia-related disorder. In: *The Tensional Network of the Human Body*, 1e (ed. R. Schelip, T. Findley, L. Chaitow, and P.A. Huijing), 233–277. Great Britain: Elsevier.

37 Dommerholt, J. (2012). Trigger point therpay. In: *The Tensional Network of the Human Body*, 1e (ed. R. Schelip, T. Findley, L. Chaitow, and P.A. Huijing), 297–475. Great Britain: Elsevier.

Section IV

Botanical and Herbal Therapies
(Section Editor – Signe Beebe)

9

Herbal Medicine – Origins and Major Systems of Herbal Therapy with Selected Evidence-based Interventions

Signe Beebe

Introduction

More and more people are seeking integration between conventional medicine and other systems of medicine for themselves and their pets. Herbal medicine, also known as botanical medicine or ethnobotanicals, is the use of plants or plant derivatives that have a medicinal or therapeutic effect on the body. The entire plant, or a part of the plant may be used; herbal practitioners use flowers, berries, leaves, stems, and roots of plants that contain multiple active constituents to produce a therapeutic effect. A common philosophy underlying the development of all traditional herbal medicines is based on the restoration and maintenance of balance (homeostasis) between the body, the mind, and the environment, with an emphasis on promotion of health and preventative care. Herbal medicine is considered to be one of the most powerful systems of medicine, as many of our most potent and effective conventional drugs are obtained from plants, and so it is considered to be the basis for the modern-day pharmaceutical industry. It is estimated that approximately one-quarter of all drugs prescribed worldwide have their basis in traditional herbal medicines [1–3].

Major Systems of Traditional Botanical/Herbal Medicines

The earliest use of medicinal plants can be traced back to the Egyptians (Edwin Smith Papyrus, Ebers Papyrus), Greeks (Theophrastus/Enquiry into Plants, Hippocrates/The Medicine of Hippokrates, Dioscorides/De Materia Medica, Galen/De simplicium medicamentorum facultatibus libri XI), Arabic (School of Salerno, Formulary of Al Kindi and Samarquandi/Experiments of Cohpon), Chinese (Shen Nong Ben Cao Jing), Indians (Brihattrayee), and British (Herbarium Apuleius). The works by Galen and Disoscorides are considered to be the two of the most influential herbals as their repeated copying and dissemination shaped Mediterranean and European medicinal plant use until the eighteenth century [4–6]. Since this time traditional herbal systems were developed in the United States, Europe, Japan, India, Africa, the Middle East, Tibet, Central and South America, and many others. There is a significant overlap in herbs used in Eastern and Western herbal systems for instance ginger, fenugreek, turmeric are used by both, however the names are different due to the traditional system in which they evolved. Some herbalists and naturopaths often consider a single herb for preventative or mild health conditions. Ayurvedic and Western herbalists tend to use single herbs or build formulas comprised of a smaller number (1–4) of herbs whereas, Kampo and TCM (Traditional Chinese Medicine) practitioners prescribe classical herbal formulas containing a larger number (5 or more) of herbs. Complex herbal formulas composed of multiple herbs are typically used for more severe medical conditions. The common belief is that by combining different herbs into a formula, the therapeutic efficacy of the herbal medicine is improved through additive or synergistic effects, and other constituents help to improve bioavailability, neutralize any adverse effects of the others [7]. The most common botanical medical systems in use today that have evolved independently from or parallel with conventional medicine include Western Herbal Medicine (WHM), Traditional Chinese Herbal Medicine (TCHM), Ayurvedic herbal medicine (one of India's traditional systems of medicine), and Kampo medicine (Japanese). Herbal medicine doctors of all systems of herbal medicine base their practice on years of historical traditional herbal medicine experience and documentation in combination with biomedical science and research.

Integrative Veterinary Medicine, First Edition. Edited by Mushtaq A. Memon and Huisheng Xie.
© 2023 John Wiley & Sons, Inc. Published 2023 by John Wiley & Sons, Inc.
Companion Website: www.wiley.com/go/memon/veterinary

Western Herbal Medicine

The term Western Herbal Medicine (WHM) is used to differentiate herbalism based on European-American traditional herbal medicine from other systems of herbal medicine such as Ayurveda, Unani, Kampo or Chinese. Western Herbal Medicine is also referred to as traditional Western herbalism, herbal or botanical medicine, and phytotherapy and is practiced in Australia, Canada, New Zealand, the United Kingdom, the United States, and Western Europe. Early Western herbal medicine traditions developed from the study of herbs used as medicine by indigenous people of that country [8]. In the US, the early schools of herbal practice were initially based on Native American herbalism from which the school of Thompsonian botanical study emanated and was soon followed by the development of Eclectic and Physiomedicalist schools [9]. Samuel Thompson (1769–1843) (Thompsonian medicine) was considered one of the first well documented physicians of the time from which emerged the "Eclectic" (from the Greek word eklego meaning to "choose or select") and Physiomedicalist physicians of the late nineteenth century. The term eclectic was used to refer to those doctors that used whatever medical treatment they determined was beneficial to their patients and included herbal medicine, homeopathy and allopathic treatments. Eclectic physicians included Wooster Beach (1794–1868) and John Scudder (1829–1894). The Eclectic botanical system eventually gave way to the Physiomedicalist practice of botanical medicine that included Alva Curtis (1797–1881) and William Cook (1832–1899). It is important to remember that there was no official "school" of medicine during the eighteenth and early to mid-nineteenth centuries and most "doctors" were largely self-trained and treated patients in their homes. The American Medical Association (AMA) was established in 1847. All of the early botanical medicine schools were developed by doctors that were unhappy with the current medical treatments of the time. Disease in the eighteenth century was considered as an entity or a demon that required violent treatments in order to drive it out to cure the affected patient [10]. These early medical treatments provided the impetus for a more natural, less aggressive method of healing. These early American medical schools, founded on the philosophy of Physio-Medicalism substituted botanical medicines for allopathic medicines and treatments were based on the belief that every living system is governed and maintained by an inherent "vital force" that can be used to heal. This belief is common to all physiomedical practices, and is similar to the concept of Qi in TCHM. Disease or illness develops when there is a disruption or imbalance of this vital force. Physiomedical practice used herbal medication to restore vitality and return the body's function to normal, to restore homeostasis, and

eliminate obstructive conditions. The ability of the body to eliminate waste and toxins is of great importance to the physiomedicalist, as it is considered that the presence of pathogenic factors obstructs the vital function of the body. The philosophy and practices of physiomedicalism are the base from which modern clinical herbal medicine is developed. Between 1836 and 1911, thirteen physio-medical colleges were developed and the last finally closed at the end of the twentieth century. Today, the written records of the Eclectics/Physiomedicalism are stored in the Lloyd library in Cincinnati, Ohio, one of the greatest botanical libraries in the Western world [6].

One of the earliest herbal texts in Britain, Banckes's Herbal, is considered the first herbal book published in English on the medicinal properties of herbs and was printed in 1525 [11, 12]. The author of this book is unknown, and the book was named after the publisher Richard Banckes. A digital scan of Banckes's Herbal is available online at the US National Library. This was followed by the Grete Herball in 1526. Nicholas Culpepper (1616–1654) a seventeenth-century physician wrote the English Physician, also known as Culpeper's Herbal, a comprehensive list of England's medicinal herbs and is one of the most enduring herbal texts ever written and is still in use and available today [13]. The first comprehensive herbal in Germany was Gart der Gesundheit, written by Dr. Johann Wonnecke von Kaub (1430–1504) and contains 435 monographs and information from Buch der Natur (Book of Nature) by Konrad von Megenberg (1309–1374) and the Physica by Hildegard of Bingen (1098–1179) [14, 15].

Cranberry has been used for hundreds of years, especially cranberry juice, to prevent and treat the development of urinary tract infection (UTI) in humans. Cranberry is commonly used in the US by veterinary herbal practitioners for prevention and treatment of recurrent UTI in dogs. Chronic urinary tract infection (UTI) is the most common infectious disease in older women, causing poor quality of life and chronic infections are a leading cause of death and associated health expenditures. Multiple studies have been conducted on the active constituents found in cranberry responsible for its ability to prevent and treat UTI [16]. Evidence suggests that cranberries decrease the recurrence of urinary tract infections and can therefore decrease the chronic use of antimicrobials and resistance to them. A systematic review and analysis were done to evaluate and provide an update on the efficacy of cranberry (Vaccinium spp.) as an adjuvant therapy for the prevention of recurrent UTI's in susceptible groups. This analysis included articles with data on the incidence of UTIs in susceptible populations using cranberry products. The meta-analysis included 23 trials with 3979 participants and reported that cranberry-based products significantly reduce the incidence of UTIs in susceptible populations [17].

A canine study was done to determine the effects of cranberry extract on the development of UTI in dogs and to determine adherence of Escherichia coli (E. coli) to Madin-Darby canine kidney (MDCK) cells [18]. Urinary tract infections in dogs are associated with poor immune defense mechanisms that allow pathogens to adhere, multiply, and persist within the urinary tract. Although other bacteria can infect the urinary tract, UTIs the most common uropathogen is Escherichia coli. The E. coli strains that cause UTIs have fimbriae that facilitate adhesion of bacteria to uroepithelial cells in the urinary tract the same as in human UTI's. This study shows that oral administration of cranberry extract prevented development of UTI by P-fimbriated E. coli and adherence to MDCK cells, which may indicate it has benefit for preventing UTIs in dogs.

Traditional Chinese Herbal Medicine

Traditional Chinese Herbal Medicine (TCHM) has a history of more than 4,000 years, and according to legend and folklore, the Divine Husbandman's Classic of the Materia Medica (*Shen Nong Ben Cao Jing)* was recorded around 250 CE (Common Era, formerly AD), the content is attributed to Shen Nong, a legendary healer thought to have lived over 2,000 years ago in China, and is the first and the oldest known herbal text in the world. This text contains information on 365 medicinal substances including details such as taste, thermal properties, dosages, and toxicity. This is the earliest record of Chinese herbal medicine, and much of its information still holds true today. Shen Nong is believed to have taught the ancient Chinese the practice of agriculture, and he dedicated his life to searching for herbal medicines to treat disease. It has been said that he traveled throughout ancient China, and personally collected and tasted each and every medicinal substance. To honor and commemorate his contributions to medicine, numerous authors and physicians compiled and published the *Shen Nong Ben Cao Jing* in his name. In addition to the *Shen Nong Ben Cao Jing*, the other seminal text on TCHM is the *Huang Di Nei Jing* (The Yellow Emperors Classic of Internal Medicine) [19]. The *Huang Di Nei Jing* is the authoritative text on Chinese medical theory and internal medicine and its contents are based in Taoist philosophy, said to have been written by the famous Chinese emperor Huangdi around 2600 BC. The Huang Di Nei Jing purports that the processes of the body follow specific natural rules and that health and disease are influenced by natural ageing processes, the environment, diet, and lifestyle choices. These two texts provide the basis for the practice of Chinese herbal medicine commonly used for the prevention and treatment of disease to this day. All systems of traditional herbal medicine are different from one another largely because of their specific medical theory and application. Chinese herbalism includes the use of animal and mineral substances; however, their primary source is plant-based [20].

Huang Qin (*Scutellaria baicalensis*) has a long history of use in TCM and is also known as Chinese Skullcap. It is known for its stress-relief, anti-oxidant, neuroprotective, blood glucose regulating, anti-microbial, anti-inflammatory, and antineoplastic properties. Two of the major chemical constituents are the flavanoids baicalein (BE) and baicalin (BA) that are isolated from the dried roots but also from the leaves of Huang Qin. Numerous studies have reported that treatment with total HQ extract or with the two main flavonoids baicalin and baicalein can prevent or decrease the toxic effects of various chemical compounds [21]. The review was done and the results indicate that the protective effects of *Scutellaria baicalensis* and its flavonoids are primarily attributed to an increase in antioxidants, inhibition of lipid peroxidation, reduction of inflammatory cytokines, and suppression of the apoptosis pathway. A research study was conducted using three canine osteosarcoma cell lines that were treated with baicalein to examine cell viability, cell cycle kinetics, anchorage-independent growth, and apoptosis [22]. Baicalein was shown to be effective in inducing apoptosis and did not prevent doxorubicin cell proliferation inhibition in all the cell lines. The mechanism for induction of apoptosis has not been fully elucidated; however, changes in mitochondrial permeability supersede the apoptotic response.

Ayurvedic Herbal Medicine

(Please see Chapter #24 for additional information on Ayurveda).

Ayurvedic medicine also called Ayurveda, is the traditional medical system of India and Nepal and is one of the oldest traditional herbal systems in the world that originated in India 5000 years ago. The term Ayurveda combines two Sanskrit words-ayur which means life and veda which means science or sacred knowledge. Ayurveda then translates to "science of life" or "sacred knowledge of life." Ayurveda and variations of it have also been practiced for centuries in Pakistan, Nepal, Bangladesh, Sri Lanka, and Tibet [23]. As with other such herbal medicine systems, it is based on theories of health and illness that treat the individual and on ways to prevent, manage, or treat health problems. Ayurveda's foundations can be traced back to the ancient schools of Hindu Philosophical teachings called Vaisheshika and the school of logic, Nyaya. These two schools eventually joined to become the nyāya–vaiśeṣika school, which helped to educate and promote the knowledge of Ayurveda throughout India [24]. The earliest known references to Ayurveda appeared in Vedic scholarly texts, and the knowledge of traditional medicines was passed from the sages to disciples and then to the common man through oral narrations and written records. The Hindu system of healing is based on the four Vedas; Yajur, Rig, Sam, and Atharva [25, 26]. The healing properties of the medicinal plants used in Ayurveda was described and recorded by the sages in the Vedas in the form of poems called Shlokas. The Rig Veda (the most well-known) describes 67 plants and 1028 Shlokas, the Atharva Veda and Yajur Veda describe 293 and 81 medicinally useful plants. The standard classical references for Ayurvedic medicine are the Brihattrayee (greater trio) namely Charaka Samhita, Sushruta Samhita, Ashtanga Sangraha/Hridaya, and Laghutrayee (lesser trio) namely Madhava Nidana, Sharngadhara Samhita, and Bhava Prakasha. The greater trio of Ayurveda texts contains the core references and standard treatises on the basics of Ayurvedic medicine in regards to pathology, diagnosis, and treatment. To promote learning the practice of Ayurvedic medicine, simpler versions were formatted over time from these seminal works, and the information from the greater trio texts were compiled in an easy to learn format, to produce the "lesser trio" of Ayurveda.

Ashwagandha (Withania sominifera) is one of the most famous rasayana (rejuvenating/adaptogenic) herbs in Ayurvedic herbal medicine. In Sanskrit, ashwagandha translates as "the smell of a horse," this description refers to its ability to give the individual that takes this herb the same strength and stamina of a horse. Its herbal name, Withania somnifera (WS) translates as "sleep inducing," which reflects its calming and relaxing properties. Ashwagandha is composed of a broad spectrum of phytochemicals having wide range of biological effects. Studies have shown that it has the ability to decrease reactive oxygen species and inflammation, modulate mitochondrial function, regulate apoptosis and improve endothelial function [27, 28]. Conventional treatment of neurological disorders is largely symptomatic, expensive and associated with adverse effects. Many Ayurvedic herbs contain bioactive constituents used for the treatment of neurological/brain disorders (anxiety, depression, autism, Parkinson's, Alzheimer's, Schizophrenia, Huntington's disease, dyslexia, addiction, amyotrophic lateral sclerosis, attention deficit hyperactivity disorder and bipolar disorders) with Ashwaganda as one of the most commonly used [29, 30]. In the last twenty years, Withaferin A, an active bio-constituent of Ashwagandha, has been identified and shown to have significant potential as an anti-cancer and immunomodulatory agent [31, 32].

Guggul is derived from *Commiphora mukul, Balsamodendron mukul and Commiphora wighti* species and belongs to the family of Burseraceae and has been used in Ayurveda herbal medicine for over 2500 years. It is highly sought after for its gummy resin that has been used since antiquity, and is cultivated commercially in India and Pakistan today. The resin of the guggul tree is known as guggulu; which means "protect from disease" in Sanskrit [33]. Gugglu contains numerous phytochemicals such as steroids, guggulsterone, phytosterol, triterpenoids, volatile oil, sesquiterpenoids, diterpenoids, and others [34]. Guggulsterone isomer is an oleo-resin and is one of the major bioactive compounds present in Commiphora species (flowering myrrh tree, Indian myrrh). Guggulsterone is one of the major active constituents that plays a central role in lowering cholesterol.

Guggulsterone has been shown to be effective in lowering lipid levels by two primary mechanisms: it upregulates the bile salt export pump, which is an efflux transporter responsible for removing cholesterol metabolites and bile acids from the liver, and it antagonizes the Farnesoid X Receptor, which is involved in the conversion of cholesterol into bile acids [35–37].

Kampo Herbal Medicine

Kampo medicine is the national herbal medicine of Japan and has its origins in Traditional Chinese Medicine and was introduced to Japan by Korea around the 5th century and adapted to Japanese culture [38]. Kampo also reads as "Kan-po," literally means "the Han (206 BCE to AD 220) method or medicine" that refers to the herbal system of China that developed during that time. Kampo is used in a Western-style medical system in Japan and medical doctors educated in Western medicine have a basic knowledge of Kampo and often prescribe it with conventional medications [39]. Kampo therapies include other components of the Chinese medical system, but rely primarily on the prescription of herbal formulas. Kampo diagnosis is similar to Chinese medicine, however, Kampo places significant emphasis on examination of the abdomen (this technique is called fukushin) which is unique to Kampo.

Kampo herbal practice differs from Chinese herbal medicine in that they rely on a different collection of herbal formulas and group of primary herbs. Kampo medicine follows a simplified prescription pattern and there is little modification of classical formulas. Chinese physicians typically work with a larger group of traditional formulas, but also make entirely new formulations using a diverse number of herbs. TCHM herbal prescriptions are modified at the herbal level, whereas in Kampo, herbal prescriptions are adapted at the formula level. A factor that has strongly influenced the practice of Kampo was the formal approval of a specific group of traditional Chinese herbals in 1971 by the Japanese Ministry of

Health that were deemed safe and effective for coverage by national health care insurance [40, 41].

Rikkunshito is a well-known Kampo herbal formula, in China this classical formula is called *Liu Jun Zi Tang* (Six Gentlemen Decoction), and is one of the most commonly tonic formula to treat disorders of the gastrointestinal system [42, 43]. Rikkunshito is mainly prescribed for patients with a deficiency pattern. In veterinary medicine it has been used to treat pancreatitis, cholangiohepatitis, cholangitis, diabetes mellitus, chronic gastritis, gastric ulcer, anorexia, poor digestion and weight loss in geriatric, weak and debilitated animals, chronic diarrhea, vomiting, inflammatory bowel disease, and for vomiting following chemotherapy or radiation therapy. The active constituents of rikkunshito include β-eudesmol (from Atractylodes rhizome), ginsenosides (from Ginseng), hesperidin (from citrus peel/Chen Pi), glycyrrhizin (from Gan Cao/licorice), and shogaol (from ginger).

The mechanisms of action of rikkunshito, include stimulation of ghrelin release, (ghrelin is a hormone secreted primarily by the stomach and plays an important role in the motility of the stomach and duodenum), causes gastric adaptive relaxation, and stimulates gastric emptying [44, 45]. In Japan, it is used as a complementary medicine for functional dyspepsia and gastroesophageal reflux disorder as well as other GI disorders and is often combined with conventional drugs. Rikkunshito is used to treat upper GI tract (esophagus, stomach, and duodenum). It is often combined with proton pump inhibitor therapy in the treatment of refractory gastroesophageal reflux disease, and has ameliorative effects on adverse GI reactions induced by a variety of conventional drugs without influencing the efficacy and bioavailability of Western drugs. A study was done in dogs to evaluate the effects of rikkunshito to evaluate the effects on functional dyspepsia. Abnormal proximal gastric relaxation is one of the causes of functional dyspepsia. The study used a barostat in eight conscious Beagles to determine the effects of rikkunshito. The results indicate that rikkunshito accelerates duodenal motility and relaxes the proximal stomach.

Summary

Herbal medicines, rather than drugs, are often used in health care by humans today, and by extension their pets. For some, herbal medicine is their preferred method of treatment. For others, herbs are used as adjunct therapy or in combination with conventional pharmaceuticals in an integrative approach to healthcare. The renewed interest in herbal products is bringing new challenges in terms of standardization, safety and associated cost effectiveness [46]. The need for identification of the active constituents of herbal medicines, and on whether whole herbs or extracted compounds are more therapeutic is clear. The identification, clarification, and treatment of herb–herb and herb–drug interactions are essential to prevent adverse effects and toxicity as polypharmacy using herbs and drugs has become increasingly common. The education of professionals and the public in the clinical use of herbal or natural products is of paramount importance to this end. Newly emerging scientific techniques (e.g. genomic testing and chemical fingerprinting techniques) and other approaches, are now available for authentication and quality control of herbal products, but questions regarding efficacy will remain until adequate amounts of scientific evidence accumulate from experimental and controlled trials. Those using or prescribing herbal medicines should be assured that the products they are buying are safe and contain what they are supposed to, whether this is a particular herb or a particular amount of a specific herbal component.

References

1 Oluyemisi, F., Henry, O., and Peter, O. (2012). Standardization of herbal medicines-a review. *Int J Biodiv Conserv* 4 (3): 101–112.

2 Veeresham, C. (2012). Natural products derived from plants as a source of drugs. *J Adv Pharm Tech Res* 3 (4): 200–201.

3 Newman, D.J. and Cragg, G.M. (2020). Natural products as sources of new drugs over the nearly four decades from 01/1981 to 09/2019. *J Natural Prod* 83 (3): 770–803.

4 Leonti, M. and Verpoorte, R. (2017). Traditional Mediterranean and European herbal medicines. *J Ethnopharmacol* 199: 161–167.

5 Petrovska, B.B. (2012). Historical review of medicinal plants' usage. *Pharmacogn Rev* 6 (11): 1–5.

6 https://www.christopherhobbs.com/library/featured-articles/history-of-western-herbalism.

7 Mills, S. and Bone, K. (2000). *Principles and Practice of Phytomedicine*. Churchill Livingstone.

8 Niemeyer, K., Bell, I.R., and Koithan, M. (2013). Traditional knowledge of Western Herbal Medicine and complex systems science. *J Herb Med* 3 (3): 112–119.

9 Haller, J.S. (1997). *Kindly Medicine: Physio-Medicalism in America, 1836–1911*. Kent State University Press.

10 Strahan, E. (2021). *Bloodletting and Germs: A Doctor in Nineteenth Century Rural New York*. Family Medicine.

11 Best, M.R. (1979). Medical use of a sixteenth century herbal; Gervase Markham and the Banckes Herbal. *Bull Hist Med* 53 (3): 449–458.

12 Barlow, H.M. (1913). Old English Herbals, 1525–1640. *Proc Royal Soc Med* 6 (SectHist Med): 108–149.

13 Culpepper, N. (2020). *The Complete Herbal*. Alpha Editions.

14 Hayer, G. (1998 October 29). Konrad von Megenberg "Das Buch der Natur". In *Konrad von Megenberg "Das Buch der Natur"*. Max Niemeyer Verlag.

15 *Hildegard von Bingen's Physica: The Complete English Translation of Her Classic Work on Health and Healing*. Simon and Schuster, 1998.

16 Blumberg, J.B., Camesano, T.A., Cassidy, A. et al. (2013). Cranberries and their bioactive constituents in human health. *Adv Nutr* 4 (6): 618–632.

17 Fu, Z., Liska, D., Talan, D., and Chung, M. (2017). Cranberry reduces the risk of urinary tract infection recurrence in otherwise healthy women: a systematic review and meta-analysis. *J Nutr* 147 (12): 2282–2288.

18 Chou, H.I., Chen, K.S., Wang, H.C. and Lee, W.M.,Effects of cranberry extract on prevention of urinary tract infection in dogs and on adhesion of Escherichia coli to Madin-Darby canine kidney cells. *Am J Vet Res* 2016 77(4): 421–427.

19 Chen, J.K. and Chen, T.T. (2009). *Chinese Herbal Formulas and Applications: Pharmacological Effects & Clinical Research*. City of Industry, CA: Art of Medicine Press.

20 Ye, X. and Dong, M.H. (2017). A review on different English versions of an ancient classic of Chinese medicine: Huang Di Nei Jing. *J Integ Med* 15 (1): 11–18.

21 Ahmadi, A., Mortazavi, Z., Mehri, S., and Hosseinzadeh, H. (2022). Scutellaria baicalensis and its constituents baicalin and baicalein as antidotes or protective agents against chemical toxicities: a comprehensive review. *Naunyn Schmiedebergs Arch Pharmacol*. doi: 10.1007/s00210-022-02258-8.

22 Helmerick, E.C., Loftus, J.P., and Wakshlag, J.J. (2014). The effects of baicalein on canine osteosarcoma cell proliferation and death. *Vet Comp Oncol* 12 (4): 299–309.

23 https://www.nhp.gov.in/origin-of-ayurveda_mtl.

24 Katoch, D., Sharma, J.S., Banerjee, S. et al. (2017). Government policies and initiatives for development of Ayurveda. *J Ethnopharmacol* 197: 25–31.

25 https://www.easyayurveda.com/2016/09/12/brihat-trayi-3-treatises-form-foundation-ayurveda.

26 Lad, V. (2002). *Textbook of Ayurveda: Fundamental Principles: Vol*. 1 New Mexico: Ayurvedic Press.

27 Mukherjee, P.K., Banerjee, S., Biswas, S. et al. (2021). Withania somnifera (L.) Dunal – modern perspectives of an ancient Rasayana from Ayurveda. *J Ethnopharmacol* 264: 113157.

28 Mandlik Ingawale, D.S. and Namdeo, A.G. (2021). Pharmacological evaluation of Ashwagandha highlighting its healthcare claims, safety, and toxicity aspects. *J Diet Suppl* 18 (2): 183–226.

29 Zahiruddin, S., Basist, P., Parveen, A. et al. (2020). Ashwagandha in brain disorders: a review of recent developments. *J Ethnopharmacol* 257: 112876.

30 Dar, N.J. and Ahmad, M. (2020). Neurodegenerative diseases and Withania somnifera (L.): an update. *J Ethnopharmacol* 256: 112769.

31 Dutta, R., Khalil, R., Green, R. et al. (2019). *Withania Somnifera* (Ashwagandha) and withaferin A: potential in integrative oncology. *Int J Mol Sci* 20 (21): 5310.

32 Kashyap, V.K., Peasah-Darkwah, G., Dhasmana, A. et al. (2022). *Withania somnifera*: progress towards a pharmaceutical agent for immunomodulation and cancer therapeutics. *Pharmaceutics* 14 (3): 611.

33 Kunnumakkara, A.B., Banik, K., Bordoloi, D. et al. (2018). Googling the Guggul (Commiphora and Boswellia) for prevention of chronic diseases. *Front Pharmacol* 9: 686.

34 Ahmad, M.A., Mujeeb, M., Akhtar, M. et al. (2020). A promising multi-purpose herbal medicinal agent. *Drug Res (Stuttg)* 70 (4): 123–130.

35 Deng, R. (2007). Therapeutic effects of guggul and its constituent guggulsterone: cardiovascular benefits. *Cardiovasc Drug Rev* 25 (4): 375–390.

36 Cui, J., Huang, L., Zhao, A. et al. (2003). Guggulsterone is a farnesoid X receptor antagonist in coactivator association assays but acts to enhance transcription of bile salt export pump. *J Biol Chem* 278 (12): 10214–10220.

37 Sabarathinam, S. and Vijayakumar, T.M. (2021). Isomers of Guggulsterone in hyperlipidemia. *Obesity Med* 22: 100326.

38 https://kampo.ca.

39 Arumugam, S. and Watanabe, K. (eds.) (2017 March 17). *Japanese Kampo Medicines for the Treatment of Common Diseases: Focus on Inflammation*. Academic Press.

40 Arai, M., Katai, S., Muramatsu, S.I. et al. (2012). Current status of Kampo medicine curricula in all Japanese medical schools. *BMC Comp Alt Med* 12 (1): 1–7.

41 Nishimura, K., Plotnikoff, G.A., and Watanabe, K. (2009). Kampo medicine as an integrative medicine in Japan. *JMAJ* 52 (3): 147–149.

42 Mogami, S. and Hattori, T. (2014). Beneficial effects of rikkunshito, a Japanese kampo medicine, on gastrointestinal dysfunction and anorexia in combination with Western drug: a systematic review. *Evid Based Complement Alternat Med (eCAM)* 2014: 1–7.

43 Inokuchi, K., Masaoka, Y., Masaoka, T., and Kanai, T. (2021). Rikkunshito as a therapeautic agent for functional dyspepsia and its prokinetic and non-prokinetic effects. *Front Pharmacol* 12: 640576.

44 Furukawa, N., Manabe, N., Kase, Y. et al. (2013). Intragastric infusion of rikkunshito (kampo) induces proximal stomach relaxation in conscious dogs. *Auton Neurosci* 179 (1–2): 14–22.

45 Yanai, M., Mochiki, E., Ogawa, A. et al. (2013). Intragastric administration of rikkunshito stimulates upper gastrointestinal motility and gastric emptying in conscious dogs. *Gastroenterol* 48 (5): 611–619.

10

Herbal Medicine Regulation, Adverse Events, and Herb-Drug Interactions
Signe Beebe

Introduction

As herbal medicines have been in use for thousands of years, herbal practitioners began written records on what specific foods and plants had healing properties that could be used to treat illness. They evaluated, defined, and recorded herbal pharmacological categories, the safety of herbs, what herbs could or could not be combined due to potential toxicity. The best growing locations for herbs was important, and instructions for the harvesting, processing, and proper storing techniques for herbs, was well-documented. In this way, the knowledge of herbal medicines was passed down from generation to generation. The therapeutic value of botanical medicines depends on the species of plant used, growing conditions, and biologically active constituents.

Herbal medicine toxicity factors include inappropriate dosing and duration of treatment, improper processing, using the wrong species of plant, use of known toxic herbs, adverse herb-drug interaction, individual patient sensitivity, adulteration and sale of herbal medications contaminated with pharmaceutical drugs, heavy metals, pesticides or other chemicals [1–3]. Herbal medicines are not considered drugs by many consumers and are considered to be safe because they are "natural" and so are often considered safer than conventional drugs, and may be administered at higher doses and for longer periods of time than is recommended. It is critical that all herbal medicine prescribed contains all the correct plant family and species before dispensing. The use of an incorrect species of plant can cause severe disease or death, (e.g., Aristolochic acid) [4].

Most herbal medicines must undergo physical and/or chemical pretreatment processing that are essential for preservation, detoxification, or enhancing efficacy. Improper processing can lead to adverse effects and toxicity. Basic processing includes washing, drying, or slicing of the plant material to clean the herbs and improve storage time. Additional processing such as sun drying, roasting, wine frying, vinegar frying, steaming, fumigation, boiling, or steaming is used to modify the therapeutic effects (detoxify, increase potency), alter bioavailability, or preserve active ingredients. Herbs contain multiple compounds, many of which may not be identified, and chemical fingerprinting is in the early stages and has not been done for most herbs. This makes standardization in terms of active constituents of herbal medicines a challenge [5, 6]. Some herbal medicines can be produced to contain a standardized amount of a key component or class of components, such as ginsenosides for ginseng products or silymarin for milk thistle products. However, even when such key compounds have been identified and a standard content is agreed upon, there is no guarantee that individual commercial products will contain this. That is because a plant's environment can significantly affect the phytochemical profiles and efficacy of the herbal medicine produced. Herbal extracts can be variable from year to year and may be significantly affected by temperature, drought, or flood as well as by geographic location. Systems have been developed, over many years, so that herbal toxicities are rare and have been largely eliminated if prescribed and taken appropriately.

Doctors using herbal medicines want to be confident that the products they are prescribing to their patients are safe and contain what is on the label whether it is a specific herb or a particular amount of an herbal component.

Quality Control of Herbal Medicines

The quality control of herbal medicines is of utmost importance for herbal prescribing as it has a direct impact on their safety and efficacy. Developed countries have specific GMP based regulatory guidelines for the production and quality control of herbal medicines and herbal-based products. GMP regulations outline the process of setting and agreeing on technical standards. Herbal manufacturers are required to follow these standards to ensure the quality, safety, efficacy, and reproducibility of herbal medicines or herbal derivatives they sell [7, 8]. One of the most important steps in GMP is record keeping on the individual species of plants used, the part of the plant used (this greatly influences the concentration of active constituents), locations and conditions of cultivation, harvesting methods, proper processing, methods of extraction of active ingredients, and storage. GMP quality control standards apply to the production of herbal medicines as well as those imported for sale and also include testing for adulteration or substitution with conventional drugs, microorganism, chemical (e.g. pesticides), and heavy metal contamination. Sanitation and hygiene of herbal medicine production is also emphasized. In addition, they perform biochemical profiling (herbal authenticity) to ensure that the herbal products are consistent [9]. Methods to identify and ensure purity of the herb involved include thin layer and high-performance thin layer chromatography (HPLC), near-infrared spectroscopy, mass spectrometry, biochromatography (combines human red cell membrane extraction and high-performance liquid chromatography (HPLC) to screen for active constituents in herbs) and most recently DNA finger printing [9, 10]. DNA barcoding, which makes use of short, standardized regions of the genome as species "barcodes" is a DNA Sanger sequencing-based targeted approach appropriate for testing single ingredient herbal products with allergic potential, known or suspected toxicity, negative interactions with other herbs, supplements or prescription medication but may also detect some undeclared species. DNA identification of herbals was recently adopted by the British and Chinese national pharmacopoeias, which provide multi-taxa identification by using the DNA of different origins extracted from complex herbal mixtures and matrices. False negatives could occur if the DNA tested was degraded or lost during post-harvest processing or manufacturing [11, 12].

Origin of Herbal Medicines

Not all herbal medicines are herbal in nature and the inclusion of certain species of plants and animals in herbal medicines is illegal. Most herbal medicines are plant-based; however, some herbal medicines contain components of animal origin (horns, insects, shells, bone, antlers, minerals, etc.). However, in the past specific species of animals have been used to produce herbal medicine products to the extent that they have become endangered (e.g., tiger bone, rhinoceroses' horn). The Convention on International Trade in Endangered Species of Wild Fauna and Flora (CITES) was instituted in 1973 and is an international agreement between

governments [13]. CITES, regulates the international trade of certain animal species, which are endangered or threatened with extinction if their exploitation is not halted. The goal of CITES is to ensure that international trade of these species of wild animals and plants does not threaten their survival. CITES regulates international trade of over 36,000 species of plants and animals, and their permit system seeks to ensure that international trade in listed species is sustainable, legal and traceable. National Laws for implementing CITES empowers government officials to act, regulates human behavior and articulates policy in relation to conservation and trade in wildlife. One of the species protected by the CITES has been detected using DNA barcoding and metabarcoding in commercial products. DNA trace of the snow leopard, which is an endangered species with the highest level of trade restriction has been identified using this method [14]. As the use of herbal medicines has become widespread for the treatment and prevention of diseases in humans, a similar trend has occurred in the veterinary field. As owners use herbal medicines for themselves, they want the same medicinal treatments for their beloved pets. It is imperative that veterinarians using herbal medicines know what herbs are potentially toxic or known to be toxic. Experienced herbalists are educated as to what these herbs are and what combinations are to be avoided. As previously described, adverse reactions or toxicity of herbal medicines occur for a variety of reasons. One of the most important and commonly seen in veterinary medicine is the use of herbal medicines without proper diagnosis by a trained herbal medicine practitioner. Experienced herbal practitioners know most diseases can be caused by several different patterns and each will have a unique treatment. Using the wrong herbal therapy for a condition can cause potential adverse effects.

Regulation for Herbal Medicines

All developed countries have regulatory bodies to ensure the quality and safety of herbal medicines and herbal products, and have developed similar GMP guidelines [15]. Regulation of herbal medicine and products in the United States, falls under the Dietary Supplement Health and Education Act (DSHEA) of 1994, any herbal medicine, supplement or herbal extract, is classified as a dietary supplement [8].This means that the herbal medicine manufacturer is responsible for determining that the dietary supplements produced are safe and any representation or claims made about them have adequate evidence to show that they are not false or misleading. GMP are used as per the FDA and are similar to those used for the manufacture of drugs [16–18]. GMP regulations in the US require that manufacturers, processors, and packagers of herbal medicines, medical devices, food products, and blood/ blood products take specific measures to ensure that their products are safe, effective and to prevent contamination and processing errors. Manufacturers or distributors of a supplement with new herbal components that was not marketed in the United States before 1994, may be required to go through a premarket review for safety data. Also, all foreign herbal medicine producers/companies must follow the FDA's GMP regulations. It is forbidden to label any herbal medicine product, sold as a dietary supplement in the United States, or suggest in any of its packaging that it can diagnose, treat, prevent, or cure a specific disease or condition without specific FDA approval.

Japan: In Japan, Kampo is regulated as part of the Japanese national health care system by the Ministry of Health, Labor and Welfare (MHLW) [8, 19]. Herbal medicines in Japan are produced under the same strict manufacturing conditions as pharmaceutical companies. The traditional use of herbal medicines is not adequate for approval as a drug. The therapeutic claims and rules of combinations of herbal ingredients are determined based on the pharmacological actions of each active constituent. If a monograph for an herbal formula is not available, the claims reported in the Japanese Pharmacopoeia are used as a guide [20]. Japanese Kampo traditionally uses fixed combinations of herbs in standardized proportions according to the Chinese classical literature. Each herbal formula is composed of the exact same components as per the MHLW. Modification of herbal formulas is not commonly practiced in Kampo as it is in TCM. The MHLW designates 210 formulas as over the counter drugs (OTC) and these herbal formulas were chosen based on the experience of doctors practicing traditional Chinese medicine. The MHLW also designated 146 formulations as National Health Insurance applicable prescription drugs [21]. An Advisory Committee for Kampo drugs was established in 1982 in close association with the MHLW in order to improve the quality control of Kampo drugs. After the institution of the Good Manufacturing Practice Law of 1986, these standards were applied to all pharmaceutical drugs but also to all Kampo drugs (herbal formulas). In 1988, the MHLW launched a new system to re-evaluate the efficacy and safety for all drugs every five years. It has three major systems for collecting adverse effects. The first involves Hospital Monitoring of adverse effects which is a voluntary process and collects data from over two thousand hospitals in Japan. The second is called the Pharmacy Monitoring System that includes over 2000 pharmacies that collect data on adverse reactions from (OTC) herbal medicines and drugs, and the third system is the Adverse Reaction Reporting from Manufacturers. These cases of adverse events are reported to the MHLW by each system, along with information obtained from medical conferences and medical journals.

Canada: In Canada, since 2003, herbal medicines and natural health products are regulated under Health Canada and must comply with the Natural Health Products Regulations [8, 22]. Any manufacturer or importer of herbal medicines and herbal supplements require a product license before they can be sold in Canada. A site license is needed for those who manufacture, pack, label, and import herbal medicines. GMP standards must be followed and require complete data on: product source, storage, handling, additives, manufacturing sites, herbal medicine composition, recommended use, microbial and chemical contaminant testing, active constituent evaluation, quantification by assay or by input. These data are then submitted to the Natural Health Product Directorate (NHPD) for evaluation. In addition, herbal medicine product license holders are required to monitor all adverse reactions associated with their products and report serious reactions to the Canadian Department of Health.

India: In India, herbal medicines have been used since the Vedic age and have been documented in Rig Veda. Initially herbal medicines were regulated under the 1940 Drug and Cosmetic Act and the Cosmetic Rules, 1945 [23]. These acts initially set the standards for Ayurvedic, Siddha and Unani medicines and the rules and regulations for their production. The Drug and Cosmetic Act describes individual monographs in their respective pharmacopoeias and has control over the licensing, formulation composition, manufacture, labeling, packing, quality, and export of herbal medications. In 2003, manufacturers were required to follow Schedule T of the act which outlines the GMP requirements for the production of herbal medicines. There are official pharmacopoeias and formularies available for the quality standards of herbal medicines sold in India. In 2014, the Ministry of AYUSH (Ayurveda, Yoga and naturopathy, Unani, Siddha, and Homeopathy) was developed and is responsible for the education, training, and research of herbal medicines in India [24, 25].

The Indian Pharmacopoeia (IP) was developed and published by the Indian Pharmacopoeia Commission (IPC) on behalf of the Ministry of Health & Family Welfare, per the requirements of the 1940 Drugs and Cosmetics Act, and Rules [26, 27]. IP is recognized as the official publications of standards for the herbal drugs manufactured and/or marketed in India. IP contains information on the analysis and specifications of herbal drugs for their authenticity, purity, and strength. The standards of the IP are enforceable by law for ensuring the quality of herbal medicine use in India. The first edition of the Indian Pharmacopoeia was published in 1955 and the latest in 2018.

Europe: In Europe, before 2004 herbal medicines were generally sold as food supplements, today they are regulated as drugs. The European Parliament and the Council of Europe provides the guidelines for the use of herbal medicines through European Directive 2004/24/EC [8, 28]. This directive states that herbal medicines require authorization by the national regulatory authorities of each European country and that these products must have a recognized level of safety and efficacy. To register an herbal medicine product, there must be sufficient evidence that the herbal product has been used as a medicinal for at least 30 years; including use in the European Union (EU) for at least 15 years and 15 years elsewhere for herbal products outside of the EU [29, 30]. This directive is limited to herbal medicinal products of pharmacological activity; food, food supplements, and cosmetics are not included. The directive defines an herbal medicinal product as "any medicinal product exclusively containing, as active ingredients, one or more herbal substances, one or more herbal preparations or one or more such herbal substances in combination with one or more such herbal preparations." Following establishment of the directive, two new herbal medicine product classifications were put forth. The first category is well-established use herbal medicinal products and the second category is traditional use herbal medicinal products. In order to sell a herbal medicinal product, manufacturers must submit data on pharmacological and toxicological testing, any existing clinical trials and all other information proving its quality, safety, and efficacy. The safety of herbal medicinal products is also evaluated on the basis of existing scientific literature data from clinical studies, case reports, and pre-clinical studies. When data on safety are not sufficient, consumers are informed of this. A Committee for Herbal Medicinal Products (HMPC) was established within the European Medicines Agency for the Evaluation of Medicinal Products to develop modern science–based public herbal monographs (European Pharmacopeia) and help simplify the registration and authorization of herbal medicinal products. The committee is composed of experts in the field of herbal medicinal products and also responds to questions relating to herbal medicines per the agency's view [31].

Training and Licensing of Herbal Practitioners

Training and licensing of herbal practitioners to ensure knowledge of herbal medicines and prevention of potential side effects is essential. While single herbs can be used for prevention or for the treatment of mild disease, most herbal practitioners use more than one herb at a time to treat most medical conditions. In other words, herbal polypharmacy or complexity, the use of multiple herbs in a formula is most commonly used [32, 33]. Appropriately constructed herbal formulas create a synergistic effect, have good efficacy for the condition treated, decrease, or prevents adverse effects, avoid herb-drug interactions and

improves treatment outcomes. The use of whole plant extracts rather than a single active constituent and a well-built formula rather than a single herb is one of the cornerstones of good herbal medicine practice. The prescription of herbal formulas is much more complex than the use of single herbs and established rules and guidelines for proper formulation must be followed closely. It is due to the complexity of multi-herb formulas and interactions of herbal constituents that makes investigating the toxicity and efficacy of herbs more difficult than for pharmaceutical drugs. Herbal medicine practitioners have tracked cases of herb-to-herb pharmacodynamic interactions for centuries, and these toxicities and interactions have been well documented [1, 34]. However, there are some situations when herbal medicines and conventional medicines interact and are incompatible. The solution to this situation is to identify/understand the pharmacokinetic and pharmacodynamic herb-drug interaction. Historically, herbs and drugs have been determined to be very different treatment modalities, that have rarely, if ever, been used together. However, the line that separates use of herbs and drugs has become blurred in recent years as the public has gained increased access to multiple treatment modalities [35–37]. It is not unusual for a client to seek care from integrative medicine doctors as well as conventional ones. As a result, a patient may easily be taking multiple drugs, herbs, supplements, and vitamins concurrently. It becomes difficult to predict whether the combination of all these substances will lead to unwanted side effects and/or interactions. It is shortsighted to assume that there will be no adverse interactions. On the other hand, it is just as unwise to abandon treatment due to fear of possible interactions. The solution to this dilemma is to understand the pharmacokinetic and pharmacodynamic herb-drug interactions in addition to historical knowledge of potential known herb toxicities. By understanding these mechanisms, one can recognize potential interactions and take proper actions to prevent their occurrence. The highest risk of clinically-significant interactions occurs between herbs and drugs that have sympathomimetic, anticoagulant, antiplatelet, diuretic, and antidiabetic effects [34, 38] Understanding synergistic and antagonistic interactions from both the herbal medicine and the pharmaceutical perspective helps practitioners anticipate and prevent, adverse reactions and/or toxicity in patients that require multiple therapeutic substances. Knowledge of dose limitations and length of therapies as well as appropriate monitoring for adverse effects is required. For any clinically relevant health effects the toxic constituents have to be both bioavailable and present in physiologically active doses. Herbal medicines, rather than drugs, are often used in health care by humans today, and by extension their pets. For some, herbal medicine is their preferred method of treatment. For others, herbs are used as adjunct therapy or in combination with conventional pharmaceuticals in an integrative approach to healthcare. The renewed interest in herbal medicine is bringing new challenges in terms of standardization, safety, and associated cost effectiveness. The need for identification of the active constituents of herbal medicines, and on whether whole herbs or extracted compounds are more therapeutic is clear. The identification, clarification, and treatment of herb-herb and herb-drug interactions are essential to prevent adverse effects and toxicity as polypharmacy using herbs and drugs has become increasingly common. Research to evaluate the quality, safety, pharmacological effects, and clinical efficacy of commonly used herbs is greatly needed, and those prescribing or using herbal medicines and products should be assured that what they are buying is safe, whether it is a specific herb or herbal extract supplement.

References

1 Xie, H. (2011). Toxicity of Chinese veterinary herbal medicines. *Am J Trad Chin Vet Med* 6 (2): 45–53.

2 Chan, K. (2003). Some aspects of toxic contaminants in herbal medicines. *Chemosphere* 52 (9): 1361–1371.

3 Liu, R., Li, X., Huang, N. et al. (2020). Toxicity of Traditional Chinese medicine herbal and mineral products. *Adv Pharmacol* 87: 301–346.

4 Yang, H.-Y., Chen, P.-C., and Wang, J.-D. (2014). Chinese herbs containing aristolochic acid associated with renal failure and urothelial carcinoma: a review from epidemiologic observations to causal inference. *BioMed Research Int* 2014: 569325, 9 pp.

5 Sahoo, N., Manchikanti, P., and Dey, S. (2010). Herbal drugs: standards and regulation. *Fitoterapia* 81 (6): 462–471.

6 Sahoo, N., Choudhury, K., and Manchikanti, P. (2009). Manufacturing of biodrugs. *BioDrugs* 23 (4): 217–229.

7 World Health Organization (2007). *WHO Guidelines on Good Manufacturing Practices (GMP) for Herbal Medicines*. World Health Organization.

8 Wachtel-Galor, S. and Benzie, I.F.F. (2011). Herbal medicine: an introduction to its history, usage, regulation, current trends, and research needs. In: *Herbal Medicine: Biomolecular and Clinical Aspects*, 2e (ed. I.F.F. Benzie and S. Wachtel-Galor). Boca Raton, FL: CRC Press/Taylor & Francis. Chapter 1.

9 Coghlan, M.L., Maker, G., Crighton, E. et al. (2015). Combined DNA, toxicological and heavy metal analyses provides an auditing toolkit to improve pharmacovigilance of traditional Chinese medicine. *Sci Rep* 105 (1): 17475.

10 de Boer, H.J., Ichim, M.C., and Newmaster, S.G. (2015). DNA barcoding and pharmacovigilance of herbal medicines. *Drug Safe* 38 (7): 611–620.

11 Raclariu, A.C., Heinrich, M., Ichim, M.C., and de Boer, H. (2020). Benefits and limitations of DNA barcoding and metabarcoding in herbal product authentication. *Phytochem Anal* 29 (2): 123–128.

12 Grazina, L., Amaral, J.S., and Mafra, I. (2020). Botanical origin authentication of dietary supplements by DNA-based approaches. *Compr Rev Food Sci Food Saf* 19 (3): 1080–1109.

13 http://cites.org/eng/disc/what.php.

14 Newmaster, S.G., Grguric, M., Shanmughanandhan, D. et al. (2013). DNA barcoding detects contamination and substitution in North American herbal products. *BMC Med* 11 (1): 1–13.

15 https://ods.od.nih.gov/About/DSHEA_Wording.aspx.

16 https://www.fda.gov/regulatory-information.

17 Bent, S. (2008). Herbal medicine in the United States: review of efficacy, safety, and regulation: grand rounds at University of California, San Francisco Medical Center. *J Gen Intern Med* 23 (6): 854–859.

18 https://web-japan.org/links/government/ministries/ministry5.html.

19 https://www.pmda.go.jp/english/rs-sb-std/standards-development/jp/0019.html.

20 Watanabe, K., Matsuura, K., Gao, P. et al. (2011). Traditional Japanese Kampo Medicine: clinical research between modernity and traditional medicine-the state of research and methodological suggestions for the future. *Evid Based Complement Alternat Med* 2011: 513842.

21 https://www.canada.ca/en/health-canada/services/drugs-health-products/natural-non-prescription.html.

22 https://data.gov.in/resource/registration-indian-medicine-and-homeopathy-practitioners-shb-2020.

23 https://www.ayush.gov.in.

24 Muthappan, S., Elumalai, R., Shanmugasundaram, N. et al. (2021). AYUSH digital initiatives: harnessing the power of digital technology for India's traditional medical systems. *J Ayurveda Integr Med* 13 (2): 100498.

25 Pharmacopoeia Commission for Indian Medicine & Homoeopathy (PCIM&H). https://pcimh.gov.in/show_content.php?lang=1&level=1&ls_id=5&lid=5.

26 https://indianpharmacopoeia.in/BookDetail.php?item_id=402&.

27 https://www.eumonitor.eu/9353000/1/j9vvik7m1c3gyxp/vitgbgift7xs.

28 Chinou, I., Knoess, W., and Calapai, G. (2014). Regulation of herbal medicinal products in the EU: an up-to-date scientific review. *Phytochem Rev* 13: 539–545.

29 Routledge, P.A. (2008). The European herbal medicines directive. *Drug-Safety* 31: 416–418.

30 https://www.ema.europa.eu/en/committees/committee-herbal-medicinal-products-hmpc.

31 Mills, S. and Bone, K. (2000). *Principles and Practice of Phytomedicine*. Churchill Livingstone.

32 Loya, A.M., González-Stuart, A., and Rivera, J.O. (2009). Prevalence of polypharmacy, polyherbacy, nutritional supplement use and potential product interactions among older adults living on the United States-Mexico border. *Drugs Aging* 26: 423–436.

33 Rivera, J.O., Loya, A.M., and Ceballos, R. (2013). Use of herbal medicines and implications for conventional drug therapy medical sciences. *Altern Integ Med* 2 (6): 1–6.

34 Chen, J. and Chen, T. (2004). *Chinese Medical Herbology and Pharmacology*. City of Industry, CA: Art of Medicine Press, 25-29 Chapter 8.

35 Farina, E.K., Austin, K.G., and Lieberman, H.R. (2014). Concomitant dietary supplement and prescription medication use is prevalent among US adults with doctor-informed medical conditions. *Journal of the Academy of Nutrition and Dietetics* 114 (11): 1784–1790.

36 Shetty, V., Chowta, M.N., Chowta, K.N. Shenoy A, Kamath A, Kamath P. et al. (2018). Evaluation of potential drug-drug interactions with medications prescribed to geriatric patients in a tertiary care hospital. *J Aging Res*. 2018 October 9;2018.

37 Watson, R.R. and Preedy, V.R. (eds.) (2008). Herb-drug interaction. In: *Botanical Medicine in Clinical Practice*. CABI. Chapters 97&98.

38 Hoffman, D. (2003). Toxicity, contra-indications and safety. In: *Medical Herbalism the Science & Practice of Herbal Medicine. Inner Tradition International*, (ed. Simon and Schuster). Rochester, Vermont: Healing Arts Press, 2003 October 24 Chapter 10.

Section V

Integrative Nutrition

(Section Editor – Laura Gaylord)

11

Novel Trends in Nutrition: Pet Food Categorization, Owner Perception and Current Marketing

Donna Raditic* and Laura Gaylord

* Corresponding author

Introduction

The rising global adoption of pets has driven the pet food market which is projected to grow from USD $115.50 billion in 2022 to USD $163.70 billion by 2029. The five main players, Mars Inc., Nestle Purina Petcare, J.M. Smucker Company, Colgate Palmolive Company, and General Mills, Inc. hold more than 60% of the pet food market [1]. Although dry commercial pet food dominates the pet food market, other unconventional pet diet types and the use of innovative ingredients are growing [2]. Pet humanization and consumers increasing concerns for the role of nutrition in pet health are demanding pet foods that they believe provides better nutrition. The pet food industry is responding with more diet types such as raw, grain free, dehydrated, freeze dried, home-prepared, and fresh refrigerated. Today's veterinarians will need to understand and address the growing diversity of pet food types as consumers want more information and education about the role of ingredients and whole diet on their pet's health and longevity.

Applying Food Processing Categorization System to Pet Foods

There is a need to apply a food categorization system to the vast array of pet foods in the marketplace. Studies of dietary effects in the human nutrition literature often use one of three food processing categorizations systems: Nova, International Food Information Council (IFIC) or University of North Carolina at Chapel Hill (UNC). These food processing categorizations systems were developed in the 1980s with the arrival of ultra-processed (UP) human foods, i.e. fractionated recombined foods with added ingredients and/or additives. For example, ready-to-eat breakfast cereals are produced with mechanical treatments (flour refining), thermal treatment to gelatinize starch, and extrusion cooking with high pressure and heat. Finally, there is addition of salt, sugar, fat and/or numerous additives and preservatives to create these convenient, ready to eat, shelf stable products. Breakfast cereals produced with these multiple treatments are now categorized as "ultra-processed foods" in food processing categorization systems. Dry pet foods are produced similar to breakfast cereals with multiple processing steps using heat and pressure and retorted or canned pet foods also undergo multiple thermal processing steps [3–6].

Nutritionist and food scientists must balance food processing to deliver safe, palatable, shelf stable foods that are also healthy and sustainable. Currently numerous published epidemiological studies have determined that populations consuming higher amounts of UP foods exhibit a higher prevalence of obesity and chronic disease. These studies utilize and support the classification systems according to the degree of processing i.e. un/minimally processed (MP), processed, and ultra-processed (UP) of human foods and ingredients [6–14].

With the increase and diversity of pet food types and the consumer demand for identifying healthy pet diets, the application of a pet food categorization system based on the level of processing is relevant. A pet food categorization system has been previously published using the level of processing to produce the final product i.e. minimally processed (MP) and ultra-processed (UP) derived from human food/ingredient categorization systems. These pet food categories, "minimally processed" (MP) and "ultra-processed" (UP) can then be combined with the traditional pet food definitions of "commercial and home-prepared diets" where appropriate [15, 16].

Integrative Veterinary Medicine, First Edition. Edited by Mushtaq A. Memon and Huisheng Xie.
© 2023 John Wiley & Sons, Inc. Published 2023 by John Wiley & Sons, Inc.
Companion Website: www.wiley.com/go/memon/veterinary

The term commercial diet (CD) infers a pet diet made by a manufacturing pet food company to be sold in the pet food market. Typically, in the United States, commercial pet diets are complete and balanced commercial products, and are intended to be fed as the main source of nutrition for designated life stages, while unbalanced products are intended to be fed supplemental to kibble, canned, or other balanced diets. For example, ultra-processed commercial diets (UPCD) are the conventional dry and retort canned pet diets that dominate the pet food market [15, 16].

The popularity of feeding minimally processed (MP), or previously known as raw meat-based diets (RMBDs) to companion dogs and cats has been increasing in popularity in recent years. Other MP diet types would include the fresh-type pet foods that are cooked and potentially pet diets that are dehydrated or freeze dried. The practice of feeding minimally processed diets can be grouped into two major types: MP commercial diets (MPCDs) or MP home-prepared diets (MPHDs). MP diets of either type may be "complete and balanced" or unbalanced [15, 16].

Pet Food Research

Utilizing a pet food processing categorizations system with these definitions is a starting point that enables studies of UP and MP diets to determine if there is a similar role of these diet types of the health, chronic diseases, and obesity in companion animals. Currently, there is a paucity of quality studies i.e. peer-reviewed meta-analysis or randomized clinical control trials evaluating UPCD compared with MPCD over a significant period measuring whole-diet effects on the health, disease, and life span of a population of dogs or cats. In fact, published peer-reviewed studies evaluating whole-diet effects are scant and more often involve veterinary therapeutic diets [17, 18]. The most evidence-based statement that can be said about pet diet impact on health and longevity would be that dogs fed to maintain a lean body condition score result in statistically significant increased life span. This finding is based on a lifetime study of 48 Labrador retrievers fed a dry UPCD, which resulted in statistically significant longer life span in the diet-restricted group as compared with the control-fed dogs. Because all dogs ate the same UPCD, this study is not evidence that UPCDs are "best nutrition" but demonstrates the benefits of restricting caloric intake [19]. However, similar to studies of human consumption of UP foods, this study could also be interpreted as evidence that the dogs consuming more UPCD had more chronic disease and a shorter life span emphasizing the role of ultra-processed foods, disease states and longevity.

Translational Studies in Food Processing: Advance Glycation End Products

Because most dogs and cats obtain consume UPCD for their entire lives, it is important to understand the effects of food processing on health. Most commercial pet foods and treats are heated to improve safety, shelf life, nutritional characteristics, texture, and nutrient digestion. When heat is applied to food, the structure of sugars and proteins are rearranged. Some of the newly formed compounds are Maillard reaction products (MRP) some termed melanoidins that improve color, flavor, and aroma, but others termed advanced glycation end products (AGEs) can lead to the loss of essential amino acids and may negatively affect animal health [20, 21].

AGEs are also formed in the body by in vivo glycation of tissue proteins, and these are termed "endogenous AGEs." Endogenous AGEs are produced and accumulate with the physiologic processes of aging and disease states. One of the first recognized endogenous AGE identified was hemoglobin A1c, a glucose-derived hemoglobin increased in diabetes mellitus. Both endogenous AGEs and dietary AGEs contribute to the body's AGE pool [22, 23]. Studies implicate that dietary AGEs that add to the total body AGEs have a role in aging and the pathogenesis of chronic disease states. AGE-associated diseases develop via two mechanisms: (i) structural alteration of intermolecular and intramolecular cross-linking of tissue proteins that change molecular properties and function, or (ii) by activation of cellular signaling pathways through receptor binding or direct activation to produce reactive oxygen species and an inflammatory response [24–26]. Receptors for AGEs termed RAGE are widely expressed on cells playing roles in oxidative stress, vasoconstriction, excessive collagen deposition, and inflammatory responses. RAGE activation, via AGE binding, may result in development of a chronic inflammatory state, which is observed in many disease states in both humans and dogs. Furthermore, dietary AGEs can impact the intestinal microbiota, compromise epithelial barrier functions, and cause immune stimulation resulting in diseases [27]. This absorption of AGEs from the diet and their accumulation into the AGE pool in the body may be one of the ways diets can impact age-related diseases in humans and animals. AGEs have been associated with age-related diseases in humans, such as diabetes mellitus, atherosclerosis, nephropathy, retinopathy, osteoarthritis, neurodegenerative diseases, and neoplasia [22, 27–29].

Similar to what has been reported in human foods, pet foods are subjected to thermal processing which facilitates the Maillard reaction and formation of AGEs [30]. Studies have measured the levels of AGES in different types of processed pet foods [20, 30–36]. Elevated levels of AGEs in tissue proteins were observed in aging dogs with diabetes mellitus, cataracts, osteoarthritis, neurodegenerative diseases, vascular dysfunction, and atherosclerosis [30–36]. Serum and urine AGEs have been measured in dogs and cats with increasing levels reported with increases in dietary AGEs intake [30–36]. These studies align with human studies of dietary AGEs intake and chronic disease states. To promote human public health and prevent chronic disease, it is currently recommended to limit the intake of UP foods containing high dietary AGEs [37–40]. As pets are now family members, some owners are looking to apply these same recommendations. Avoiding UPCDs may be applicable to consumers looking to feed some or all MP diets. As more is learned about the role of AGEs in processed foods, whether for human or pet consumption, food manufacturers will face the challenge to produce foods with lower AGE content while still being palatable, shelf stable, and safe [41–44].

Pet Food Safety

Health risks for both UPCDs and MPCDs include bacterial pathogens, nutritional imbalances, aflatoxins, and other toxic contaminations which have been previously summarized as pet food recalls or "contamination incidents" that are reported by the Food and Drug Administration (FDA) Pet Food Recalls and/or publications [15]. Currently, the American Animal Hospital Association (AAHA), American Veterinary Medical Association (AVMA), and other veterinary organizations discourage the practice of feeding MP due to pathogenic risks to dogs, cats, and humans. It is important to note that historically bacterial-contaminated pet foods were recognized as a risk to humans from large outbreak in 2006–2008 with Mars Petcare's dry UPCDs that was linked to human infections with Salmonella [45, 46] and again in 2012 with human Salmonella infections that occurred across the USA and Canada from Diamond Pet Foods dry UPCDs [41]. Following these outbreaks, the Center for Veterinary Medicine's Veterinary Laboratory Investigation Response Network began testing UPCDs as well as MP diets, exotic animal feeds, and treats. As a result of these outbreaks and surveillances, in July 2013, the FDA set forth Compliance Policy Guide Sec.690.800 Salmonella in Food for Animals [46], establishing a policy of zero tolerance for Salmonella in pet food in the USA, which is more stringent than policies for human food. This means in the USA, all commercial pet diets whether UP or MP are held to the same standard (e.g., zero tolerance policy).

European organizations like European Pet Food Industry (FEDIAF) which is like AAFCO in the USA, has taken a different approach to pathogens in pet food by providing MP diet handling and food safety information and education to the public to help mitigate risk [16]. FEDIAF recognizes recognize that pet owners are likely to continue feeding MP diets despite discouragement of such practices from any regulatory or veterinary authority and therefore has been proactive with campaigns to educate pet owners on proper food safety and handling techniques to mitigate risk [16].

There are numerous reports and publications of raw or MP diets and their potential risk to human and pet health containing bacterial pathogens. Commonly, it is not clear if these publications involve MP commercial diets with established pathogen control (e.g., high pressure processing) or if they include both MPCD, MPHD and/or animal meat treats. It is important to know that a MPHD, if made from meats from the human food supply in many countries, would be expected to harbor pathogens, as these meats are sold with the intent of being cooked. Based on this overview of pet food safety, it would seem most prudent for the veterinary medical communities need to provide to clear directives and protocols to prevent potential pathogen cases in relation to public and animal health regardless of diet type [15, 16].

Understanding Consumers and the Pet Food Market

Veterinarians should understand that stating UP is better nutrition than MP is not supported by published peer-reviewed studies nor is it clear that MP diets represent better nutrition. Veterinarians are integrating their clinical experiences when recommending UPCDs, but there is a need to add client values to evidence based medicine decision making, especially for owners interested in MP diets. Recommending only UPCD as a nutritional standard of care may be eroding pet owner confidence in veterinarians. Surveys of pet owners feeding MP diets indicate they tend to obtain nutrition information from sources other than veterinarians and may view their veterinarian less favorably [48–50]. These surveys suggest determinants of pet food purchases more often involve humanization and the desire to feed healthy, quality diets that are less processed [50–52]. To improve pet owner confidence, today's veterinarians need to understand many owners are not looking to feed a wolf, but instead are trying to provide healthy, less processed diets to a family member.

A review of consumer survey is provided for veterinarians to understand consumer perspectives on diet selection and the pet food market. A survey of owners found that for those feeding MP diets, more than half "learned about feeding raw animal products for pets" from the internet and family/friend while only 8% from "my veterinarian." The survey also reported that pet owners perceived that nutrition was not discussed at most veterinary visits and owners feeding MP diets had a "lower trust in veterinary advice" than pet owners feeding UPCDs. MP feeders were mostly female (89%), 41 years of older (61%) and interestingly, more educated with 54% of owners feeding MP having some advanced degree [50]. Another survey of 218 dog owners feeding MP diets reported 60% of owners chose MP diets from information on the internet, 19% books or magazines, 12% encouraged by breeders with only 8% by veterinarians [48]. Connolly et al. reporting on the feeding practices of dog breeders found that only 49% consulted with their veterinarian about nutrition. Breeders feeding HD compared to breeders feeding CD viewed their veterinarian less favorably [49]. A telephone survey of 449 cat and 621 dog owners reported an interaction between feeding practices i.e., feeding a CD versus a non-CD and species i.e., dog or cat for the statement "I do not trust my veterinarians to provide sound nutritional advise." When cat and dog owners were analyzed separately there were significant differences between commercial and non-commercial responses with CD feeders agreeing more strongly than non -CD feeders [53].

Pet foods reviews often discuss why pet owners select MP diet types despite veterinarian recommendations to feed only UPCDs. Owner motivations for feeding MP diets have been reported as "symbolic of inclusion of the pet in the owner's family and culture, empowerment, claims of nutritional superiority of these diets, owner perception that they are providing a more natural diet, and a founding premise that these are the diets that wild, non-domesticated dog and cat species ate" [54–56]. The trend of humanization is evidenced in a survey of 2,181 pet owners where 87% had a high level of bonding with their pet and 53.1% reported giving equal or more priority (43.7%) to buying healthy food *for their pet* compared with themselves. The study concluded that pet owners assess the healthfulness, freshness, and ingredients of a pet food when making pet food decisions [52]. An internet survey reported the most common reason for cat owners to feed MP diets was that they "try not to consume processed foods and do not want their cat to consume one either" while for MP dog owners, 77.4% responded "feeding a raw diet is healthier" [50]. A survey of pet owners in Brazil reported that 69% of owners chose MP diets believing them to be more natural and 18% believed them to be healthier [51].

A recent observational study of pet feeding practices reported on changes from 2008 to 2018 noting "it appears the practice of feeding non- commercial and unconventional foods, either as the sole source of nutrition or in conjunction with a conventional diet, is higher now than has been previously reported". The authors report that these changes may be from an overall distrust of the pet food industry, pet humanization, and trends in animal nutrition shadowing trends in human nutrition, with increasing consumer interest in "natural" and "holistic" foods [57]. This aligns with the growing MP market which not only includes raw pet foods previously RMBD, but other MPCDs such as cooked fresh food, dehydrated, and freeze-dried type diets and home prepared or MPHDs. The growth of MPCDs is exemplified in Mars Pet Care January 2022 acquisition of Nom Nom, a wholefood fresh food company for $1 billion [58]. Although there is no formal data on MPHD, the authors have seen a significant increase for "home-prepared diet recipes" as Board Certified Veterinary Nutritionists®.

Consumers also want to know about pet food ingredients and have options to select diets with ingredients they believe to be healthier for their pet. This resulted in an increase in "grain-free" pet foods, typically UPCD becoming popular in the pet food market. Consumers seem to believe that grain-free diets are better for their pets because they assume they are more "natural, carbohydrate-free," and less likely to result in health problems such as allergies. The UPCD grain free marketed was rapidly growing however, more recently it has been impacted by its association with canine dilated cardiomyopathy (DCM) [59]. In addition, the FDA in 2018 alerted about the reports of dogs with DCM that were eating pet foods containing peas, lentils, other legume seeds, or potatoes, that are more common in diets labeled as "grain-free." It is not yet known if or how these ingredients are truly linked to cases of DCM and there is much controversy about the FDA investigation, DCM research and the pet food industry [60, 61].

Other pet food niches and definitions that veterinarians should be aware of because of consumer interest include the following [60]:

Human grade: According to the Association of American Feed Control Officials a pet food is considered "human grade" if a human can also consume it. All ingredients of the product must be edible to the human being and the product must be manufactured, packaged, and maintained according to the federal norms that regulate the manufacture of food.

Non-genetically modified (No-GMO): Consumers who avoid giving their pets genetically modified food. Consumers believe that non-GMO food ingredients are healthier for their dogs and cats, believing that fewer synthetic pesticides, herbicides or fertilizers are used in non-GMO crops.

Organic Pet foods: These are considered organic they should be in accordance with USDA's National Organic Program which states that an organic food is that produced through approved methods that integrate cultural, biological, and mechanical practices that promote the cycling of resources and balance, conserving biodiversity.

Synthetic fertilizers, sewage sludge, irradiation, and genetic engineering cannot be used.

Natural: Defined by the Association of American Feed Control Officials, food or ingredient derived solely from plant, sources of animal origin or extracted, in its natural state or subject to physical processing, thermal processing, rendering, purification, extraction, hydrolysis, enzymolysis or fermentation, but not being produced by or subject to a chemically synthetic process and which does not contain additives or processing aids which are chemically synthetic.

Sustainable: For many, commercial pet foods are formulated to provide nutrients in excess of the recommended minimum, using ingredients that compete directly with human food. Therefore, there is a need to produce high quality, safe, and affordable food using environmentally friendly ingredients. These foods need to use culturally acceptable raw materials by pet owners, to be nutritious and palatable to pets. The challenge is to combine consumer demand and provide natural nutrition for pets, reducing the impact on the environment.

Plant-based (PB) diet: This is considered a novel feeding trend practiced by approximately 2% [62] of dog owners (around one million dog owners in the USA alone). Note that there exists some disagreement among both pet keepers and pet health professionals, it is generally accepted that dogs can thrive when fed nutritionally complete and balanced diets devoid of animal ingredients [63].

Summary

The pet food industry responds to consumer demands by producing different diet types. Commercial diets should meet pet food safety standards first and foremost. A pet food categorization based on processing will not only benefit veterinarian – client nutrition discussions, but it is also needed to improve pet nutrition research. Beyond marketing and safety there is a dire need for research and assessment of whole diet effects on pet health and longevity.

References

1 Pet food market size, growth, trends (2029). Industry Analysis (fortunebusinessinsights.com). https://www.fortunebusinessinsights.com/industry-reports/pet-food-market-100554 (accessed 21 September 2022).

2 Niche pet food formats poised for growth in pet specialty. Pet Food Processing. https://www.petfoodprocessing.net/articles/14594-niche-pet-food-formats-poised-for-growth-in-pet-specialty (accessed 21 September 2022).

3 Gibney, M.J. (2018). Ultra-processed foods: definitions and policy issues. *Curr Dev Nutr* 3 (2): 1–7.

4 Alam, M.S., Kaur, J., Khaira, H. et al. (2016). Extrusion and extruded products: changes in quality attributes as affected by extrusion process parameters: a review. *Crit Rev Food Sci Nutr* 56 (3): 445–475.

5 Bleiweiss-Sande, R., Chui, K., Evans, E.W. et al. (2019). Robustness of food processing classification systems. *Nutrients* 11 (6): 1344.

6 Monteiro, C.A., Cannon, G., Moubarac, J.C. et al. (2018). The UN decade of nutrition, the NOVA food classification and the trouble with ultra-processing. *Public Health Nutr* 21 (1): 5–17.

7 Fardet, A. (2018). Characterization of the degree of food processing in relation with its health potential and effects. *Adv Food Nutr Res* 85: 79–129.

8 Hall, K.D., Ayuketah, A., Brychta, R. et al. (2019). Ultra-processed diets cause excess calorie intake and weight gain: an inpatient randomized controlled trial of Ad Libitum food intake. *Cell Metab* 30: 67–77.e63.

9 Monteiro, C.A., Levy, R.B., Claro, R.M. et al. (2010 Nov). A new classification of foods based on the extent and purpose of their processing. *Cad Saúde Pública* [Internet] 26 (11). Available from: https://doi.org/10.1590/S0102-311X2010001100005.

10 Monteiro, C.A., Levy, R.B., Claro, R.M. et al. (2011). Increasing consumption of ultra-processed foods and likely impact on human health: evidence from Brazil. *Public Health Nutr* 14: 5-13.

11 Monteiro, C.A. (2009 May). Nutrition and health. The issue is not food, nor nutrients, so much as processing. *Public Health Nutr* 12 (5): 729–31. doi:10.1017/S1368980009005291. PMID: 19366466.

12 Adams, J. and White, M. (2015). Characterisation of UK diets according to degree of food processing and associations with socio-demographics and obesity: cross-sectional analysis of UK National Diet and Nutrition Survey (2008–12). *Int J Behav Nutr Phys Act* 12 (1): 160. https://doi.org/10.1186/s12966-015-0317-y.

13 Baraldi, L.G., Martinez Steele, E., Canella, D.S. et al. (2018). Consumption of ultra-processed foods and associated sociodemographic factors in the USA between 2007 and 2012: evidence from a nationally representative cross-sectional study. *BMJ Open* 8: e020574.

14 Elizabeth, L., Machado, P., Zinöcker, M. et al. (2020). Ultra-processed foods and health outcomes: a narrative review. *Nutrients* 12.

15 Raditic, D.M. (2021). Insights into commercial pet foods. *Vet Clin North Am Small Anim Pract* 51: 551–562. doi: 10.1016/j.cvsm.2021.01.013.

16 Cammack, N.R., Yamka, R.M., and Adams, V.J. (2021). Low number of owner-reported suspected transmission of foodborne pathogens from raw meat-based diets fed to dogs and/or cats. *Front Vet Sci* 8: 741575. doi: 10.3389/fvets.2021.741575.

17 Davies, M. (2016). Veterinary clinical nutrition: success stories: an overview. *Proc Nutr Soc* 75 (3): 392–397.

18 de Godoy, M.R., Hervera, M., Swanson, K.S. et al. (2016). Innovations in canine and feline nutrition: technologies for food and nutrition assessment. *Annu Rev Anim Biosci* 4: 311–333.

19 Lawler, D.F., Larson, B.T., Ballam, J.M. et al. (2008). Diet restriction and ageing in the dog: major observations over two decades. *Br J Nutr* 99 (4): 793–805.

20 Oba, P.M., Hwisa, N., Huang, X. et al. (2022 Nov 1). Nutrient and Maillard reaction product concentrations of commercially available pet foods and treats. *J Anim Sci* 100 (11): skac305. doi:10.1093/jas/skac305. PMID: 36082767; PMCID: PMC9667973.

21 Twarda-Clapa, A., Olczak, A., Białkowska, A.M. et al. (2022). Advanced Glycation End-Products (AGEs): formation, chemistry, classification, receptors, and diseases related to AGEs. *Cells* 11.

22 Uribarri, J., del Castillo, M.D., de la Maza, M.P. et al. (2015). Dietary advanced glycation end products and their role in health and disease. *Adv Nutr* 6 (4): 461–473.

23 Poulsen, M.W., Hedegaard, R.V., Andersen, J.M. et al. (2013). Advanced glycation endproducts in food and their effects on health. *Food Chem Toxicol* 60: 10–37.

24 Nowotny, K., Schroter, D., Schreiner, M., and Grune, T. (2018). Dietary advanced glycation end products and their relevance for human health. *Ageing Res Rev* 47: 55–66.

25 ALjahdali, N. and Carbonero, F. (2019). Impact of Maillard reaction products on nutrition and health: current knowledge and need to understand their fate in the human digestive system. *Crit Rev Food Sci Nutr* 59 (3): 474–487. doi:10.1080/10408398.2017.1378865. Epub 2017 Oct 20. PMID: 28901784.

26 Delgado-Andrade, C. (2014). Maillard reaction products: some considerations on their health effects. *Clin Chem Lab Med* 52 (1): 53–60.

27 Teodorowicz, M., Hendriks, W.H., Wichers, H.J., and Savelkoul, H.F.J. (2018 Sep 13). Immunomodulation by processed animal feed: the role of maillard reaction products and Advanced Glycation End-Products (AGEs). *Front Immunol* 9 (2088): 1–15. doi:10.3389/fimmu.2018.02088. PMID: 30271411; PMCID: PMC6146089.

28 Teissier, T. and Boulanger, É. (2019). The receptor for advanced glycation end-products (RAGE) is an important pattern recognition receptor (PRR) for inflammaging. *Biogerontology* 20 (3): 279–301.

29 Hudson, B.I. and Lippman, M.E. (2018). Targeting RAGE signaling in inflammatory disease. *Annu Rev Med* 69: 349–364.

30 van Rooijen, C., Bosch, G., van der Poel, A.F. et al. (2013). The Maillard reaction and pet food processing: effects on nutritive value and pet health. *Nutr Res Rev* 26 (2): 130–148.

31 Rutherford, S.M., Rutherford-Marwick, K.J., and Moughan, P.J. (2007). Available (ileal digestible reactive) lysine in selected pet foods. *J Agric Food Chem* 55: 3517–3522.

32 van Rooijen, C., Bosch, G., van der Poel, A.F. et al. (2014). Reactive lysine content in commercially available pet foods. *J Nutr Sci* 3: e35.

33 van Rooijen, C., Bosch, G., van der Poel, A.F. et al. (2014). Quantitation of Maillard reaction products in commercially available pet foods. *J Agric Food Chem* 62 (35): 8883–8891.

34 van Rooijen, C., Bosch, G., Butre′, C.I. et al. (2016). Urinary excretion of dietary Maillard reaction products in healthy adult female cats. *J Anim Sci* 94 (1): 185–195.

35 Palaseweenun, P., Hagen-Plantinga, E.A., Schonewille, J.T. et al. (2020). Urinary excretion of advanced glycation end products in dogs and cats. *J Anim Physiol Anim Nutr (Berl)* 105 (1): 149–156.

36 Bridglalsingh, S. (2020). Influence of four differently processed diets on plasma levels of advanced glycation end products (AGEs), serum levels of receptors for advanced glycation end products (RAGE), serum and urine metabolome, and fecal microbiome in healthy dogs [PhD dissertation]. Athens (GA): University of Georgia.

37 Kim, Y., Keogh, J.B., Deo, P. et al. (2020). Differential effects of dietary patterns on advanced glycation end products: a randomized crossover study. *Nutrients* 12 (6): 1767.

38 ALjahdali, N. and Carbonero, F. (2019). Impact of Maillard reaction products on nutrition and health: current knowledge and need to understand their fate in the human digestive system. *Crit Rev Food Sci Nutr* 59 (3): 474–487. doi:10.1080/10408398.2017.1378865. Epub 2017 Oct 20. PMID: 28901784.

39 Sharma, C., Kaur, A., Thind, S.S. et al. (2015). Advanced glycation end-products (AGEs): an emerging concern for processed food industries. *J Food Sci Technol* 52 (12): 7561–7576.

40 Uribarri, J., Woodruff, S., Goodman, S. et al. (2010). Advanced glycation end products in foods and a practical guide to their reduction in the diet. *J Am Diet Assoc* 110 (6): 911–916.e12.

41 Cooke, J. (2017). Dietary reduction of advanced glycation end products: an opportunity for improved nutrition care. *J Ren Nutr* 27 (4): e23–e26.

42 Lin, J.A., Wu, C.H., and Yen, G.C. (2018). Perspective of advanced glycation end products on human health. *J Agric Food Chem* 66 (9): 2065–2070.

43 Wautier, M.P., Tessier, F.J., and Wautier, J.L. (2014). Advanced glycation end products: a risk factor for human health. *Ann Pharm Fr* 72 (6): 400–408.

44 Williams, P.A., Hodgkinson, S.M., Rutherford, S.M. et al. (2006). Lysine content in canine diets can be severely heat damaged. *J Nutr* 136: 1998S–2000S.

45 Behravesh, C.B., Ferraro, A., Deasy, M., 3rd et al. (2010). Human Salmonella infections linked to contaminated dry dog and cat food, 2006–2008. *Pediatrics* 126 (3): 477–483.

46 Kukanich, K.S. (2011). Update on Salmonella spp contamination of pet food, treats, and nutritional products and safe feeding recommendations. *J Am Vet Med Assoc* 238 (11): 1430–1434.

47 Kukanich, K.S. (2013 July). Compliance Policy Guide Sec. 690.800 Salmonella in food for animals. U.S. Department of Health and Human Services Food and Drug Administration; Center for Veterinary Medicine Office of Regulatory Affairs. https://www.fda.gov/regulatory-information/search-fda-guidance-documents/cpg-sec-690800-compliance-policy-guide-salmonella-food-animals.

48 Morelli, G., Bastianello, S., Catellani, P. et al. (2019). Raw meat-based diets for dogs: survey of owners' motivations, attitudes and practices. *BMC Vet Res* 15 (1): 74.

49 Connolly, K.M., Heinze, C.R., and Freeman, L.M. (2014). Feeding practices of dog breeders in the United States and Canada. *J Am Vet Med Assoc* 245 (6): 669–676.

50 Morgan, S.K., Willis, S., and Shepherd, M.L. (2017). Survey of owner motivations and veterinary input of owners feeding diets containing raw animal products. *PeerJ* 5: e3031.

51 Viegas, F.M., Ramos, C.P., Xavier, R.G.C. et al. (2020). Fecal shedding of Salmonella spp., Clostridium perfringens, and Clostridioides difficile in dogs fed raw meat-based diets in Brazil and their owners' motivation. *PLoS One* 15 (4): e0231275.

52 Schleicher, M., Cash, S.B., and Freeman, L.M. (2019). Determinants of pet food purchasing decisions. *Can Vet J* 60 (6): 644–650.

53 Michel, K.E., Willoughby, K.N., Abood, S.K. et al. (2008). Attitudes of pet owners toward pet foods and feeding management of cats and dogs. *J Am Vet Med Assoc* 233 (11): 1699–1703.

54 Michel, K.E. (2006 Nov). Unconventional diets for dogs and cats. *Vet Clin North Am Small Anim Pract* 36 (6): 1269–1281, vi–vii. doi:10.1016/j.cvsm.2006.08.003. PMID: 17085234.

55 Freeman, L.M., Chandler, M.L., Hamper, B.A., and Weeth, L.P. (2013 Dec 1). Current knowledge about the risks and benefits of raw meat–based diets for dogs and cats. *J Am Vet Med Assoc* 243 (11): 1549–1558. doi:10.2460/javma.243.11.1549. PMID: 24261804.

56 Parr, J.M. and Remillard, R.L. (2014). Handling alternative dietary requests from pet owners. *Vet Clin North Am Small Anim Pract* 44 (4): 667–688, v.

57 Dodd, S., Cave, N., Abood, S. et al. (2020). An observational study of pet feeding practices and how these have changed between 2008 and 2018. *Vet Rec* 186: 643.

58 Mars to Acquire Petfood Brand Nom Nom. ProFood World https://www.profoodworld.com/industry-news/news/22017833/mars-to-acquire-petfood-brand-nom-nom (accessed 21 September 2022).

59 Yamka, R. (2019). 'BEG' pet food and DCM, part 2: is veterinary bias at play? *'BEG' pet food and DCM, part 2: Is veterinary bias at play?* Pet Food Industry.

60 Viana, L.M., Mothé, C.G., and Mothé, M.G. (2020). Natural food for domestic animals: a national and international technological review. *Res Vet Sci* 130: 11–18.

61 Did industry funding influence an FDA investigation into canine heart disease and grain-free dog food?. 100Reporters https://100r.org/2022/07/did-industry-funding-influence-an-fda-investigation-into-canine-heart-disease-and-grain-free-dog-food (accessed 23 September 2022).

62 Dodd, S., Adolphe, J., and Verbrugghe, A. (2018). Plant-based diets for dogs. *J Am Vet Med Assoc* 253 (11): 1425–1432.

63 FEDIAF (2017). Are vegetarian diets for cats and dogs safe? https://europeanpetfood.org/wp-content/uploads/2022/02/fediaf_Vegetarian_diets_4_1.pdf.

12

Integrative Nutrition in Select Conditions: Obesity, Performance, Physical Rehabilitation

Laura Gaylord* and Donna Raditic

* Corresponding author

Introduction

"Let food be thy medicine and medicine be thy food." This quote from Hippocrates, referred to as the "father of medicine," speaks to the importance of nutrition as the foundation for good health. Utilizing an integrative approach in veterinary nutrition allows the veterinary practitioner to tailor a comprehensive nutrition plan for each pet as an individual utilizing current as well as developing knowledge on nutrition and supplements employed for both nutritional and therapeutic purposes. Veterinary nutritionists will rely on conventional nutrition data from the National Research Council (NRC) text "Nutrient Requirements for Dogs and Cats" [1] as a meta-analysis of all the scientific knowledge concerning the nutrition of dogs and cats, the annual Official Publication (OP) from the Association of American Feed Control Officials (AAFCO) [2] for recommendations for commercial pet foods, and the compilation of peer-reviewed scientific research on nutrition and disease condition management for designing optimal nutrition plans. Integrative veterinary medicine, however, may incorporate conventional nutritional strategies for patient management along with evidence-informed practices that are considered alternative or complementary – these may be practices that are based on the best evidence available, even when such evidence does not meet the strictest criteria for efficacy and safety. Pet owners are seeking integrative approaches to pet care with ever higher demand and often for pets with chronic disease states [3, 4]. Although clinical studies on integrative veterinary nutrition are few in number, opportunities exist for integrative practices concerning obesity management, performance nutrition, and nutrition for enhancing physical rehabilitation which may include conventional nutritional knowledge along with the inclusion of strategic nutrients or therapeutic supplements.

Obesity

In 2020, the American Animal Hospital Association declared that pet obesity has become an epidemic [5] and current statistics confirm that >60% of dogs and cats are overweight or obese [6]. In contrast, only 39% of dog owners and 45% of cat owners consider their pet overweight or having obesity [7]. Obesity is associated with an increase in disease risk including joint/mobility disorders, diabetes mellitus, endocrine disease, respiratory disease, cardiovascular disease, liver dysfunction, and even urinary tract disorders [8]. Ultimately, being overweight/obese will lead to a reduced quality of life and a shortened lifespan [8, 9]. Naturally, both pet owners and veterinarians are seeking nutritional or supplemental strategies to help prevent as well as treat overweight/obese body conditions. Assessing body condition and body weight should be an essential part of integrative veterinary practice.

Even though we classify dogs as omnivores, natural feeding studies in domesticated dogs showed that when dogs are given a choice of foods with varying protein, fat, and carbohydrate levels they will choose diets with higher protein and fat content and less carbohydrates (33% of the energy derived from protein, 7% from carbohydrate, and more than 60% from fats). [10] Consistent with cats as true carnivores, similar studies in cats demonstrate they will choose a diet that is 52% protein, 36% fat, and only 12% carbohydrate when allowed to choose their preferred foods [11]. Trends in integrative veterinary nutrition focus on a return to a more "natural" diet often with higher protein/fat content and fewer carbohydrates. These diets may be raw, cooked, air dried, freeze dried, less processed, homemade, commercial, or the standard diet of kibble or canned food marketed to include more "whole food" type ingredients. The term "natural" as defined by the Association of

Integrative Veterinary Medicine, First Edition. Edited by Mushtaq A. Memon and Huisheng Xie.
© 2023 John Wiley & Sons, Inc. Published 2023 by John Wiley & Sons, Inc.
Companion Website: www.wiley.com/go/memon/veterinary

American Feed Control Officials (AAFCO), however, is often unsatisfactory in integrative practice seeking less processed diets as it may also be applied to common highly processed kibble or canned foods. Choosing a "natural diet" does not guarantee that it will be successful in weight management or weight loss, in fact, the macronutrient content and/or energy density of the food may facilitate unintentional overfeeding of calories unless strict portion control is employed. Reducing meal volume may result in a loss of satiety for some pets; which makes calorie restriction difficult. No matter what diet type is employed, ultimately weight loss will require establishing a calorie deficit to induce reduction of body fat stores.

During weight loss, the nutrition plan should utilize diets fortified in nutrients to avoid potential nutrient deficiencies that may occur with food restriction in attempt to limit calorie intake. Research indicates that higher protein diets can spare lean body mass while restricting calories [12, 13]. Both protein and fiber contribute a satiety effect promoting a sense of fullness which may aide in prevention of begging behaviors [14, 15]. In one study, it was shown that a higher protein, medium carbohydrate diet may be a good solution for weight loss as it may preserve lean body mass, improve insulin sensitivity and result in a lower post-prandial glucose and insulin concentration compared to a diet with moderate protein and higher carbohydrate content [16]. Diets with sufficient content of the amino acids leucine and pyridoxine may also encourage lipolysis while maintaining lean tissue mass [17].

Diets selected for weight management should be evidence based and should be higher protein, higher fiber, and formulated for caloric restriction with higher nutrient levels. Diets should be fed in a calorie controlled manner to create a calorie deficit promoting a safe rate of weight loss at around 1–2% body weight per week. Co-morbidities should always be considered during diet selection in case contraindications are present that require limiting protein, fiber, or other select nutrient levels in the diet.

Spay/Neuter

Spaying and neutering are advocated for virtually all dogs and cats; however, this intervention does have potential consequences on body weight. It is in fact the largest risk factor for obesity in dogs and cats [18, 19]. 85% of dogs and 93% of cats are spayed and neutered [20]. Spaying and neutering will increase appetite even within three days of the procedure while decreasing metabolic rates up to 30% in dogs and 24% in cats [21–23]. Recognizing that most of our veterinary patients are or will be spayed and neutered mandates that diets recommended should consider weight management and obesity prevention as a priority.

L-Carnitine

L-carnitine is a nutrient that may offer benefits during weight loss. Carnitine serves as an essential cofactor in the transfer of long chain fatty acids within cells from the cytosol into the mitochondria where they will undergo beta oxidation in production of energy. Increasing intakes of dietary L-carnitine may promote the oxidation of long chain fatty acids [24]. Lower blood carnitine concentrations were found in overweight dogs compared to lean dogs in two studies [25, 26]. This finding could indicate a carnitine insufficiency related to spontaneous adiposity and altered lipid metabolism in overweight dogs. A carnitine supplemented diet was shown to support weight loss and improve body condition [27]. L-carnitine may also support muscular function during exercise. In one study, supplementing L-carnitine had positive benefits in Labrador retrievers for activity intensity, body composition, muscle recovery, and oxidative capacity [28]. Currently, optimal L-carnitine dosing for weight management or support of muscle mass is not known; however, multiple therapeutic weight loss diets include this nutrient.

Omega 3 Fatty Acids

Regulation of energy expenditure occurs through uncoupling proteins located in the mitochondria. Novel therapies could target these molecules for prevention and treatment of obesity in animals. As polyunsaturated fatty acids play a role in regulating gene expression of uncoupling proteins, the omega-3 fatty acids can enhance their expression. The results of a single unpublished grade II study suggests that increased consumption of dietary omega-3 fatty acids may be beneficial in overweight dogs subjected to caloric restriction [29]. Further studies are needed, however, to define the role and benefit of omega-3 fatty acids in weight loss in addition to optimal dosing.

Obesity is well known to create a state of inflammation and heightened state of oxidation within the body, for both humans as well as dogs [30–32]. Cats fed a diet enriched in omega-3 fatty acids when obese were found to have less insulin secretion and were postulated to have a lower risk of developing diabetes mellitus [33]. In dogs, the omega-3 fatty acids eicosapentanoic acid (EPA) and docosahexanoic acid (DHA) may reduce the overall inflammatory state as they reflect increased adiponectin and decreased leptin. Current evidence suggests a positive, dose-dependent relationship between omega-3 fatty acid intake and circulating levels of adiponectin [34]. Supplementing EPA and DHA in diets may be a strategy to reduce inflammation in the body associated with obesity.

Other Nutraceuticals Used for Obesity Management

Low grade evidence, defined as that extrapolated from clinical opinions, descriptive studies, studies in other species, pathophysiology justifications, or reports by expert committees exists for other nutraceuticals for weight management including DHEA (use limited due to toxicity), pyruvate, amylase inhibitors, conjugated linoleic acid, phytoestrogens, diacylglycerol, chromium, and vitamin A supplementation [35]. Use of these supplements, however, cannot be recommended without further research.

Performance Nutrition

For the working dog or canine athlete, genetics, inherent behavior, and musculoskeletal conformation are the major determinants of performance; however, nutrition and training play key roles in maximizing outcomes. Nutritional studies are lacking for dogs enrolled in agility, field trials, and detection work, and thus, much information is derived from data collected in studies on endurance dogs (sled dogs) and sprinting dogs (racing greyhounds). In general, energy intakes must increase to meet demands from activity and modifications of the nutrient composition of the food and feeding schedule accordingly may improve performances.

Energy and Performance

Exercise relies on energy production or specifically ATP produced from substrates such as carbohydrates, fats, or protein. The energy available in any particular diet is reported as kilocalories (kcal) or kilojoules (kJ) per cup and will be available on packages or in product guides. The National Research Council (NRC) has established energy requirements for dogs based on the available scientific research (130 x metabolic body weight MBW = [(kg body weight)^0.75] [1]; however, active dogs will require more calories depending on the type of exercise or work performed. Racing greyhounds have been reported to require a minimal increase (5–10% more) while endurance dogs require much more (up to an eight fold increase) [36]. Other factors to consider affecting energy needs include ambient temperature, thermal stress, and terrain traversed. The increased energy needs during such activities may not be recognized by owners, making underfeeding a potential issue especially if participating in multiple-day events. Conversely, overfeeding or overtreating is a concern, especially in events with frequent rewards for behaviors. Increased food intake will also increase fecal mass and needs for defecation, which can negatively affect performance.

Nutrients for Energy: Fats and Carbohydrates

Animals performing at maximal speeds immediately during exercise (sprinting) will deplete ATP reserves quickly and then rely on easily accessible energy from glucose generated via glycogenolysis from glycogen stores (liver, muscle). Fatty acid oxidation begins within minutes but does not peak until after 30 minutes or longer. Dogs may utilize either fats or carbohydrates during longer duration, lower intensity exercise. Earlier studies have shown that dogs perform equally well on diets containing almost no carbohydrate (1 g/1000 kcal) as compared with two diets with increasing carbohydrate content in moderate-intensity working sled dogs [37, 38]. In general, dogs participating in longer duration, endurance type activities will benefit from higher fat intakes with up 50–70% of calories (metabolizable energy (ME)) from fats and then only 10–15% of calories from carbohydrates [36, 39]. In times of extreme demand, fats may be utilized to provide even up to 85% of ME calories [36]. It is important to note that acclimation is needed even over several weeks' time to a higher fat diet to avoid adverse gastrointestinal consequences (steatorrhea) and the diet is only fed for a limited time. Sprinting dogs such as racing greyhounds may benefit from diets with carbohydrate content between 30–50% of ME calories which is similar to many commercial kibble foods available [40]. It is important to note that many canine athletes are more likely intermediate between these and perform for a shorter duration and intensity, thus diets chosen for these dogs should reflect the intensity and duration of performance. Those participating in longer duration endurance might incorporate more fats and those with sprinting activities could utilize more carbohydrates.

Meal timing may optimize availability of nutrients and it is recommended to feed the canine athlete at least four hours prior to exercise, one meal with in two hours post-exercise and then, if needed, small amounts during exercise for longer events. The largest meal should be after exercise has been completed. Providing sufficient water throughout the event and after is essential to prevent dehydration and facilitate normal heat dissipation/cooling during events [41].

Protein for the Working Dog

Proteins (amino acids) are not stored within the body as other nutrients; rather they are oxidized for energy, incorporated into tissue protein, or converted to fatty acids/glycerol then stored as adipose or glycogen. Amino acids will contribute only a small amount of energy (5–15%) during exercise which is derived from the branched chain amino acids (leucine, isoleucine, and valine). Animal protein sources (meat, organ tissues) have the highest content of essential amino acids and the highest digestibility. Dietary protein will help maintain muscle mass and total body proteins, serum albumin, and hematocrit [36]. Based on studies in sled dogs, it has been recommended to feed performance dogs diets that contain approximately 30% protein (metabolizable energy; 70–80 grams protein/1000 kcal) from highly digestible animal based protein [40]. Plant-based proteins exclusively fed may not be sufficient, as dogs fed on a diet of soy protein versus fish or meat-meal based diets had decreased hematocrits and increased red cell fragility after three weeks of feeding according to one study [42]. Endurance athletes will require more protein for exercise (30%+ protein ME or higher) while diets selected for sprinting or intermediate athletes are sufficient with at least 24% protein (ME calories; 60 grams protein/1000 kcal).

Dietary Fiber in the Working Dog Diet

Dietary fiber will increase fecal moisture and bulk leading to increased defecation and body weight during performance. Alternatively, fibers may improve the gastrointestinal microbiome, stool quality, and reduce risk of stress-induced diarrhea. Strategic use of different fiber types (soluble vs insoluble) may have advantages for different dogs. Most commercial diets will contain a mix of fiber types utilizing ingredients such as whole grains (barley, oats, sorghum) or by adding specific supplements. Fiber content in commercial foods is usually reported only as "crude fiber" which represents only the insoluble fiber content. Addition of psyllium husk fiber, a mucilage with water binding properties that acts as an insoluble fiber and mildly fermentable fiber, has been used as a strategy to prevent stress induced diarrhea. A starting dose of 4 grams powder (1 tsp) daily (not to exceed 4 tsp/day for a 20–30 kg canine athlete) has been recommended [36, 43].

Physical Rehabilitation

Key nutritional factors that should be evaluated during physical rehabilitation include dietary protein, fatty acid composition, and caloric intake. Nutrition can be useful to modify tissue responses to injury and during recovery. No specific diets are marketed for physical rehabilitation; however, diets formulated for management of osteoarthritis or dermatologic conditions may include selectively optimized nutrients such as protein or omega-3 fatty acids that may benefit the rehabilitation patient. Diets should be evaluated for nutrient content by comparing them on an "energy basis" (grams or milligrams per 1000 or 100 kcal). Nutritional information is best obtained by referencing a current product guide or contacting the manufacturer directly.

Macronutrients in Physical Rehabilitation

Protein

Protein intake is important to address increased rates of protein turnover in injured tissues during inflammation, recovery, and repair. The amino acid leucine has been noted to reduce proteolysis during exercise in dogs during muscular activity [44]. Human data suggests that leucine stimulates skeletal muscle protein synthesis which may aide dogs in recovery [45]. Leucine may also aide in maintenance of muscle mass for convalescing dogs [17]. It has been suggested to feed diets that contain >75 g protein/1000 kcal to prevent relative deficiencies of select amino acids [46]. It is critical to assess the protein content in commercial pet foods as there is wide variability across diets. Commercial diets formulated for growth, athletic performance, working dogs, or recovery diets may be suitable.

Fats/Fatty Acids

Dogs (or cats) enrolled in physical rehabilitation will most often have a condition associated with inflammation such as osteoarthritis, obesity, tissue injury, etc. Increased intakes of the omega-3 fatty acids (eicosapentaenoic acid (EPA; 20:5n3) and docosahexaenoic acid (DHA; 22:6n3) may decrease the presence of pro-inflammatory mediators within the body due to their inhibition of the arachidonic cascade thereby reducing pro-inflammatory metabolites (prostaglandins, thromboxane, and leukotrienes) [47]. EPA and DHA are also precursors to inflammation resolving mediators thereby hastening the resolution of inflammation [48]. Other mediators down regulated by EPA and DHA include the matrix metalloproteinases (MMPs), interleukins (IL-1, IL-2), cyclooxygenase (COX-2) and tumor necrosis factor-alpha, which enhances their effect [49, 50]. EPA and DHA are derived from metabolic conversion of alpha-linolenic acid (ALA), however, this bioconversion is very limited in dogs and cats and therefore EPA and DHA must be supplied through diet [51, 52]. Doses recommended to achieve anti-inflammatory benefits in one study noted the most improvement with foods containing >7.5 g/1000 kcal [53], however, supplementation to this level may be impractical and require a large amount of capsules or liquid added to any diet. Commercial diets containing 1–3 g/1000 kcal have also demonstrated clinical improvements. Recommended dosing by body weight to achieve anti-inflammatory benefits for treatment of osteoarthritis is 310 mg combined EPA + DHA/kg (body weight^0.75) or approximately 150 mg EPA + DHA/kg/day [54]. Use of EPA and DHA supplementation or selection of diets with their inclusion may facilitate reduction of other medications such as nonsteroidal anti-inflammatory drugs [55, 56]. Anecdotally, high amounts of fish oil added to a diet may cause untoward gastrointestinal side effects for some dogs. A slow titration of any added dose is recommended, and the additional calories contributed should be considered in the total daily diet.

Energy/Caloric Restriction

While convalescing, dogs and cats will require less energy intake. During hospitalization, calories are most often reduced to provide the Resting Energy Requirement (RER) (BW(kg)^0.75 x 70) and no more to avoid inappropriate weight gain. Cage confinement reduces calorie needs up to 25–30% [46]. During a weight loss program, the goal rate of weight loss is generally 1–2% body weight per week; however, slower rates (0.5–1%) may be utilized to prevent losses in lean body mass or if co-morbidities prohibit aggressive caloric restriction. Diets should be selected to facilitate a negative energy balance without creating nutrient deficiencies (especially protein) during rehabilitation. Selecting diets that are higher protein, higher fiber, lower in fat and caloric density will provide benefits for the patient needing weight loss during physical rehabilitation.

Exercise for Weight Loss

Underwater treadmill therapy can increase energy expenditure. Heathy dogs walking on an underwater treadmill at elbow height water level were shown to use 1.9 kcal/kg^0.75 per kilometer [46]. Unfortunately, there is a lack of evidence for best recommendations for pet owners regarding exercise programs that will lead to safe and efficient weight reduction [57]. Studies evaluating use of exercise for achieving weight loss for overweight/obese dogs have not shown significant benefits over caloric restriction. In one study, bodyweight decreased significantly with the dietary caloric restriction (–12%; P = 0.028) but not with the physical activity intervention (–2%, P = 0.107) [58]. Although exercise may not accelerate weight loss, when used in combination with caloric restriction it may help to preserve lean body mass which can improve metabolism and musculoskeletal function [57]. An additional study reported that active dogs would reach their target ideal body weights quicker or were able to be fed additional calories/day and achieve the same rate of loss during the weight loss program [59]. Thus, while exercise is important in improving musculoskeletal fitness and lean body mass, dietary modification with selection of appropriate diets and implementing caloric restriction must be foremost when weight loss is needed.

Other Nutraceuticals for Physical Rehabilitation

While numerous nutraceuticals are available in the current nutraceutical market for dogs and cats, few have robust clinical evidence for efficacy as part of a multi-modal plan for dogs or cats undergoing physical rehabilitation. An exception to this may be use of the omega-3 fatty acids EPA and DHA previously discussed which have numerous clinical studies documenting their anti-inflammatory benefits. Several other nutraceuticals may be considered for individual patients. Often nutraceuticals contain several nutrients in the same product.

Glucosamine/Chondroitin

Efficacy of glucosamine/chondroitin nutraceuticals has not been well established, with studies providing mixed results. Two high quality, prospective, randomized studies evaluated the use of glucosamine/chondroitin and documented opposite results. One study showed a benefit after 70 days, whereas another 60-day trial found no improvement [60, 61]. Anecdotally, many practitioners report they may be useful as part of a multi-modal support plan for a patient with osteoarthritis. A recent meta-analysis evaluating canine and feline therapeutic diets and nutraceuticals for osteoarthritis has concluded no benefit can be confirmed from glucosamine/chondroitin nutraceuticals [62].

Undenatured Collagen Type II

Benefits of undenatured collagen type II (UCII) may be due to its unique form and mechanism. UCII works to stimulate T helper tolerance leading to a diminished immune response to byproducts of cartilage degradation in the joint space resulting in lessened inflammation [63]. Placebo controlled studies demonstrated some benefit when compared to nonsteroidal anti-inflammatory medications when used alone or in combination with other nutraceuticals [64]. Extended dosing (>90 days) is often required to document clinical benefit. Use of the undenatured form as UCII is important as many collagen type products are available.

Green-Lipped Mussel (Perna canaliculus)

Green-lipped mussel (GLM) is marketed for the treatment of osteoarthritis in dogs and can provide an alternate dietary source of glucosamine, omega-3 fatty acids, and trace minerals. Three prospective, randomized studies evaluated GLM for the treatment of osteoarthritis in dogs and showed a positive effect; however, one study indicated no effect was noted at a lower dosing [65–68]. GLM was supplemented separately or as an inclusion in a diet, but its direct mechanism of action is yet to be fully defined. It is suspected that it works similarly to fish oil supplements providing the omega-3 fatty acids EPA and DHA with resulting reduction in pro-inflammatory mediators.

Boswellic Acid (*Boswellia serrata*)

Boswellia is derived from frankincense and has shown benefits in treating osteoarthritis in humans through randomized, double-blind, placebo controlled studies [69]. A resin extract (AKBA (3-O-acetyl-11-keto-beta boswellic acid)) has anti-inflammatory effects and has been shown to support structural integrity of joints and connective tissues. Products marketed for canine osteoarthritis will contain this ingredient often in combination with other nutrients having potential benefits for osteoarthritis [70–72].

Turmeric/Curcumin

Curcumin is a polyphenol extract from the familiar yellow spice turmeric and has thousands of years of use in both culinary as well as traditional Chinese and Ayurvedic medicine. Curcuminoid extracts have shown both anti-inflammatory and antineoplastic effects including decreases in inflammatory cytokines (IL-6, IL-8, COX-2, PGE_2, iNOS, MMP-3, MMP-9) and inhibition of NF-κB and TNF-α signaling in both *in vitro* and *in vivo* studies. When taken orally, however, curcumin has very poor absorption and bioavailability (<1%) [73]. Absorption can be improved, however, when given in combination with a fat source (phospholipids). One study in dogs with osteoarthritis showed decreased gene expression for inflammatory mediators when taking curcumin compared to non-steroidal anti-inflammatory medications. In combination with other nutraceuticals, curcumin has also shown a reduction in pain indicators for dogs with osteoarthritis [74].

Avocado/Soybean Unsaponifiables (ASU)

Only limited canine studies are available examining use of ASU in dogs with osteoarthritis. Within articular chondrocytes, monocytes, and macrophages, ASU can suppress TNF-α, IL-1β, COX-2, iNOS gene expression, and prostaglandin E_2 and nitric oxide production [75]. In two canine studies, ASU increased extracellular matrix production (type II collagen, proteoglycan) within chondrocytes and reduced development of early cartilage and subchondral bone lesions associated with osteoarthritis compared to placebo-treated dogs [73, 74].

Elk Velvet Antler

The mechanism of action of elk velvet antler is poorly understood but postulated to provide molecules such as parathyroid hormone-related peptide and retinoic acid (RA) that may stimulate fibroblasts, chondrocytes, osteoblasts, and osteoclasts resulting in joint repair. One randomized, blinded, placebo-controlled, parallel group clinical trial for osteoarthritis was evaluated where gait analysis via force plate, clinical signs assessed by an orthopedic surgeon, performances in daily life activities and vitality assessed by the owners, and blood analyses were analyzed. The study documented positive efficacy data from both objective and subjective outcome measures [75].

Other nutraceuticals such as gelatin hydrolysate or protein fractions from hyperimmunized cow milk have been preliminarily studied in dogs but additional information is needed on their efficacy.

Summary

Integrative nutrition in obesity, performance, and physical rehabilitation should focus on providing an optimized diet and supplemental therapies tailored for the individual dog (or cat) and consider the unique needs each. Selection of diets and nutraceuticals should be evidence based whenever possible; however, research is limited to guide veterinarians in the decision-making process. Veterinarians should continue to review available research studies and apply current evolving knowledge to each patient's situation to decide which diets and nutraceuticals might be useful.

References

1 McReynolds, T. (2020). Pet obesity is an epidemic. NEWStat®. https://www.aaha.org/publications/newstat/articles/2020-02/pet-obesity-is-an-epidemic/#:~:text=AAHA%20AAHA%20publications%20NEWStat%C2%AE%202020-02%20Pet%20obesity%20is,of%20a%20new%20report%20from%20Banfield%20Pet%20Hospital (accessed September 26, 2022).

2 Larsen, J.A. and Villaverde, C. (2016). Scope of the problem and perception by owners and veterinarians. *Vet Clin North Am Small Anim Pract* 46: 761–772.

3 Prevention AfPO (2021). Press release & summary of the pet owner: pet food, nutrition, & weight management survey 2021. https://petobesityprevention.org/2021 (accessed September 26, 2022).

4 Shepherd, M. (2021). Canine and feline obesity management. *Vet Clin North Am Small Anim Pract* 51: 653–667.

5 Prevention AfPO (2018). Press release and summary of the pet obesity veterinary clinic prevalence survey & pet owner: pet food, nutrition, & weight management survey. https://petobesityprevention.org/2018 (accessed September 26, 2022).

6 Hewson-Hughes, A.K., Hewson-Hughes, V.L., Colyer, A. et al. (2013). Geometric analysis of macronutrient selection in breeds of the domestic dog, Canis lupus familiaris. *Behav Ecol* 24: 293–304.

7 Hewson-Hughes, A.K., Hewson-Hughes, V.L., Miller, A.T. et al. (2011). Geometric analysis of macronutrient selection in the adult domestic cat, *Felis catus. J Exp Biol* 214: 1039–1051.

8 des Courtis, X., Wei, A., Kass, P.H. et al. (2015). Influence of dietary protein level on body composition and energy expenditure in calorically restricted overweight cats. *J Anim Physiol Anim Nutr (Berl)* 99: 474–482.

9 Blanchard, G., Nguyen, P., Gayet, C. et al. (2004). Rapid weight loss with a high-protein low-energy diet allows the recovery of ideal body composition and insulin sensitivity in obese dogs. *J Nutr* 134: 2148s–2150s.

10 Bissot, T., Servet, E., Vidal, S. et al. (2010). Novel dietary strategies can improve the outcome of weight loss programmes in obese client-owned cats. *J Feline Med Surg* 12: 104–112.

11 Weber, M., Bissot, T., Servet, E. et al. (2007). A high-protein, high-fiber diet designed for weight loss improves satiety in dogs. *J Vet Intern Med* 21: 1203–1208.

12 André, A., Leriche, I., Chaix, G. et al. (2017). Recovery of insulin sensitivity and optimal body composition after rapid weight loss in obese dogs fed a high-protein medium-carbohydrate diet. *J Anim Physiol Anim Nutr* 101: 21–30.

13 Murphy, M., Bartges, J.W., Zemel, M.B. et al. (2020). Effect of a leucine/pyridoxine nutraceutical on caloric intake and body composition of obese dogs losing weight. *Front Vet Sci* 7: 555.

14 Kutzler, M.A. (2020). Possible relationship between long-term adverse health effects of gonad-removing surgical sterilization and luteinizing hormone in dogs. *Animals (Basel)* 10.

15 Martin, L.J., Siliart, B., Dumon, H.J. et al. (2006). Hormonal disturbances associated with obesity in dogs. *J Anim Physiol Anim Nutr (Berl)* 90: 355–360.

16 Association APP. (2018). The 2017–2018 APPA National pet owners survey debut.

17 Jeusette, I., Detilleux, J., Cuvelier, C. et al. (2004). Ad libitum feeding following ovariectomy in female Beagle dogs: effect on maintenance energy requirement and on blood metabolites. *J Anim Physiol Anim Nutr (Berl)* 88: 117–121.

18 Jeusette, I., Daminet, S., Nguyen, P. et al. (2006). Effect of ovariectomy and ad libitum feeding on body composition, thyroid status, ghrelin and leptin plasma concentrations in female dogs. *J Anim Physiol Anim Nutr (Berl)* 90: 12–18.

19 Kanchuk, M.L., Backus, R.C., Calvert, C.C. et al. (2003). Weight gain in gonadectomized normal and lipoprotein lipase-deficient male domestic cats results from increased food intake and not decreased energy expenditure. *J Nutr* 133: 1866–1874.

20 Hall, J.A. and Jewell, D.E. (2012). Feeding healthy beagles medium-chain triglycerides, fish oil, and carnitine offsets age-related changes in serum fatty acids and carnitine metabolites. *PLoS One* 7: e49510.

21 Qu, W., Chen, Z., Hu, X. et al. (2022). Profound perturbation in the metabolome of a canine obesity and metabolic disorder model. *Front Endocrinol (Lausanne)* 13: 849060.

22 Söder, J., Höglund, K., Dicksved, J. et al. (2019). Plasma metabolomics reveals lower carnitine concentrations in overweight Labrador Retriever dogs. *Acta Vet Scand* 61.

23 Floerchinger, A.M., Jackson, M.I., Jewell, D.E. et al. (2015). Effect of feeding a weight loss food beyond a caloric restriction period on body composition and resistance to weight gain in dogs. *J Am Vet Med Assoc* 247: 375–384.

24 Varney, J.L., Fowler, J.W., McClaughry, T.C. et al. (2020). L-Carnitine metabolism, protein turnover and energy expenditure in supplemented and exercised Labrador Retrievers. *J Anim Physiol Anim Nutr* 104: 1540–1550.

25 Ishioka, K., Sagawa, M., Okumura, M. et al. (2004). Treatment of obesity in dogs through increasing energy expenditure by mitochondrial uncoupling proteins. *J Vet Intern Med* 18: 431.

26 Cortese, L., Terrazzano, G., and Pelagalli, A. (2019). Leptin and immunological profile in obesity and its associated diseases in dogs. *Int J Mol Sci* 20.

27 Kawai, T., Autieri, M.V., and Scalia, R. (2021). Adipose tissue inflammation and metabolic dysfunction in obesity. *Am J Physiol Cell Physiol* 320: C375–C391.

28 Vendramini, T.H.A., Macedo, H.T., Amaral, A.R. et al. (2020). Gene expression of the immunoinflammatory and immunological status of obese dogs before and after weight loss. *PLoS One* 15: e0238638.

29 Wilkins, C., Long, R.C., Jr., Waldron, M. et al. (2004). Assessment of the influence of fatty acids on indices of insulin sensitivity and myocellular lipid content by use of magnetic resonance spectroscopy in cats. *Am J Vet Res* 65: 1090–1099.

30 Gray, B., Steyn, F., Davies, P.S. et al. (2013). Omega-3 fatty acids: a review of the effects on adiponectin and leptin and potential implications for obesity management. *Eur J Clin Nutr* 67: 1234–1242.

31 Roudebush, P., Schoenherr, W.D., and Delaney, S.J. (2008). An evidence-based review of the use of nutraceuticals and dietary supplementation for the management of obese and overweight pets. *J Am Vet Med Assoc* 232: 1646–1655.

32 Council NR. (2006). *Nutrient Requirements of Dogs and Cats*. Washington, DC: The National Academies Press.

33 Wakshlag, J. and Shmalberg, J. (2014). Nutrition for working and service dogs. *Vet Clin North Am Small Anim Pract* 44: 719–740, vi.

34 Kronfeld, D.S., Hammel, E.P., Ramberg, C.F., Jr. et al. (1977). Hematological and metabolic responses to training in racing sled dogs fed diets containing medium, low, or zero carbohydrate. *Am J Clin Nutr* 30: 419–430.

35 Hammel, E.P., Kronfeld, D.S., Ganjam, V.K. et al. (1977). Metabolic responses to exhaustive exercise in racing sled dogs fed diets containing medium, low, or zero carbohydrate. *Am J Clin Nutr* 30: 409–418.

36 Case, L.P., Daristotle, L., Hayek, M.G. et al. (2011). Chapter 24 – Performance. In: *Canine and Feline Nutrition*. 3e (ed. L.P. Case, L. Daristotle, and M.G. Hayek, et al.), 243–260. Saint Louis: Mosby.

37 Center, S., Wakshlag, J., Cullen, J. et al. (2021). Possible diet-related increase in copper-associated liver disease in dogs. *Vet Rec* 189: 117.

38 Hand, M.S., Thatcher, C.D., Remillard, R.L. et al. (2011). *Small Animal Clinical Nutrition*, 5e. Mark Morris Institute.

39 Yamada, T., Tohori, M., Ashida, T. et al. (1987). Comparison of effects of vegetable protein diet and animal protein diet on the initiation of anemia during vigorous physical training (sports anemia) in dogs and rats. *J Nutr Sci Vitaminol (Tokyo)* 33: 129–149.

40 Leib, M.S. (2000). Treatment of chronic idiopathic large-bowel diarrhea in dogs with a highly digestible diet and soluble fiber: a retrospective review of 37 cases. *J Vet Intern Med* 14: 27–32.

41 Hamada, K., Matsumoto, K., Okamura, K. et al. (1999). Effect of amino acids and glucose on exercise-induced gut and skeletal muscle proteolysis in dogs. *Metabolism* 48: 161–166.

42 Drummond, M.J. and Rasmussen, B.B. (2008). Leucine-enriched nutrients and the regulation of mammalian target of rapamycin signaling and human skeletal muscle protein synthesis. *Curr Opin Clin Nutr Metab Care* 11: 222–226.

43 Shmalberg, J. (2015). Canine rehabilitative nutrition. *Tod Vet Pract* 5: 87–90.

44 Shahidi, F. and Ambigaipalan, P. (2018). Omega-3 polyunsaturated fatty acids and their health benefits. *Annu Rev Food Sci Technol* 9: 345–381.

45 Weylandt, K.H., Chiu, C.Y., Gomolka, B. et al. (2012). Omega-3 fatty acids and their lipid mediators: towards an understanding of resolvin and protectin formation. *Prostaglandins Other Lipid Mediat* 97: 73–82.

46 Hansen, R.A., Ogilvie, G.K., Davenport, D.J. et al. (1998). Duration of effects of dietary fish oil supplementation on serum eicosapentaenoic acid and docosahexaenoic acid concentrations in dogs. *Am J Vet Res* 59: 864–868.

47 Zainal, Z., Longman, A.J., Hurst, S. et al. (2009). Relative efficacies of omega-3 polyunsaturated fatty acids in reducing expression of key proteins in a model system for studying osteoarthritis. *Osteoarthr Cartil* 17: 896–905.

48 Bauer, J.E. (2016). The essential nature of dietary omega-3 fatty acids in dogs. *J Am Vet Med Assoc* 249: 1267–1272.

49 Bauer, J.E. (2006). Metabolic basis for the essential nature of fatty acids and the unique dietary fatty acid requirements of cats. *J Am Vet Med Assoc* 229: 1729–1732.

50 Fritsch, D., Allen, T.A., Dodd, C.E. et al. (2010). Dose-titration effects of fish oil in osteoarthritic dogs. *J Vet Intern Med* 24: 1020–1026.

51 Bauer, J.E. (2011). Therapeutic use of fish oils in companion animals. *J Am Vet Med Assoc* 239: 1441–1451.

52 Fritsch, D.A., Allen, T.A., Dodd, C.E. et al. (2010). A multicenter study of the effect of dietary supplementation with fish oil omega-3 fatty acids on carprofen dosage in dogs with osteoarthritis. *J Am Vet Med Assoc* 236: 535–539.

53 Roush, J.K., Cross, A.R., Renberg, W.C. et al. (2010). Evaluation of the effects of dietary supplementation with fish oil omega-3 fatty acids on weight bearing in dogs with osteoarthritis. *J Am Vet Med Assoc* 236: 67–73.

54 Ratsch, B.E., Levine, D., and Wakshlag, J.J. (2022). Clinical guide to obesity and nonherbal nutraceuticals in canine orthopedic conditions. *Vet Clin North Am Small Anim Pract* 52: 939–958.

55 Chapman, M., Woods, G.R.T., Ladha, C. et al. (2019). An open-label randomised clinical trial to compare the efficacy of dietary caloric restriction and physical activity for weight loss in overweight pet dogs. *Vet J* 243: 65–73.

56 Wakshlag, J.J., Struble, A.M., Warren, B.S. et al. (2012). Evaluation of dietary energy intake and physical activity in dogs undergoing a controlled weight-loss program. *J Am Vet Med Assoc* 240: 413–419.

57 McCarthy, G., O'Donovan, J., Jones, B. et al. (2007). Randomised double-blind, positive-controlled trial to assess the efficacy of glucosamine/chondroitin sulfate for the treatment of dogs with osteoarthritis. *Vet J* 174: 54–61.

58 Moreau, M., Dupuis, J., Bonneau, N.H. et al. (2003). Clinical evaluation of a nutraceutical, carprofen and meloxicam for the treatment of dogs with osteoarthritis. *Vet Rec* 152: 323–329.

59 Barbeau-Grégoire, M., Otis, C., Cournoyer, A. et al. (2022). A 2022 systematic review and meta-analysis of enriched therapeutic diets and nutraceuticals in canine and feline osteoarthritis. *Int J Mol Sci* 23.

60 Yoshinari, O., Moriyama, H., and Shiojima, Y. (2015). An overview of a novel, water-soluble undenatured type II collagen (NEXT-II). *J Am Coll Nutr* 34: 255–262.

61 D'Altilio, M., Peal, A., Alvey, M. et al. (2007). Therapeutic efficacy and safety of undenatured type II collagen singly or in combination with glucosamine and chondroitin in arthritic dogs. *Toxicol Mech Methods* 17: 189–196.

62 Bui, L.M. and Bierer, R.L. (2001). Influence of green lipped mussels (Perna canaliculus) in alleviating signs of arthritis in dogs. *Vet Ther* 2: 101–111.

63 Bierer, T.L. and Bui, L.M. (2002). Improvement of arthritic signs in dogs fed green-lipped mussel (Perna canaliculus). *J Nutr* 132: 1634s–1636s.

64 Pollard, B., Guilford, W.G., Ankenbauer-Perkins, K.L. et al. (2006). Clinical efficacy and tolerance of an extract of green-lipped mussel (Perna canaliculus) in dogs presumptively diagnosed with degenerative joint disease. *N Z Vet J* 54: 114–118.

65 Hielm-Björkman, A., Tulamo, R.M., Salonen, H. et al. (2009). Evaluating complementary therapies for canine osteoarthritis part I: green-lipped mussel (Perna canaliculus). *Evid Based Complement Alternat Med* 6: 365–373.

66 Yu, G., Xiang, W., Zhang, T. et al. (2020). Effectiveness of Boswellia and Boswellia extract for osteoarthritis patients: a systematic review and meta-analysis. *BMC Complement Med Ther* 20: 225.

67 Caterino, C., Aragosa, F., Della Valle, G. et al. (2021). Clinical efficacy of Curcuvet and Boswellic acid combined with conventional nutraceutical product: an aid to canine osteoarthritis. *PLoS One* 16: e0252279.

68 Martello, E., Bigliati, M., Adami, R. et al. (2022). Efficacy of a dietary supplement in dogs with osteoarthritis: a randomized placebo-controlled, double-blind clinical trial. *PLoS One* 17: e0263971.

69 Reichling, J., Schmökel, H., Fitzi, J. et al. (2004). Dietary support with Boswellia resin in canine inflammatory joint and spinal disease. *Schweiz Arch Tierheilkd* 146: 71–79.

70 Kotha, R.R. and Luthria, D.L. (2019). Curcumin: biological, pharmaceutical, nutraceutical, and analytical aspects. *Molecules* 24.

71 Comblain, F., Barthélémy, N., Lefèbvre, M. et al. (2017). A randomized, double-blind, prospective, placebo-controlled study of the efficacy of a diet supplemented with curcuminoids extract, hydrolyzed collagen and green tea extract in owner's dogs with osteoarthritis. *BMC Vet Res* 13: 395.

72 Au, R.Y., Al-Talib, T.K., Au, A.Y. et al. (2007). Avocado soybean unsaponifiables (ASU) suppress TNF-alpha, IL-1beta, COX-2, iNOS gene expression, and prostaglandin E2 and nitric oxide production in articular chondrocytes and monocyte/macrophages. *Osteoarthr Cartil* 15: 1249–1255.

73 Altinel, L., Saritas, Z.K., Kose, K.C. et al. (2007). Treatment with unsaponifiable extracts of avocado and soybean increases TGF-beta1 and TGF-beta2 levels in canine joint fluid. *Tohoku J Exp Med* 211: 181–186.

74 Boileau, C., Martel-Pelletier, J., Caron, J. et al. (2009). Protective effects of total fraction of avocado/soybean unsaponifiables on the structural changes in experimental dog osteoarthritis: inhibition of nitric oxide synthase and matrix metalloproteinase-13. *Arthritis Res Ther* 11: R41.

75 Moreau, M., Dupuis, J., Bonneau, N.H. et al. (2004). Clinical evaluation of a powder of quality elk velvet antler for the treatment of osteoarthrosis in dogs. *Can Vet J* 45: 133–139.

Section VI

Physical Rehabilitation
(Section Editor – Janice Huntingford)

13

Introduction to Rehabilitation

*Ronald B. Koh and Janice Huntingford**

* Corresponding author

Introduction

Physical rehabilitation is a rapidly expanding field within veterinary medicine. Initially it was considered an alternative therapy but is quickly emerging as an essential service for small animal practice as more clients treat their pets as family members, and pets are living longer and developing more chronic conditions that would benefit from rehabilitation [1]. The American Association of Rehabilitation Veterinarians (AARV) defines physical rehabilitation as "the diagnosis and management of patients with painful or functionally limiting conditions, particularly those with injury or illness related to the neurologic and musculoskeletal systems" [2]. Rehabilitation focuses on improving the function and quality of life in animals with arthritis or neurologic disorders as well as those recovering from surgical procedures [2]. The overall goal of rehabilitation is to decrease pain, reduce edema, promote tissue healing, restore gait and mobility to its prior activity level, regain strength, prevent further injury, and promote optimal quality of life [3]. Typically, a multimodal approach Integrating pharmacological and non-pharmacological intervention is utilized by rehabilitation therapists to manage patients during their recovery. Formal education in rehabilitation is required before incorporating these techniques into practice settings. In addition to certificate programs, Veterinary Sports Medicine and Rehabilitation is now a recognized specialty with over 200 diplomates in many countries. (See Table 13.1 for list of formal education for rehabilitation).

Anatomy

Knowledge of canine and feline anatomy is critical to develop rehabilitation plans safely and effectively. A working knowledge of boney landmarks, the origin, insertion and function of muscles and neurology is critical for this discipline. A discussion of anatomy is beyond the scope of this book, however many books, and websites thoroughly review anatomy for the practitioner. Formal rehabilitation courses teach working anatomy for rehabilitation veterinarians.

Assessments

Accurate orthopedic, neurological, and physical examinations are required for successful rehabilitation. Box 13.1 summarizes an Integrated Patient Evaluation. In some cases, further diagnostics may be required. These may include radiographs, musculoskeletal ultrasound, magnetic resonance imaging (MRI), computed tomography (CT), arthrocentesis and laboratory tests. All therapists should be able to perform a thorough physical examination and understand underlying diseases and appropriate treatment. Failing to properly diagnose the patient can result in aggravation of pre-existing conditions or prescribing inappropriate treatments.

Box 13.1 Integrative Patient Evaluations
All patients should have the following examinations
Medical history
Physical Examination
TCVM Examination
Posture Examination
Gait/Movement (Lameness) Examination
Orthopedic Examination
Neurological Examination

Medical History

The medical history should consist of general information and history of presenting problem. Signalment, species, diet,

Integrative Veterinary Medicine, First Edition. Edited by Mushtaq A. Memon and Huisheng Xie.
© 2023 John Wiley & Sons, Inc. Published 2023 by John Wiley & Sons, Inc.
Companion Website: www.wiley.com/go/memon/veterinary

Table 13.1 Resources on animal physical rehabilitation.

a) Institutes that offer animal physical rehabilitation training and certification programs (listed alphabetically):

    1) Canine Rehabilitation Institute: caninerehabinstitute.com

    2) Chi University: chiu.edu

    3) Curacore: curacore.org

    4) Healing Oasis Wellness Center: healingoasis.edu

    5) University of Tennessee: utvetce.com

b) Non-profit organizations that promote the art and science of veterinary rehabilitation:

    1) American Association of Rehabilitation Veterinarians (AARV): rehabvets.org

    2) American College of Veterinary Sports Medicine and Rehabilitation (ACVSMR): vsmr.org

c) Advanced certification in veterinary rehabilitation:

    1) American College of Veterinary Sports Medicine and Rehabilitation (ACVSMR): vsmr.org

    2) Academy of Physical Rehabilitation Veterinary Technicians (APRVT): aprvt.com

vaccination status, allergies, pre-existing problems, pre-existing surgeries or injuries and activity level of the patient should be noted. The history of the presenting problem should be thoroughly documented. An important part of the history is the patient's diet. Animals in rehabilitation have an increased need for protein to strengthen and build muscle and heal from injury [4]. The therapist should be able to evaluate the suitability of the patient's diet with consideration for rehabilitation, weight loss if appropriate, and determine the optimum number of calories required for health and healing.

Physical Examination

A complete physical examination should be performed on all rehabilitation patients. This would include current body weight and Body Condition Score (BCS) as well as vitals and pain score. The ability to assess pain in an individual patient is essential before beginning any form of rehabilitation. Patients with significant pain cannot perform therapeutic exercise as effectively, and rehabilitation becomes unpleasant for the patient, client, and therapist if the exercises make the patient uncomfortable [5]. To avoid this, each patient should be pain scored appropriately. Several validated pain scales exist for scoring both acute and chronic pain (See Chapter 18). The rehabilitation team should select one acute and one chronic pain scale and use these appropriately with each patient. Both pharmacologic and non-pharmacologic therapies may be instituted for pain control throughout rehabilitation [6]. For more information on animal pain consult www.ivapm.org.

TCVM Examination

Many integrative practitioners are trained in Traditional Chinese Veterinary Medicine (TCVM). TCVM emphasizes individualized treatment by using a unique theory and terminology to diagnose and treat a wide range of health problems in animals. Two concepts that are unique and fundamental to TCVM are *Qi* (usually translated as "vital energy") and Yin and Yang [7]. *Qi* flows through the body to maintain proper functioning of body systems towards health and wellbeing. Yin and Yang are the harmony of all the opposite and complementary forces that make up *all* aspects and phenomena of *life*, and when they are in balance, the body is in harmonious and healthy state. Disharmony or imbalance of *Qi* and/or Yin and Yang cause disease and illness. Additionally, the Wu Xing or Five Elements is another unique theory that is central to the practice of TCVM. It describes stages of the constantly moving cycle between Yin and Yang in nature and is used to explain the body's physiology [7]. The Five Elements include Wood, Fire, Earth, Metal and Water. Each Element is associated with a number of characteristics, such as certain body organs, a color, a taste, an emotion, a constitution, and a season of the year (Table 13.2) [7]. Prior to treatment, a TCVM practitioner will complete a detailed assessment based on the four diagnostic methods to evaluate the patient's condition, including observing (tongue, mental attitude, appearance and color of feces and urine), hearing/smelling (vocal, odor of body, feces, and urine), asking (history, diet, and environmental interaction), and touching/palpating (pulse, integument, nails, muscle, meridians, and acupoints) [7]. The practitioner will then determine a TCVM pattern diagnosis based on examination findings, followed by formulation of an individualized treatment plan that may include acupuncture, herbal therapy, food therapy, and Tui-na (Chinese Medical Massage).

Posture Examination

Abnormalities in posture may give you clues to both neurological and orthopedic problems.

Table 13.2   Characteristics of the Five Elements ([7]. Xie, H and Preast V 2013 / Jing Tang).

	Wood	Fire	Earth	Metal	Water
Season	Spring	Summer	Late Summer	Fall	Winter
Organs	Liver (LIV)	Heart (HT)	Spleen (SP)	Lung (LU)	Kidney (KID)
	Gallbladder (GB)	Pericardium (PC)	Stomach (ST)	Large Intestine (LI)	Bladder (BL)
		Small Intestine (SI)			
		Triple Heater (TH)			
Constitution	Competitive, confident, dominant, aggressive	Lively, playful, affectionate, sensitive	Friendly, relaxed, laid back, slow response to a stimulus	Aloof, quiet, independent, obey the rules	Careful, timid, fearful, self-contained

Table 13.3   Common postural abnormalities (Adapted from [8]. Duerr, Felix, 2013).

Clinical Abnormality	Orthopedic Condition	Neurological Condition
Dropped hock	Calcaneal Tendon (Achilles) Injury	Diabetic Neuropathy in cats
	Gastrocnemius muscle injury	Peripheral nerve issues
	Lumbosacral Disease	
Fixed Extension of Limb		Myopathies, LMN disease or UMN spasticity
Flexion of limb	Joint or Muscles Disease causing pain eg arthritis, ruptured CCL	Nerve root signature pain
Head tilt		Vestibular disease
Kyphosis	Back/ muscle pain, arthritis	IVDD
Lordosis	Muscle weakness	Spinal disease
Ventral Neck flexion	Muscle weakness	Pain, Hypokalemia in cats, Myasthenia gravis, hyperthyroidism

Table 13.3 lists common postural abnormalities and possible diagnoses.

Gait/Movement /Lameness Examination

All rehabilitation patients should have an assessment of gait and movement and a lameness evaluation to determine which limb or limbs are affected. This gait examination should be performed prior to manipulation. Remember that patients may have orthopedic or neurological lameness [9, 10] Before watching a patient ambulate, assessment of symmetry is critical. Static stance analyzers, pressure walkways or force plates can objectively measure the amount of weight placed on each limb. Slow motion video may also be helpful [9]. Figure 13.1 demonstrates an abnormal posture.

A gait examination should occur on a flat surface with good footing ideally in an area free of distractions. Observing the patient at a walk, trot, while circling and while going over obstacles or up and down stairs can give the examiner

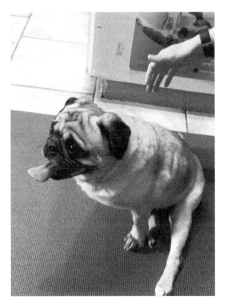

Figure 13.1   A common posture for a dog with T3-L3 Myelopathy.

vital information [9]. Examine the patient from three directions: Walking towards you, walking away from you and from the side. Observe the length of the swing phase, stance phase and the position of the contact point. When an animal is lame, the swing and stance phases are shortened, thereby reducing the length of time spent on the affected limb. In general, the hind foot follows in the track of the fore foot. If the animal abducts or adducts the limb during the gait cycle, this should be noted. Look for alterations in joint range of motion (ROM); a decreased ROM may indicate pain or restriction in the joint whereas an increased ROM may indicate a ligament problem such as Achilles tendon rupture. Ataxia and dragging toes in indicative of neurological lameness [9, 10] See Table 13.4 for more tips on forelimb and hindlimb lameness diagnosis.

Orthopedic Examination

A thorough orthopedic examination involves palpation of all the musculoskeletal structures – palpating all bones, muscles, tendons, ligaments and moving all joints. See Figure 13.2 and Figure 13.3. Evaluation should start in the standing position and the limbs should be palpated simultaneously to determine asymmetry and compare painful reactions. Specific orthopedic tests for common diseases are listed in Table 13.5.

Hind Limb Evaluation

Flex and extend all joints from the toes to the hip. The stifle should be assessed for patellar luxation, medial buttress, pain on extension (early cruciate disease), joint effusion and direct and indirect drawer. Hip extension pain can indicate hip dysplasia, arthritis, iliopsoas injury, or lumbosacral disease or cruciate disease. Some authors believe that dogs who lack pain on hip abduction do not have hip

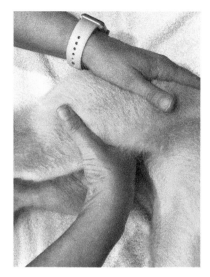

Figure 13.2 Orthopedic exam includes palpation of all joints.

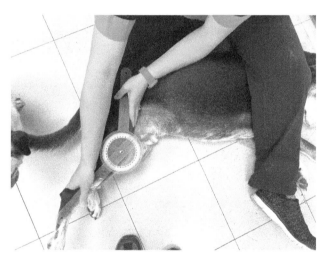

Figure 13.3 Goniometry is used to determine Range of Motion of all joints.

Table 13.4 Clinical diagnosis of hindlimb and forelimb lameness [10]. Lorinson K, et al., 2019 / VBS GmbH.

Hind limb	● Weight is shifted forward by extending the neck and lowering the head.
	● Tail movement may be altered from the normal horizontal to vertical. The tail may be raised when the painful limb contacts the ground.
	● Shortened strike link
	● Hemi pelvis on affected side is more dorsal (hip hike)
	● Pelvis tilted to side in unilateral hip disease and dog uses lateral bending of the spine to reduce hip motion.
	● Bilateral hip disease–pelvis swivels from side to side when viewed from behind
	● If the hind limbs are wider than the fore, then bilateral hind-limb problems should be suspected.
	● Observe patient when sitting to determine if one leg is held extended on sitting (positive sit test for stifle disease or severe coxofemoral arthritis)
Forelimb	● Patient lifts his head when affected limb contacts the ground and dips head when sound limb contacts the ground
	● If the forelimbs are held wider than the hind, then bilateral forelimb problems may be present.

Table 13.5 Orthopedic tests for common diseases by location (Adapted from [9]. Duerr, F, von Pfeil DJF, 2020).

Location/Problem	Test
Hip/Femur	Ortolani – for juvenile hip dysplasia
	Abduction – for hip pathology
	Pain on hip extension – can be associated with hip pathology, iliopsoas injury, lumbosacral disease, sacroiliac dysfunction, or cruciate disease
	Long bone pain – Panosteitis, OSA
Stifle	Direct and indirect drawer for cruciate disease
	Medial buttress/effusion/pain on extension-cruciate disease
	McMurray Test – medial or lateral meniscus
	Patellar luxation
Tarsus	Flat footed hyperflexion – Full Achille's tendon tear
	Crab clawed stance – this occurs when all of the Achille's tendons are disrupted except the Superficial Digital Flexor
Shoulder/Humerus	Increased abduction angle – Medial shoulder instability
	Shoulder ROM – painful on extension in OCD
	Biceps Tendon – Biceps tendon test
	Humerus pain – panosteitis, OSA
Elbow	Hyperextension – medial compartment pain can be elbow dysplasia
	Campbell's test – collateral ligaments

pathology [9]. Long bone palpation is very important due to the incidence of osteosarcoma.

Front Limb Evaluation

Digital palpation is as for the hind limb. Long bone palpation should be done to assess for primary bone tumors found most commonly on the humerus and distal radius. Medial compartment of the elbow should be palpated for elbow dysplasia. Shoulder abduction angles should be included along with shoulder palpation. NOTE: it is often difficult to separate shoulder from elbow pain so radiographs of both joints should be taken if pain is found in either [11].

Neurological Examination

A neurological examination should be performed on each patient. Figure 13.4 shows common instruments used for a neurological examination. Start with the patient standing and the doctor behind the patient. Perform conscious proprioception tests on all 4 limbs. Palpate entire spine for pain and assess neck using cooking stretches. Do a brief cranial nerve examination particularly checking for Horner's syndrome as this may indicate disc disease or brachial plexus problems. Lie the patient in lateral recumbency and perform withdrawal reflexes, patellar and gastrocnemius reflex tests and crossed extensor test. Extension of the contralateral limb when testing withdrawal is a positive crossed extensor reflex, and indicates an upper motor neuron (UMN) lesion

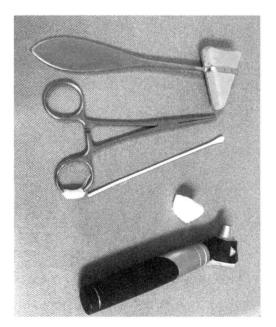

Figure 13.4 Instruments required for a basic neurological examination.

when present. The crossed extensor test is of note because if the test is positive, it is helpful for anatomical localization. A positive crossed extensor test in the hind limbs only is indicative of a T3-L3 lesion whereas positive crossed extensor tests front, and hind indicates a C1-C5 lesion [12].

Rehabilitation Based on Tissue Healing

Stages of Tissue Healing

First and foremost, rehabilitation programs, whether from a conservative or surgical management, must be based on the basic science and stages of tissue healing. The phases of rehabilitation closely match the stages of healing [13, 14]. The therapist must have a thorough understanding of sequence of the various stages of the healing process in order to develop and implement an effective and safe rehabilitation program.

The healing process consists of the inflammatory stage, reparative (fibroblastic) stage, and remodeling (maturation) stage [13, 14]. These processes are continuum and overlap one another with no definitive beginning or end points. Each tissue type (skin, muscle, tendon, ligament, bone, etc.) will follow a predictable sequence and time frame of healing, however the amount of time spent in each stage may vary depending on the type of tissue injury

[13]. Therefore, a rehabilitation program should be individualized and primarily based on recognizing the stages of tissue healing, the type of injured tissue, and the clinical signs of an individual patient. It must also be stressed that inappropriate therapy selected at any stage could possibly inhibit its healing progress or inflict further injury which may further jeopardize the patient's recovery. Table 13.6 shows the healing stages of tissue corresponding the phases of rehabilitation and summarizes interventions.

Phases of Rehabilitation

As mentioned above, the phases of rehabilitation closely follow the stages of tissue healing and should be well understood by the therapist to have a better understanding of the process that each patient must go through before advancing to the next level. Each rehabilitation phase has specific goals to accomplish prior to progressing to the next phase, rather than being based on a time frame of the injury. Table 13.4

Table 13.6 The 3 stages of tissue healing corresponding the 3 phases of rehabilitation and its proposed rehabilitation intervention.

Healing Stage	Rehabilitation Phase	Rehabilitation Goals	Rehabilitation Intervention
Inflammatory stage (Time 0 to 7 days post surgery/injury)	Acute or Inflammatory phase	• Protect healing tissues	• Confinement/immobilization • Pain medication • Manual therapy
		• Relieve pain • Reduce inflammation and edema • Maintain joint ROM	• Cryotherapy, ES[a], PBM[a], PEMF, acupuncture • PROM, assisted standing and walking, weight shifting
Reparative (Proliferative) stage (Up to 6 weeks post injury)	Subacute or Transition/Motion phase	• Promote weight bearing	• Promote tissue strength • Manual therapy
		• Re-education of muscle	• Heat therapy, ES[a], PBM[a], PEMF, TUS[a], acupuncture
		• Regain range of motion • Regain flexibility and strength	• Muscle reeducation, gait patterning, and exercises to improve weight bearing, balancing, and active ROM
Remodeling (Maturation) stage	Chronic or Strength and Function phase	• Restore full ROM and flexibility	• Protect healing tissues • Manual therapy • Exercises to improve muscle and core strength, proprioception, endurance, and functional activities
		• Improve muscle mass and strength • Improve • proprioception • Regain endurance and conditioning • Controlled functional activities	• ES[a], PBM[a], PEMF, TUS[a], ESW[a], acupuncture as needed

Abbreviations: ES, electrical stimulation; PBM, photobiomodulation; PEMF, pulsed electromagnetic field therapy; TUS, therapeutic ultrasound; ESW, extracorporeal shockwave therapy; ROM, range of motion.

[a] Settings are varied depending on injury type, tissue type, and injured tissue region.

Adapted from Kirkby Shaw K et al. 2020 with modifications [13].

shows the characteristics of each rehabilitation phase and its proposed rehabilitation intervention.

Many formal rehabilitation programs start in the reparative phase as this phase emphasizes weight bearing and regaining range of motion, flexibility and strength. This phase starts once the pain and edema are under controlled. At this time, connective tissue is still immature, but it begins to gain tensile strength and can sustain a certain amount of stress or load, which is necessary to regain strength [14]. Weight bearing and joint motion should be encouraged as soon as possible to attain an optimal outcome. It has been shown that joint immobilization or failure to bear weight on a limb can lead to deleterious changes in cartilage, bone, and muscle [13, 14].

Over the next 2 weeks, the patient receiving proper rehabilitation treatment should gradually progresses from non-weight bearing to full weight bearing by approximately 4 weeks. Prior to exercises, manual therapy with soft tissue and joint mobilizations should be performed to improve flexibility and stimulate proprioceptors within the joint. Weight bearing and balancing exercises such as weight shifting on a flat ground or an uneven surface (such as pillow, mattress, or balancing disc), rocker board, side-stepping, circling, and figure-8 can be initiated 2–3 times per day. All joints in the affected limb should be placed through pain-free range of motion exercises such as sit-to-stand, lie-to-stand, high-five, obstacle courses, and Cavaletti rails [5, 15]. In this phase, therapeutic modalities can be progressed from cryotherapy to thermotherapy to promote circulation to the injured tissue. Neuro-muscular electrical stimulation (NMES) can be used to stimulate muscle contraction and for muscle reeducation if the animal is not weight bearing. Photobiomodulation, acupuncture, and pulsed electromagnetic field therapy can be continued to relieve pain and enhance healing. To advance to the next phase, the patient should have consistent full weight bearing at walk and pain-free range of motion [5, 15]. Figure 13.5 shows a dog receiving Photobiomodulation therapy.

The final phase of the rehabilitation process is the strength/function phase. This phase is the longest spanning from months to years depending on the type of injured tissue. For examples, bone is normally expected to regain full strength in approximately 12 weeks, but tendon and ligament are generally less vascular, and may take up to 1 year or longer to resume full strength [13]. Depending on the severity of the injury and the type of job of the animal, this phase may be approached by subdividing into an early phase that focuses on strength and stability, a mid-phase that emphases endurance, and a late phase that targets functional skills and activities. The transition from one phase to the next phase should be gradual to prevent reinjury. For the most part, pain and swelling will dictate the rate of progression. Any exacerbation of pain or swelling during or after a specific exercise or activity indicates that the load is too great for the level of tissue strength. The

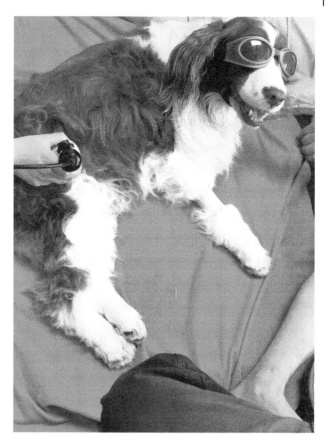

Figure 13.5 A dog receiving Photobiomoduation therapy.

therapist must assess the patient frequently during the early period of this phase and make proper adjustment of the rehabilitation program accordingly based on the patient pain and functional status. It is also important to know that some patients may never achieve preinjury level of function and activity. Therefore, every rehabilitation protocol or program should be individualized to the specific needs of the patient and owner, and it should also follow general tissue healing principles outlined above [13].

Reduced strength, muscle atrophy, and poor proprioception that results from a period of immobility are generally a concern in this rehabilitation phase. Controlled strengthening exercises are the keys to increase muscle mass and strength, such as 3-leg standing, diagonal-leg standing, sit-to-stand, lie-to-stand, incline or decline walking, hydrotherapy, etc. Proprioception training includes balance exercises and Cavaletti rails should also be instituted. If soft tissue flexibility is reduced or joint motion remains restricted, soft tissue and joint mobilization techniques should be considered, respectively. Therapeutic modalities such as photobiomodulation, acupuncture, electrostimulation and pulsed electromagnetic field therapy can be used as needed for chronic pain [16]. Thermotherapy and therapeutic ultrasound prior to exercises help increasing circulation and improving extensibility of soft tissues, thus reducing joint stiffness, and leading to increased

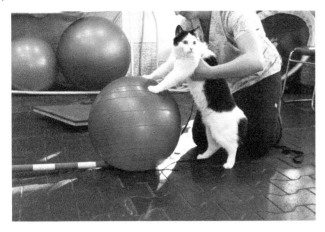

Figure 13.6 Exercise therapy is key to recovery.

ROM [17] Extracorporeal shockwave therapy is beneficial for managing chronic tendinopathy or chronic pain in osteoarthritis [17]. Figure 13.6 shows a dog exercising.

As the patient becomes stronger, the frequency, duration, and intensity of strengthening exercises should be gradually increased, with an increase of emphasis toward endurance and re-conditioning training. The degree of endurance training will differ based on the expected activity level of the patient following therapy. The last step of this phase is to gradually return to normal function and activity, so that the patient can safely perform routine activities, such as playing, chasing, running, and jumping [13].

Summary

Integrative rehabilitation can also be used to improve pain, mobility, and quality of life in geriatric patients or patients with ongoing or progressive medical conditions. Rehabilitation should begin as soon as the patient stabilizes to minimize the deleterious impacts of rest and immobilization. The optimal rehabilitation plan involves a thorough patient assessment to identify musculoskeletal or neurological impairment, discover the TCVM pattern, address pain and then utilizes a combination of rehabilitation therapies (acupuncture, manual therapy, therapeutic exercise, and therapeutic modalities), supplements, herbals, and pharmaceuticals. Lastly, re-assessment at regular time intervals is required to monitor the patient's progress.

References

1 Kramer, A., Hesbach, A.L., and Sprague, S. (2018 April 23). Introduction to canine rehabilitation. In: Zink, C. & Van Dyke, J. B. (eds), *Canine Sports Medicine and Rehabilitation*, 96–119.

2 AARV (American Association of Rehabilitation Veterinarians). What is rehabilitation? http://rehabvets.org/what-is-rehab.lasso (accessed 8 August 2022).

3 Marcellin-Little, D.J., Levine, D., and Millis, D.L. (2021 November 1). Multifactorial rehabilitation planning in companion animals. *Adv Small Anim Care* 2: 1–0.

4 Wakshlag, J.J. (2018 April 23). The role of nutrition in canine performance and rehabilitation. In:Zink, C. & Van Dyke, J. B. (eds) *Canine Sports Medicine and Rehabilitation*, 72–95.

5 Huntingford, J.L. and Bale, J. (2017 September 14). Therapeutic exercises Part 1: land exercises. In: Goldberg, M.E, & Tomlinson, J. E. (eds.), *Physical Rehabilitation for Veterinary Technicians and Nurses*, 286.

6 Frye, C., Carr, B.J., Lenfest, M., and Miller, A. (2022). Canine geriatric rehabilitation: considerations and strategies for assessment, functional scoring, and follow up. *Front Vet Sci* 9.

7 Xie, H. and Preast, V. (2013). *Traditional Chinese Veterinary Medicine: Fundamental Principles*, 2e. Jing Tang Press, 1–43, 249–302.

8 Duerr, F. (2013). The 5 minute orthopedic exam. *North American Veterinary Conference, Proceedings of the NAVC Conference: January 19–23, 2013*, Orlando, FL.

9 Duerr, F. and von Pfeil, D.J.F. (2020). The Orthopedic Examination. Canine lameness Wiley-Blackwell, 31–40.

10 Lorinson, K., Lorinson, D., Millis, D.L. et al. (2019). Examination of the physiotherapy patient. In: Bockstahler, B., Wittek, K., Levine, D., Maieri, J., Millis, D. (eds), *Essential Facts of Physical Medicine, Rehabilitation and Sports Medicine in Companion Animals*, 1e. VBS GmbH, 83–106.

11 Canapp, S.O., Jr. and Kirkby, K. (2013 April 11). Disorders of the canine forelimb: veterinary diagnosis and treatment. In:Zink, C. & Van Dyke, J. B. (eds) *Canine Sports Medicine and Rehabilitation*, 223–249.

12 Drum, M.G. (2010 January 1). Physical rehabilitation of the canine neurologic patient. *Vet Clin Small Anim Pract* 40 (1): 181–193.

13 Kirkby Shaw, K., Alvarez, L., Foster, S.A. et al. (2020 January). Fundamental principles of rehabilitation and musculoskeletal tissue healing. *Vet Surg* 49 (1): 22–32.

14 Henderson, A. and Millis, D. (2014). Tissue Healing: Tendons, Ligaments, Bones, Muscles and Cartilage. In: *Canine Rehabilitation and Physical Therapy*, 2e (ed. D.L. Millis and D.Levine), 79–91. Elsevier.

15 Hanks, J., Levine, D., and Bockstahler, B. (2015 January). Physical agent modalities in physical therapy and rehabilitation of small animals. *Vet Clin North Am Small Anim Pract* 45 (1): 29–44.

16 Saunders, D.G., Walker, J.R., and Levine, D. (2014). Joint mobilization. In: *Canine Rehabilitation and Physical Therapy*, 2e (ed. D.L. Millis and D. Levine), 447–463. Elsevier.

17 Gamble, L.J. (2022 May 11). Physical rehabilitation for small animals. *Vet Clin Small Anim Pract* 52 (4): 997-1019.

14

Common Therapeutic Modalities in Animal Rehabilitation

Part I

Ronald B. Koh* and Janice Huntingford

* Corresponding author

Introduction

The use of therapeutic modalities, also known as electrophysical agents, is widespread in the field of veterinary medicine including physical rehabilitation, sports medicine, integrative medicine, pain medicine, geriatric medicine, and palliative and hospice medicine. They are noninvasive therapies used to complement other therapeutic interventions and together lead to optimal therapeutic outcomes for patients. Therapeutic modalities are essential components of a complete rehabilitation program in veterinary medicine to assist in controlling pain and inflammation, and regaining joint range of motion, flexibility, muscular strength, and balance, thus enhancing a full functional recovery. In general, therapeutic modalities can be categorized as thermal, mechanical, or electromagnetic. Thermal agents include thermotherapy and cryotherapy agents. Mechanical agents include traction, compression, water, and soundwaves. Electromagnetic agents include electromagnetic fields, photobiomodulation, and electrical currents. Some therapeutic agents fall into more than one category. Water and ultrasound, for example, can have mechanical and thermal effects. This chapter with three parts focuses on the therapeutic modalities most commonly used in animal rehabilitation in the United States, including cryotherapy, thermotherapy, photobiomodulation, and electrical therapy. Part I focuses on the discussion of thermal energy modalities. Photobiomodulation and electrical therapy are discussed in Parts II and III respectively. The clinical application of these therapeutic interventions is based on their history of clinical use and research data supporting their efficacy. However, there is still a great need for high-quality, randomized, double-blinded placebo-controlled clinical studies to determine their therapeutic efficacy in veterinary patients.

Cryotherapy

Cryotherapy, the therapeutic use of cold, has clinical applications in rehabilitation. Cryotherapy is applied to the skin but can decrease tissue temperature deep to the area of application in order to control pain, decrease inflammation and edema, and reduce spasticity [1]. Animal models have demonstrated that tissue cooling can have significant beneficial effects on postoperative or post-injury pain, inflammation, and swelling by reducing or delaying infiltration of white blood cells and subsequent inflammatory cytokines within injured tissue [2–4].

The means by which cold or heat is delivered to the target tissue is attributed to the following physical mechanisms: conduction, convection, radiation, conversion, and evaporation [5]. Soft tissues such as adipose tissue, skeletal muscle, bone, and blood have different levels of thermal conductivity, therefore they do not conduct temperature changes in the same way [6]. Adipose tissue acts as insulation to underlying tissues limiting the degree of temperature change in deeper tissues. Blood and muscle contain relatively high-water contents, thus they readily absorb and conduct thermal energy or temperature changes.

Cryotherapy exerts its therapeutic effects by influencing hemodynamic, neuromuscular, and metabolic processes within the body [7].

a) Hemodynamic Effects: Cold applied to the tissue causes vasoconstriction, increased blood viscosity, and decreased capillary permeability resulting in reduction in blood flow [8]. Decreased blood flow impedes the movement of fluid from the capillaries to the interstitial tissue, thereby controlling bleeding, edema, and fluid loss after acute trauma or surgery. Cooling of the tissue also reduces inflammation and edema by decreasing the production

Integrative Veterinary Medicine, First Edition. Edited by Mushtaq A. Memon and Huisheng Xie.
© 2023 John Wiley & Sons, Inc. Published 2023 by John Wiley & Sons, Inc.
Companion Website: www.wiley.com/go/memon/veterinary

and release of vasodilator mediators, such as histamine and prostaglandins, resulting in reduced vasodilation [9].

b) Neuromuscular Effects: The use of cold has a variety of effects on neuromuscular function, including decreasing nerve conduction velocity, elevating the pain threshold, altering muscle force generation, decreasing spasticity, and facilitating muscle contraction [7]. When tissue temperature is decreased, nerve conduction velocity decreases, thus increase the pain threshold and decrease the sensation of pain [10]. Along with decreased blood flow, these physiological changes lead to some therapeutic effects such as a reduction in pain and muscle spasm, and the prevention of edema. When applied appropriately, cryotherapy can temporarily decrease spasticity of muscles by decreasing gamma motor neuron activity and afferent spindle activity because of decreased muscle temperature [11].

c) Metabolic Effects: Cold decreases the rate of metabolic reactions in treated tissues, thereby decreases the rate of reactions related to the acute inflammatory process [12]. The cooling of the tissue also inhibits enzymatic effects related to inflammation, and minimizes the release of histamine, which reduces tissue inflammation and damage [13].

Indications of Cryotherapy

Knowledge of the physiological effects of cold helps to identify the benefits of the use of cryotherapy as an adjunctive treatment intervention in rehabilitation, such as managing edema, pain, and abnormal muscle tone, etc., that are related to mobility and function. The therapeutic effect of cryotherapy is believed to occur when tissue temperature reaches 59 to 66.2°F (15 to 19°C).

a) Inflammation Control: Cryotherapy can be used to control acute inflammation, thereby accelerating recovery from injury or surgery [7]. Application of cold slows the rate of chemical and metabolic reactions that occur during the acute inflammatory phase, as well as directly reduces the heat associated with inflammation by decreasing the temperature of the area to which it is applied.

b) Edema Reduction: The decrease in blood flow associated with vasoconstriction in cryotherapy prevents the accumulation of fluid and metabolites in the injured area, thus reducing edema. Cryotherapy in combination with compression have been reported to be more effective than compression alone for the management of edema [14].

c) Pain Reduction: Cryotherapy is commonly used to decrease pain. The mechanism is likely due to increased pain threshold and decreased pain sensation as a results of decreased nerve conduction velocity by cryotherapy [10].

d) Reduction of Muscle Spasticity: Several studies indicate that spasticity can be reduced by cryotherapy [15]. The reduction of spasticity may be a result of direct cooling of the muscle decreasing activities of gamma motor neurons and afferent spindles [11].

Applications of Cryotherapy

Cryotherapy can be applied in several ways: reusable ice packs, ice cubes wrapped in a towel, ice cups, cold compression devices, cold water-circulating blankets, cold immersion, vapocoolant sprays, or contrast baths. Selection of the type depends on the desired effects, depth of penetration desired, stage of tissue healing, treatment area, and treatment goals. In animal rehabilitation, cold packs are a simple and effective method for cooling tissue in patients. There are commercially available cold packs, as well as cold packs that can easily be made at home or in the clinic. Ice packs can be made using a plastic bag or towel and crushed ice or ice cubes. They may be applied either directly to the skin or can be used with a wet or dry interface. Water has a higher conductivity than air, therefore wet cryotherapy may work better than dry cryotherapy.

Cryotherapy is usually recommended during the acute inflammatory phase of healing (which is typically lasts 48 to 72 hours after injury or surgery) to avoid delaying tissue healing. Following surgery or injury, applying cryotherapy to the incision or surrounding injured area for 10 to 15 minutes every 4 to 12 hours daily for the first three days is recommended. In general, cryotherapy should be applied for no longer than 20 minutes and at least an hour apart between treatments to avoid further tissue damage. Although cryotherapy is a relatively safe intervention, its use is contraindicated in some circumstances, and it should be applied with caution in animals. If the patient's condition is worsening or is not improving after two or three treatments, the treatment approach should be reevaluated and changed. Figure 14.1.1 shows a dog is receiving cryotherapy post radiation to reduce pain and edema in the left shoulder affected by osteosarcoma. Precautions and contraindications of cryotherapy are as follows:

Precautions for the use of cryotherapy:

- Very young and very old patients
- Small animals or extremities
- Poor temperature regulation
- Over the superficial main branch of a nerve
- Over an open wound
- Poor sensation
- Hypertension

Contraindications for the use of cryotherapy:

- Hypothermia
- Cold hypersensitivity (cold-induced urticaria reported in humans)

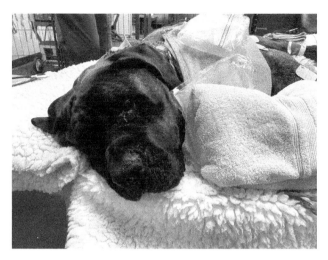

Figure 14.1.1 A dog is receiving cryotherapy post radiation to reduce pain and edema in the left shoulder affected by osteosarcoma.

- Cold intolerance
- Over-regenerating peripheral nerves
- Over an area with circulatory compromise or peripheral
- Vascular disease

Thermotherapy

Thermotherapy or heat therapy is the application of heat sources or thermal agents over skin surface areas for heating superficial and deep soft tissues to increase blood flow, relieve pain, increase tissue elasticity, and promote healing in the injured area. Like cold, heat has therapeutic effects on pain, soft tissue extensibility, and wood healing because of its influence on hemodynamic, neuromuscular, and metabolic processes in the body [7]. Thermotherapy causes vasodilation which increases tissue oxygenation and transport of metabolites, and increases rate of enzymatic and biochemical reactions that may facilitate tissue healing [5]. The use of heat also alters tissue viscoelastic properties which results in increased soft tissue extensibility, decreased stiffness, and improved range of motion [5].

a) Hemodynamic Effects: Heat stimulates the cutaneous thermoreceptors that are connected to the cutaneous blood vessels, causing the release of bradykinin which relaxes the smooth muscle walls resulting in vasodilation [16]. Vasodilation increase the rate of blood flow to the treated area. The increased blood flow reduces edema and accelerates wound healing by improving perfusion of the wound and peri-wound tissue and increasing oxygen tension of the wound [17]. Increasing tissue temperature to therapeutic levels (104°F to 111.2°F; 40°C to 45°C) can facilitate the release of oxygen from the blood's hemoglobin, thus improving tissue nutrition [18].

b) Neuromuscular Effects: Increased tissue temperature with thermotherapy increases nerve conduction velocity and decreases the conduction latency of sensory and motor nerves [19]. Both effects may contribute to the reduced pain perception. Thermotherapy has also been shown to reduce muscle spasm by affecting the nerve firing rate (frequency) [20]. Muscle relaxation occurs because of a decreased firing rate of the gamma efferents, thus lowering the threshold of the muscle spindles and increasing afferent activity. There is also a decrease in firing of the alpha motor neuron to the extrafusal muscle fiber, resulting in muscle relaxation and decrease in muscle tone [18, 21]. Lastly, several studies demonstrate that the application of thermotherapy can increase the pain threshold by activation of the spinal gating mechanism [22]. Heated tissues increase the activity of the cutaneous thermoreceptors which have an immediate inhibitory gating effect on the transmission of the sensation of pain at the spinal cord level.

c) Metabolic Effects: The heating of tissue increases the rate of enzymatic biological reactions when a tissue is heated from 102°F to 109°F (39°C to 43°C), with the reaction rate increasing by approximately 13% for every 1.0°C (1.8°F) increase in temperature [23]. The enzymatic activity rate decreases and the protein constituents of enzymes begin to denature at temperature of 45°C (113°F) [24]. Increased enzymatic activity can lead to increase in metabolic rate and oxygen uptake which may contribute to acceleration of tissue healing in conjunction with the increased rate of blood flow caused by thermotherapy [25]. The use of heat also stimulates fibroblast proliferation [26], accelerates endothelial cell proliferation [27], and improves phagocytic activity of inflammatory cells [28], thus promoting tissue healing after injury.

Indications of Thermotherapy

The main benefits of thermotherapy include pain relief, reduction of edema, decreased of muscle stiffness or spasm, and increased tissue flexibility. In animal rehabilitation, thermotherapy is commonly used as an adjunctive intervention technique to facilitate the accomplishment of the treatment goals.

a) Pain Reduction: Thermotherapy is well recognized for the alleviation or management of pain mainly through via the gate-control mechanism. Heat has also been shown to elevate the pain threshold, and increase nerve conduction velocity [22, 29].

b) Reduction of Muscle Guarding: Muscle guarding (muscle tonus) is a protective response in muscle after intensive exercise, injury, or trauma. However, intensive muscle guarding could lead to muscle spasms, stiffness, pain, and reduced range of motion. Thermotherapy relaxes muscle and improves the efficacy of stretching by reducing muscle tonus (guarding) through the reduction of gamma motor neuron excitability and muscle spindle sensitivity [30].

c) Increased Tissue Extensibility: Shortening of connective tissue is common in aging, injured, or immobilized animals, which may result in decreased range of motion and impaired function. Heat therapy has been shown to increase tissue extensibility and improve flexibility and range of motion in rehabilitation [31]. Heat increases viscoelastic properties of collagen in connective tissues, specifically muscle, tendon, and joint capsule, thus enhancing the efficacy of stretching, reducing muscle spasms, and alleviating pain [32]. Furthermore, the use of heat therapy before stretching reduces muscle irritation and spams to enhance tissue flexibility and range of motion. Stretching is best applied immediately after removal of the heat source.

Applications of Thermotherapy

Thermotherapy can be performed in the form of either superficial or deep (penetrating) heating agents. Common examples of superficial thermotherapy are heat packs, whirlpools, hot tubs and Jacuzzis, and paraffin baths, with heat packs being the most common thermotherapy used in animals. Heat can be induced in the deeper tissues through electrotherapy, including ultrasound, phonophoresis, and diathermy heat, with ultrasound being commonly used in animals. The selection of the appropriate heating agent is based on the size and location of the area to be treated, depth of affected tissue, and treatment goals. Cautions must be taken when using electric heating pads or infrared lamp on animals as they pose a higher risk of burns. Never place electric heating pads under anesthetized, immobilized, or paralyzed animals without close monitoring.

There are also two different types of thermotherapy: dry heat and moist heat. Dry heat includes dry heating packs, hot water bottles, gel packs, and electric heating pads which may work best for local or small areas of pain. Moist heat includes items such as steamed towels, damp heat packs, or hot baths. In general, moist heat is preferred over dry heat as it heat conducts better and penetrates deeper to reach muscles, ligaments, and joints. It is, however, important to remember that superficial heat therapy does not sufficiently raise the temperature of deeper muscle and other tissues. Warm compresses significantly increase tissue temperature of the lumbar region (>2°C or >35.6°F) at 0.5 cm and 1 cm depths but heating was minimal at 1.5 cm depth [5]. Exercise is the best means to increase blood flow to skeletal muscle [33].

Heat therapy should be avoided during the acute inflammatory phase of healing (within 48 to 72 hours after injury) when inflammation, swelling, or bruising is present, and the skin is warm or hot to touch or in an area of recent bleeding. Heat applied too early potentiate swelling, inflammation, and pain. Thermotherapy is better used during the subacute and chronic phases of the healing process known as the proliferative and remodeling phase, respectively. During these phases, the benefits of using heat therapy include relieving pain, increases blood flow, reducing muscle spasms or tightness, increasing flexibility and range of motion, and enhancing tissue healing.

Before treatment, the therapist should test the temperature of the heat therapy agent by placing the item on back of the therapist's neck to check to make sure it is not hot or too warm. A thin towel or other material (e.g., shirt or pillowcase) is commonly placed between the heat source and the skin. Slightly moist towel may increase the conductivity of heat. During treatment, the patient should be repeatedly monitored for its comfort level, and the skin observed for excessive response, such as redness, blistering, signs of burning, and red mottled skin. Risk of burn increases with decrease in the amount of subcutaneous fat because fat serves as an insulator. Thermotherapy generally last from 10 minutes to a maximum of 15 minutes each session. The treatment may be repeated three or four times daily or as needed depending on severity of injury, stage of tissue healing, area of the injured tissue, and desired outcome. Thermotherapy agents typically heat the skin and subcutaneous tissues to a depth of 1 to 2 cm. For deeper tissues (>2 cm depth), therapeutic ultrasound with continuous frequency is recommended. The most desired effects of heat are achieved when the temperature is increased between 2 and 4°C in the tissues. Temperature of tissue that is greater than 45°C (113°F) can be painful and cause irreversible damage.

Precautions and contraindications of cryotherapy are as follows:

Precautions for the use of thermotherapy:

- Very young and very old patients
- Small animals or extremities
- Pregnancy
- Obesity
- Impaired circulation
- Poor thermal regulation
- Cardiac insufficiency
- Over the superficial main branch of a nerve
- Over an open wound
- Poor or impaired sensation
- Hypertension

Contraindications for the use of cryotherapy:

- During acute phase of tissue healing with swelling and inflammation
- Acute bleeding
- Fever or hyperthermia
- Heat hypersensitivity or intolerance
- Over tumor or malignancy
- Over-regenerating peripheral nerves
- Over an area with circulatory compromise or peripheral
- Vascular diseases

Conclusion

Thermal energy modalities are commonly used in animal rehabilitation. They are applied to connective, muscle, and soft tissues to cause either a tissue temperature to decrease or increase in order to achieve a therapeutic effect. Cryotherapy reduces blood flow, decreases nerve conduction velocity, increases pain threshold, inhibit muscle spasticity, and decreases enzymatic activity rate. These effects of cryotherapy are used clinically to control or reduce inflammation, pain, edema, and muscle spasm. Thermotherapy, on the contrary, increases blood flow, increases nerve conduction velocity, reduces muscle guarding, increases extensibility, and increases the enzymatic activity rate. These effects of thermotherapy are used clinically to control pain, relax muscles, increase soft tissue flexibility and stretching, and accelerate healing. Subcutaneous fat acts as a major thermal barrier between the skin and deeper soft tissues, adjustment of treatment duration is required with overweight and obese patients. There remains an ongoing need for more sufficiently powered high-quality randomized control trials on the effects of cold and heat therapy.

References

1 Malanga, G.A., Yan, N., and Stark, J. (2015 January). Mechanisms and efficacy of heat and cold therapies for musculoskeletal injury. *Postgrad Med* 127 (1): 57–65.

2 Kwiecien, S.Y. and McHugh, M.P. (2021 August). The cold truth: the role of cryotherapy in the treatment of injury and recovery from exercise. *Eur J Appl Physiol* 121 (8): 2125–2142.

3 Vieira Ramos, G., Pinheiro, C.M., Messa, S.P. et al. (January 4, 2016). Cryotherapy reduces inflammatory response without altering muscle regeneration process and extracellular matrix remodeling of rat muscle. *Sci Rep* 6: 18525.

4 Takagi, R., Fujita, N., Arakawa, T. et al. (2011 February). Influence of icing on muscle regeneration after crush injury to skeletal muscles in rats. *J Appl Physiol (1985)* 110 (2): 382–388.

5 Dragone, L., Heinrichs, K., Levine, D. et al. (2014). Superficial thermal modalities. In: *Canine Rehabilitation and Physical Therapy*, 2e (ed. D.L. Millis and D. Levine), 312–327. Elsevier.

6 Lowdon, B.J. and Moore, R.J. (1975 October). Determinants and nature of intramuscular temperature changes during cold therapy. *Am J Phys Med* 54 (5): 223–233.

7 Cameron, M.H. (2013). *Physical Agents in Rehabilitation: From Research to Practice*, 4e. St. Louis, MO: Elsevier/Saunders, 129–163.

8 Yarnitsky, D. and Ochoa, J.L. (1991 August). Warm and cold specific somatosensory systems. Psychophysical thresholds, reaction times and peripheral conduction velocities. *Brain* 114 (Pt 4): 1819–1826.

9 Wolf, S.L. (1971 February). Contralateral upper extremity cooling from a specific cold stimulus. *Phys Ther* 51 (2): 158–165.

10 Lee, J.M., Warren, M.P., and Mason, S.M. (1978 January). Effects of ice on nerve conduction velocity. *Physiotherapy* 64 (1): 2–6.

11 Wolf, S.L. and Letbetter, W.D. (1975 June 20). Effect of skin cooling on spontaneous EMG activity in triceps surae of the decerebrate cat. *Brain Res* 91 (1): 151–155.

12 McMaster, W.C. (1977 May–June). A literary review on ice therapy in injuries. *Am J Sports Med* 5 (3): 124–126.

13 Olson, J.E. and Stravino, V.D. (1972 August). A review of cryotherapy. *Phys Ther* 52 (8): 840–853.

14 Rexing, J., Dunning, D., Siegel, A.M. et al. (2010 Janaury). Effects of cold compression, bandaging, and microcurrent electrical therapy after cranial cruciate ligament repair in dogs. *Vet Surg* 39 (1): 54–58.

15 Bleakley, C., McDonough, S., and MacAuley, D. (2004 January–February). The use of ice in the treatment of acute soft-tissue injury: a systematic review of randomized controlled trials. *Am J Sports Med* 32 (1): 251–261.

16 Bickford, R.H. and Duff, R.S. (1953 November). Influence of ultrasonic irradiation on temperature and blood flow in human skeletal muscle. *Circ Res* 1 (6): 534–538.

17 Rabkin, J.M. and Hunt, T.K. (1987 February). Local heat increases blood flow and oxygen tension in wounds. *Arch Surg* 122 (2): 221–225.

18 Lehmann, J.F. and de Lateur, B.J. (1990). Therapeutic heat. In: *Therapeutic Heat and Cold*, 4e (ed. J.F. Lehman). Baltimore: Williams and Wilkins.

19 Currier, D.P. and Kramer, J.F. (1982). Sensory nerve conduction: heating effects of ultrasound and infrared radiation. *Physiother Canada* 34: 241–246.

20 Fountain, F.P., Gersten, J.W., and Senger, O. (1960 July). Decrease in muscle spasm produced by ultrasound, hot packs, and infrared radiation. *Arch Phys Med Rehabil* 41: 293–298.

21 Prentice, W.E., Jr. (January 1, 1982). An electromyographic analysis of the effectiveness of heat or cold and stretching

for inducing relaxation in injured muscle. *J Orthop Sports Phys Ther* 3 (3): 133–140.

22 Benson, T.B. and Copp, E.P. (1974 May). The effects of therapeutic forms of heat and ice on the pain threshold of the normal shoulder. *Rheumatol Rehabil* 13 (2): 101–104.

23 Hocutt, J.E., Jr, Jaffe, R., Rylander, C.R., and Beebe, J.K. (1982 September–October). Cryotherapy in ankle sprains. *Am J Sports Med* 10 (5): 316–319.

24 Miller, M.W. and Ziskin, M.C. (1989). Biological consequences of hyperthermia. *Ultrasound Med Biol* 15 (8): 707–722.

25 Barcroft, J. and King, W.O. (December 23, 1909). The effect of temperature on the dissociation curve of blood. *J Physiol* 39 (5): 374–384.

26 Xia, Z., Sato, A., Hughes, M.A., and Cherry, G.W. (2001). Stimulation of fibroblast growth in vitro by intermittent radiant warming. *Wound Repair Regen* 8 (2): 138–144.

27 Hughes, M.A., Tang, C., and Cherry, G.W. (2003). Effect of intermittent radiant warming on proliferation of human dermal endothelial cells in vitro. *J Wound Care* 12 (4): 135–137.

28 Price, P., Bale, S., Crook, H., and Harding, K.G. (2000). The effect of radiant heat dressing on pressure ulcers. *J Wound Care* 9 (4): 201–205.

29 Coseutino, A.B. et al. (1983). Ultrasound effects on electroneuromyographic measure in sensory fibers in the median nerve. *Phys Ther* 63: 1789.

30 Fischer, E. and Solomon, S. (1965). Physiological responses to heat and cold. In: *Therapeutic Heat and Cold*, 2e (ed. S. Licht), 126–169. Baltimore, MD: Waverly Press.

31 Lehmann, J.F., Masock, A.J., Warren, C.G., and Koblanski, J.N. (1970 August). Effect of therapeutic temperatures on tendon extensibility. *Arch Phys Med Rehabil* 51 (8): 481–487.

32 Lentell, G., Hetherington, T., Eagan, J., and Morgan, M. (1992). The use of thermal agents to influence the effectiveness of a low-load prolonged stretch. *J Orthop Sports Phys Ther* 16 (5): 200–207.

33 Heinrichs, K. (2014). Superficial thermal modalities. In: *Canine Rehabilitation and Physical Therapy*, 2e (ed. D.L. Millis and D. Levine), 321–327. Elsevier.

Part II

Ronald B. Koh and Janice Huntingford*

Corresponding author

Photobiomodulation

Photobiomodulation (PBM), photobiomodulation therapy (PBMT), uses non-ionizing light sources in the visible and infrared spectrum (such as lasers, LEDs, and broadband light), is a rapidly growing treatment modality used for a variety of medical conditions in companion animals. PBMT is painless, noninvasive, and easily administered in a primary care setting to accelerate healing in a number of tissues, provides analgesia, and decreases inflammation through modulation of immune and inflammation responses [1]. PBMT has been used in human and veterinary medicine to improve wound healing, treat snake bites, decrease pain and inflammation resulting from musculoskeletal conditions, improve neurologic function after trauma or injury, treat stomatitis and other oral inflammation conditions, treat intraoperative and postoperative inflammation, and enhance healing of sport-related injuries [2].

Since its development, PBMT has been referred to by many names; terms such as cold laser, low-level laser therapy, phototherapy, and low-level light therapy appear in the literature. According to the American Society for Laser Medicine and Surgery (ASLMS), photobiomodulation (PBM) and PBMT are accurate and specific terms for its effective and important therapeutic application of light. Hence, the term photobiomodulation therapy was added to the Medical Subject Headings (MeSH) database in 2015, and it is defined as "a form of light therapy that utilizes nonionizing forms of light sources, including lasers, light-emitting diodes (LEDs), and broadband light, in the visible and infrared spectrum."[3]

Mode of Actions of Photobiomodulation

Evidence suggests that PBMT has a wide range of effects at cellular and subcellular levels, including increasing reactive oxygen species (ROS), adenosine triphosphate (ATP), and nitric oxide (NO) [4, 5]. Increased ROS activates the endogenous antioxidant enzyme systems; increased ATP supplies cells with energy for reparation; increased NO promotes angiogenesis, modulates the inflammatory and immune responses, and mediates vasodilation [5]. To produce such effects, the light energy or photons must be absorbed by a target cell, specifically intracellular chromophores within the mitochondria, to promote a cascade of biochemical events that affect tissue function. The primary chromophores are *cytochrome c oxidase in mitochondria*. Cytochrome c *oxidase* absorbs light energy or photons in the spectrum of 500 to 1000 nm (the therapeutic window of PBMT), and breaks the bond with NO, which allows bonding with oxygen and production of cytochrome c oxidase at an optimal rate [5, 6]. Cytochrome c oxidase is responsible for the production of ATP. Additional electrons are accepted by oxygen to produce ROS [7].

The overall clinical effects of PBMT can be summarized as follows:

1) <u>Promote Adenosine Triphosphate Production</u>: The primary function of mitochondria is to generate ATP as the energy source for all other cellular functions. Laser light energy ranges from 500 to 1000 nm have been shown to improve mitochondrial function and increase their production of ATP by up to 70% [4, 5, 8]. Increased ATP production by PBMT is thought to be the primary

contributor to many of the clinical benefits of PBMT, particularly enhancement of tissue healing.

2) Promote Collagen Production: PBMT, particularly red laser light (632.8 nm), enhances tissue healing by promoting a more than threefold collagen synthesis through the stimulation of mRNA production that codes for procollagen [9, 10]. In addition, PBMT improves tissue healing process by upregulating fibroblast populations and enhancing collagen organization for soft tissue and bone regeneration [11, 12], likely due to the result of PBM-induced osteogenesis and angiogenesis [13].

3) Modulate Inflammation: PBMT with light energy ranges from 500 to 1000 nm can modulate inflammation and is associated with decreased levels of prostaglandin-F_2 (PGE_2) and tumor necrosis factor-alpha (TNF-a), and increased levels of interleukin-1a (IL-1a), and interleukin-8 (IL-8) [14–17]. PBMT has also been shown to reduce cyclooxygenase 2 (COX2), bradykinin production, and neutrophils in joint fluid to relieve joint pain and hence increase joint mobility and function [14].

4) Promote Vasodilation: PBMT such as red light (632.8 nm) can induce vasodilation, particularly of the microcirculation, mediated by the release of nitric oxide [18, 19]. Vasodilation could accelerate tissue healing by increasing oxygen and nutrient deliveries from the irradiated area.

5) Alter Nerve Conduction Velocity and Regeneration: Some studies have shown PBMT increases peripheral nerve conduction velocities, decreases distal sensory latencies, accelerates nerve regeneration, and reduces nerve scarring in response to laser stimulation [20–25]. In addition, laser irradiation has been found to induce axonal sprouting and outgrowth in cultured nerves and in in-vitro brain cortex [26, 27]. In a prospective study in dogs with T3–L3 myelopathy, dogs that received low level laser therapy (LLLT) regained ambulation within 3–5 days, whereas those in the control group required a median of two weeks to regain ambulation [28]. The functional improvement likely due to axonal remyelination and blood vessels migrating into injured spinal cord followed LLLT [29].

6) Inhibit Bacterial Growth: PBMT red laser light (632.8 or 670 nm) has shown to inhibit bacterial growth on photosensitized *Staphylococcus aureus (S. aureus)* and *Pseudomonas aeruginosa (P. aeruginosa)* [30]. Red laser light with 630 nm was also found to be more effective than 660, 810, or 905 nm laser light in inhibiting the growth of *P. aeruginosa*, *S. aureus*, and *Escherichia coli* [31]. Shorter-wavelength blue light (405 nm or 405 nm combined with 470 nm) had a dose-dependent bactericidal effect on *S. aureus* and *P. aeruginosa*, reducing bacterial colonies by approximately 62% to 95% [32, 33]. Based on overall results of research on the effects of laser light on bacterial growth, wavelengths of 405 to 670 nm (visible red to blue) are most effective in inhibiting bacterial growth.

Classifications of Photobiomodulation

Lasers are classified into four major hazard classes (1, 2, 3a/b, and 4) based on the power outputs [34]. Class 1, 2, and 3a lasers have single-diode power outputs of less than 5 milliwatt (mW) and are not used for therapeutic purposes. Class 3b lasers have power outputs ranging between 5 and 500 mW and Class 4 lasers, which have power outputs greater than 500 mW are used for therapeutic purposes [34]. These lasers pose eye hazards. The class IV lasers are high powered lasers that include surgical lasers. This class of laser devices has various surgical applications, most notably making precise surgical incisions with less scarring and damage to surrounding tissue. The type of lasers used in rehabilitation should not be confused with high powered lasers used in surgical applications. Table 14.2.1 describes laser classifications [34]. Figure 14.2.1 shows example of common Class 4 laser units used veterinary medicine.

Parameters of Photobiomodulation

For PBMT to be effective, the irradiation parameters, including the wavelength and energy delivered, power density, pulse structure, delivery to the appropriate anatomical location, and appropriate treatment frequency, need to be within the biostimulatory dose windows [34–37]. When used with appropriate parameters, the light energy can penetrate tissues sufficiently to activate cellular processes. Fundamental PBMT parameters and definitions are summarized in Table 14.2.2 [38, 39]. It includes the three most important parameters that are discussed here.

1) Wavelength: A PBMT will emit light in the 620- to 1200-nm range, often called the therapeutic window [34].

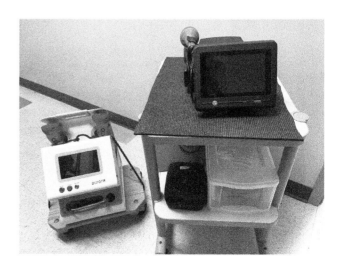

Figure 14.2.1 Aurora laser therapy system (left) and Companion CTX therapy laser are Class 4 laser units that are commonly used in veterinary medicine.

Table 14.2.1   Laser classifications.

Class	Description
1	• Not hazardous to the eyes and requires no eye protection. • Examples: laser printers and CD players.
2	• Limited to 1 mW of power. • No protective eyewear is needed, but extended viewing is not recommended. • Examples: point-of-sale scanners.
3a (also known as 3r)	• Have output of up to 5 mW. • Only an optical hazard if focused or viewed for an extended period of time. • Examples: laser pointers.
3b	• Have output greater than 500 mW. • Can burn skin or cause permanent eye damage. • Protective eyewear must be worn when operating these devices. • Examples: therapeutic class 3b lasers.
4	• Have output greater than 500 mW. • Can burn skin or cause permanent eye damage. • Protective eyewear must be worn when operating these devices. • May represent a fire risk. • Examples: therapeutic class 4 lasers (up to 25W).

Adapted from Riegel, R. J., & Godbold, J. C. 2017.

Table 14.2.2   Fundamental PBMT parameters and definitions.

Term	Definition
Coherent	Photons travel in the same phase in time and space
Collimated	Light divergence is minimized over a distance
Duty cycle	Percentage of total emission time to total treatment time in a pulsed laser
Fluence, J/cm2	Energy absorbed per area treated
Frequency, Hz	Number of waveforms in a defined time interval
Irradiance. W/cm2	Power intensity
Joule	Energy unit used to measure dose or rate of energy delivery
Monochromatic	Light of 1 wavelength
Spot size	Radius of the laser beam
Watt	Unit of power measured as 1 J/second
Wavelength, nm	Distance between crests of electromagnetic waves

Hz = hertz; J = joule; nm = nanometer; PBMT = photobiomodulation therapy; W = watt.
Adapted from Hochman, L. 2018.

Wavelengths that minimize scattering and reflection as well as absorption by unwanted chromophores will provide optimal penetration into the tissue and ensure a better therapeutic result [2]. Melanin, hemoglobin, and oxyhemoglobin chromophores absorb shorter wavelengths (600 to 800 nm), making these wavelengths better for superficial areas. Wavelengths above 1000 nm are primarily absorbed by water, making tissue penetration difficult. Surgical lasers, such as the CO_2 laser, produce wavelengths around 10,600 nm, which are strongly absorbed by water and therefore can be used for surgical applications [2, 14]. Wavelengths of 800 to 1000 nm can achieve appropriate depth of penetration to treat most musculoskeletal conditions [14].

2) <u>Dosage</u>: Dosage applied to the tissue is another important consideration regarding PBMT. Dosage is expressed as the amount of energy (joules [J]) delivered to a certain surface area (cm^2). The size of the patient, body type, coat length and color, skin color, and depth of the condition to be treated must be taken into consideration when calculating the correct dose [2, 14, 38]. In general, the larger the patient, the larger the dose required for a therapeutic effect. Many of the newer PBMT units have preset protocols for treating various conditions. The operator inputs parameters such as size, coat length and color, and area and condition treated, and the unit uses this input to calculate the fluence required.

At this time, optimal treatment doses have yet to be identified. The World Association of Laser Therapy (WALT) recommends a dose of $4–6 J/cm^2$ [40]. In general, dose ranging from 1 to $5 J/cm^2$ is probably optimal for wound healing or superficial lesions, whereas a higher dose ranging from 8 to $10 J/cm^2$ or higher may be an appropriate range for osteoarthritis, deep lesions, pain conditions, and other chronic ailments [2, 41]. It is worth noting that excessive PBMT dosing has been shown to delay wound healing and reduce fibroblast metabolism in certain injury types [42, 43], indicating that a lower-level energy or power densities may be more appropriate in some cases. Examples of proposed treatment doses are as follows:

- Superficial tissue: $1–5 J/cm^2$
- Deep tissue: $8–10 J/cm^2$
- Chronic condition: $10–20 J/cm^2$

3) <u>Power and Duration</u>: Penetration depends on wavelength and tissue type, not laser power (watts [W]) or laser intensity (irradiance) at the tissue surface (W/cm^2) [34]. Using a higher-powered laser delivers more photons to the penetration depth and also determines the time needed to deliver the energy. Lower-powered lasers must be used for a longer time to achieve the same dose. Very low-powered lasers will have no measurable results even when used for long periods of exposure [2, 14].

Applications of Photobiomodulation

In animal rehabilitation, PBMT is commonly used for pain relief, reduction of inflammation and edema, and accelerated tissue regeneration in many species. It is also being clinically applied for various medical conditions. Conditions that may benefit from PBMT include:

- Acute or chronic pain
- Musculoskeletal disorders: osteoarthritis, dysplasia, tendinopathy, myopathy
- Neurological conditions: spinal pain, intervertebral disc disease, degenerative myelopathy, neuropathy
- Soft tissue injuries
- Postoperative wound

Prior to treatment, the patient and the therapist need to wear protective eyewear when operating the laser device. If needed, the patient's eyes can be protected by covering them with a dark cloth or towel. The patient is comfortable and appropriately positioned, providing good access to the area being treated. If that area is a joint, ensure access to all sides of the joint. Treatment techniques will vary according to the condition treated, the tissue treated, and the type of laser used. In general, clipping the area will allow the best penetration of light to the underlying tissues; however, if clipping is not possible then the dosage needs to be adjusted (increased). Be cautious not to overheat the coat or skin if using lasers with higher wattage or wavelengths less than 900 nm.

Treatment technique will also vary with the laser used. Lower-powered lasers (less than 0.5 W) can use a point-to-point method in which a dose is delivered for up to 30 seconds in 1 location before the probe is moved. This method can be more time-consuming, depending on which joint is being treated and whether multiple joints are involved. Higher-powered lasers (1 to 25 W) use a scanning method that delivers the dose over a large area, ensuring that the handpiece is moving during treatment. It is important to remember that the higher the power the more heat it delivers. Thus, caution must be exercised to ensure that the laser does not burn the haircoat or skin of the patient. The therapy can be delivered with a contact or off-contact method, depending on the unit. The contact method allows for tissue compression and can cause deeper penetration. The off-contact method is frequently used over bony prominences or excessively painful areas.

The frequency of treatment can vary greatly, from every 1 to 2 days to once a week, depending on the severity of the lesion. Several PBM therapy sessions (up to 10 sessions) may be necessary over a few weeks to elicit a successful outcome. For acute or chronic painful conditions, it is useful to begin with an induction phase of treatment with more frequent treatments (usually daily or 2 to 3 times weekly treatment for 2 to 3 weeks) until a significant effect is noticed, followed by transition phase with less frequent treatment sessions (such as once a week for 2 to 3 weeks). Finally, the treatment frequency in the maintenance phase varies with the individual patient and treated conditions, ranging from once every 1 to 6 weeks of PBMT. For instance, an old Labrador retriever with severe osteoarthritis in multiple joints may need PBMT once every 1 to 2 weeks for long term pain management. In general, a total of 4 to 6 treatments within 2 to 3 weeks are needed to observe improvement, although 8 to 10 sessions may be needed for patients with chronic condition, multiple joint involvement, or severe disease. Be sure that clients are aware that each patient responds differently to PBMT. Figure 14.2.2 to 14.2.4 shows patients undergoing PBMT for treating different conditions.

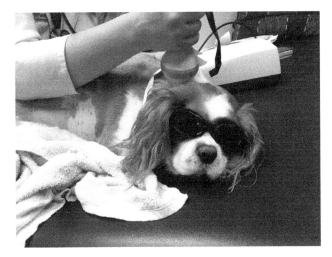

Figure 14.2.2 A Cavalier King Charles Spaniel was receiving PBMT for the treatment of his cervical pain from syringomyelia caused by Chiari-like malformation. Note the protective eyewear and minimal restraint.

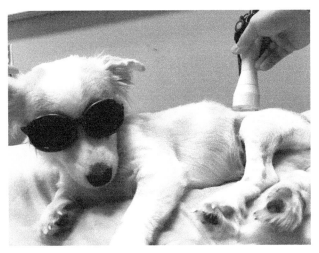

Figure 14.2.4 A dog was receiving PBMT as an adjunct treatment to control pain, reduce edema, and accelerate wound healing post-surgery for his left pelvis and hip fractures.

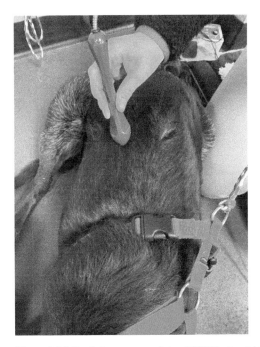

Figure 14.2.3 A dog was receiving PBMT to treat his back pain caused by degenerative intervertebral disc disease.

Precautions and Contraindications of Photobiomodulation

Overall, photobiomodulation therapy is a safe and effective treatment to be used throughout the healing stages of injured tissue aimed at controlling pain, reducing inflammation and edema, and enhancing tissue healing in animals. The only absolute clinical contraindication for PBM therapy is direct or reflected exposure through the pupil on to the retina. The animal's eyes can be protected by covering them with a dark cloth or towel. Another well-known contraindication for PBM therapy is in the presence of known or suspected neoplasia, due to the ability of PBMT to enhance cell proliferation which can contribute to aggression in certain cancer types [41]. Because PBMT increases microcirculation in tissue, treatment of actively hemorrhaging lesion should be avoided. Contraindications and precautions of PBMT are as follows:

Precautions for the use of PBMT:

- Dark skin or haircoat (melanin increases light absorption)
- Active epiphyses
- Hemorrhage
- Bacterial infection
- Hyperpigmentation and tattoos
- Implants

Absolute Contraindications for the use of PBMT

- Eye exposure
- Pregnancy (over the pregnant uterus)
- Tumor/Cancer (over the tumor site)
- Over the thyroid gland
- Pediatric joint epiphysis
- Immuno-suppressed patients
- Photosensitive patients

Conclusion

PBMT has become highly popular both in the veterinary clinic settings and for use at home by pet owners. While future research for determining efficacy and treatment parameters is critically needed in veterinary medicine, there is strong scientific evidence showing that PBMT can induce significant photobiologic effects in the body of humans and lab animals, and that it provides therapeutic effects for the treatment of pain, inflammation, edema, and wound healing. Thus, PBMT is a valuable modality that can be used to treat a variety of diseases and conditions in veterinary patients. For PBMT to be effective, the therapist needs to have clear understanding of irradiation parameters, including the wavelength and energy delivered, power density, pulse structure, delivery to the appropriate anatomical location, and appropriate treatment frequency, as they greatly affect the overall therapy prediction and outcomes.

References

1 Chung, H., Dai, T., Sharma, S.K. et al. (2012). The nuts and bolts of low-level laser (light) therapy. *Ann Biomed Eng* 40 (2): 516–533.

2 Pryor, B. and Millis, D.L. (2015). Therapeutic laser in veterinary medicine. *Vet Clin North Am Small Anim Pract* 45 (1): 45–56.

3 Anders, J.J., Lanzafame, R.J., and Arany, P.R. (2015). Low-level light/laser therapy versus photobiomodulation therapy. *Photomed Laser Surg* 33 (4): 183–184.

4 Lubart, R., Eichler, M., Lavi, R. et al. (2005). Low-energy laser irradiation promotes cellular redox activity. *Photomed Laser Surg* 23: 3–9.

5 Prindeze, N.J., Moffatt, L.T., and Shupp, J.W. (2012). Mechanisms of action for light therapy: a review of molecular interactions. *Exp Biol Med (Maywood, NJ)* 237: 1241–1248.

6 Millis, D.L. and Saunders, D.G. (2014). Laser therapy in canine rehabilitation. In: *Canine Rehabilitation and Physical Therapy*, 2e (ed. D.L. Millis and D. Levine), 359–380. Elsevier.

7 Hawkins, D., Houreld, N., and Abrahamse, H. (2005 November). Low level laser therapy (LLLT) as an effective therapeutic modality for delayed wound healing. *Ann N Y Acad Sci* 1056: 486–493.

8 Silveira, P.C., Streck, E.L., and Pinho, R.A. (March 1, 2007). Evaluation of mitochondrial respiratory chain activity in wound healing by low-level laser therapy. *J Photochem Photobiol B* 86 (3): 279–282.

9 Carney, S.A., Lawrence, J.C., and Ricketts, C.R. (November 28, 1967). The effect of light from a ruby laser on the metabolism of skin in tissue culture. *Biochim Biophys Acta* 148 (2): 525–530.

10 Lam, T.S., Abergel, R.P., Castel, J.C. et al. (1986). Laser stimulation of collagen synthesis in human skin fibroblast cultures. *Laser Life Sci* 1: 61–77.

11 Tam, S.Y., Tam, V.C., Ramkumar, S. et al. (2020). Review on the cellular mechanisms of low-level laser therapy use in oncology. *Frontiers in Oncology* 10: 1255.

12 Khadra, M., Rønold, H.J., Lyngstadaas, S.P. et al. (2004 June). Low-level laser therapy stimulates bone–implant interaction: an experimental study in rabbits. *Clinical Oral Implants Research* 15 (3): 325–332.

13 Bai, J., Li, L., Kou, N. et al. (2021). Low level laser therapy promotes bone regeneration by coupling angiogenesis and osteogenesis. *Stem Cell Research & Therapy* 12 (1): 1–8.

14 Miller, L.A. (2017). Musculoskeletal disorders and osteoarthritis. In: *Laser Therapy in Veterinary Medicine: Photobiomodulation* (ed. R.J. Reigel and J.C. Godbold Jr.), 132–149. Ames, IA: John Wiley and Sons.

15 Bjordal, J.M., Lopes-Martins, R.A., and Iversen, V.V. (2006 January). A randomised, placebo controlled trial of low level laser therapy for activated Achilles tendinitis with microdialysis measurement of peritendinous prostaglandin E2 concentrations. *Br J Sports Med* 40 (1): 76–80; discussion 76–80.

16 Yu, H.S., Chang, K.L., Yu, C.L. et al. (1996 October). Low-energy helium-neon laser irradiation stimulates interleukin-1 alpha and interleukin-8 release from cultured human keratinocytes. *J Invest Dermatol* 107 (4): 593–596.

17 Aimbire, F., Albertini, R., Pacheco, M.T. et al. (2006 February). Low-level laser therapy induces dose-dependent reduction of TNF alpha levels in acute inflammation. *Photomed Laser Surg* 24 (1): 33–37.

18 Schindl, A., Heinze, G., Schindl, M. et al. (2002 September). Systemic effects of low-intensity laser irradiation on skin microcirculation in patients with diabetic microangiopathy. *Microvasc Res* 64 (2): 240–246.

19 Lindgård, A., Hultén, L.M., Svensson, L., and Soussi, B. (2007 March). Irradiation at 634 nm releases nitric oxide from human monocytes. *Lasers Med Sci* 22 (1): 30–36.

20 Anders, J.J., Geuna, S., and Rochkind, S. (2004 March). Phototherapy promotes regeneration and functional recovery of injured peripheral nerve. *Neurol Res* 26 (2): 233–239.

21 Alayat, M.S.M., Basalamah, M.A., Elbarrany, W.G.E.A. et al. (2021 July). Efficacy of multi-wave locked system laser therapy on nerve regeneration after crushing in Wister rats. *J Phys Ther Sci* 33 (7): 549–553.

22 Araujo, T., Andreo, L., Tobelem, D.D.C. et al. (November 9, 2022). Effects of systemic vascular photobiomodulation using LED or laser on sensory-motor recovery following a peripheral nerve injury in Wistar rats. *Photochem Photobiol Sci.* 2022 Nov 9.

23 Reis, C.H.B., Buchaim, D.V., Ortiz, A.C. et al. (August 2, 2022). Application of fibrin associated with photobiomodulation as a promising strategy to improve regeneration in tissue engineering: a systematic review. *Polymers (Basel)* 14 (15): 3150.

24 Muniz, X.C., de Assis, A.C.C., de Oliveira, B.S.A. et al. (2021 October). Efficacy of low-level laser therapy in nerve injury repair-a new era in therapeutic agents and regenerative treatments. *Neurol Sci* 42 (10): 4029–4043.

25 Li, B. and Wang, X. (2022 March). Photobiomodulation enhances facial nerve regeneration via activation of PI3K/Akt signaling pathway-mediated antioxidant response. *Lasers Med Sci* 37 (2): 993–1006.

26 Wollman, Y., Rochkind, S., and Simantov, R. (1996 October). Low power laser irradiation enhances migration and neurite sprouting of cultured rat embryonal brain cells. *Neurol Res* 18 (5): 467–470.

27 Wollman, Y. and Rochkind, S. (1998 July). In vitro cellular processes sprouting in cortex microexplants of adult rat brains induced by low power laser irradiation. *Neurol Res* 20 (5): 470–472.

28 Draper, W.E., Schubert, T.A., Clemmons, R.M. et al. (2012). Low-level laser therapy reduces time to ambulation in dogs after hemilaminectomy: a preliminary study. *J Small Anim Pract* 53: 465–469.

29 Rochkind, S. (2004). The role of laser phototherapy in nerve tissue regeneration and repair: research development with perspective for clinical application. In: *Proceedings of the World Association of Laser Therapy*, 94–95. Sao Paulo, Brazil. Cited in Millis, D.L., Francis, D., and Adamson, C. (2005). Emerging modalities in veterinary rehabilitation. *Vet Clin Small Anim* 35: 1335–1355.

30 DeSimone, N.A., Christiansen, C., and Dore, D. (1999 September). Bactericidal effect of 0.95-mW helium-neon and 5-mW indium-gallium-aluminum-phosphate laser irradiation at exposure times of 30, 60, and 120 seconds on photosensitized Staphylococcus aureus and Pseudomonas aeruginosa in vitro. *Phys Ther* 79 (9): 839–846. Erratum in: Phys Ther 1999 Nov;79(11):1082.

31 Nussbaum, E.L., Lilge, L., and Mazzuli, T. (2002). Effects of 630-, 660-, 810- and 905-nm laser irradiation delivering radiant exposure of 1–50 J/cm^2 on three species of bacteria in vitro. *J Clin Laser Med Surg* 20: 325–333.

32 Guffey, J.S. and Wilborn, J. (2006 December). Effects of combined 405-nm and 880-nm light on Staphylococcus aureus and Pseudomonas aeruginosa in vitro. *Photomed Laser Surg* 24 (6): 680–683.

33 Guffey, J.S. and Wilborn, J. (2006 December). In vitro bactericidal effects of 405-nm and 470-nm blue light. *Photomed Laser Surg* 24 (6): 684–688.

34 Riegel, R.J. and Godbold, J.C., Jr. (2017). Fundamental information. In: *Laser Therapy in Veterinary Medicine: Photobiomodulation* (ed. R.J. Riegel and J.C. Godbold Jr.), 9–18. Ames, IA: John Wiley and Sons.

35 Huang, Y.Y., Chen, A.C., Carroll, J.D., and Hamblin, M.R. (2009). Biphasic dose response in low level light therapy. *Dose.Response* 7: 358–383.

36 Sommer, A.P., Pinheiro, A.L., Mester, A.R. et al. (2001). Biostimulatory windows in low-intensity laser activation: lasers, scanners, and NASA's light-emitting diode array system. *J Clin Laser Med Surg* 19: 29–33.

37 Gavish, L. and Houreld, N.N. (2018 November 10). Therapeutic efficacy of home-use photobiomodulation devices: a systematic literature review. *Photobiomodul Photomed Laser Surg.* 2019 Jan; 37 (1): 4–16.

38 Hochman, L. (2018). Photobiomodulation therapy in veterinary medicine: a review. *Top Companion Anim Med* 33 (3): 83–88.

39 Jenkins, P.A. and Carroll, J.D. (2011). How to report low-level laser therapy (LLLT)/photomedicine dose and beam parameters in clinical and laboratory studies. *Photomed Laser Surg* 29: 785–787.

40 Bjordal, J.M. (2012 February). Low level laser therapy (LLLT) and World Association for Laser Therapy (WALT) dosage recommendations. *Photomed Laser Surg* 30 (2): 61–62.

41 Riegel, R.J. (2018). *Laser Therapy in Veterinary Medicine: Photobiomodulation*. Chichester, West Sussex: John Wiley & Sons Inc, 77–112.

42 Bjordal, J.M., Couppé, C., Chow, R.T. et al. (2003). A systematic review of low level laser therapy with location-specific doses for pain from chronic joint disorders. *Australian Journal of Physiotherapy* 49 (2): 107–116.

43 Alves, A.C., de Paula Vieira, R., Leal-Junior, E.C. et al. (2013). Effect of low-level laser therapy on the expression of inflammatory mediators and on neutrophils and macrophages in acute joint inflammation. *Arthritis Research & Therapy* 15 (5): 1–1.

Part III

Ronald B. Koh* and Janice Huntingford

* Corresponding author

Electrical Stimulation

Electrical stimulation (ES) or electrical therapy is a common therapeutic modality in animal rehabilitation that can be applied to injured tissues or immobilized muscles to decrease pain, reduce spasticity, increase blood flow, improve range of motion and muscle strength, re-educate muscle, prevent muscle atrophy, promote wound healing, and facilitate absorption of anti-inflammatory or analgesic drugs to the injured area (iontophoresis) [1].

An understanding of the clinical use of ES requires an understanding of the types of current parameters of electricity to achieve certain therapeutic effects [2]. The characteristics of electrical currents can be described as parameters. The terminology used to describe these parameters is complex and can be confusing. Followings are descriptions and explanations of commonly available and often adjustable electrical current parameters used for clinical electrical stimulation. Other parameters have been explored but are not in common use, nor are they generally commercially available today. More research is needed to better understand the clinical relevance and application of these additional parameters.

a) Waveform

In general, there are three types of electrical current waveforms: direct current (DC), alternating current (AC), and pulsed current (PC). DC is a continuous one-directional flow of ions. It is most used for iontophoresis and for stimulating contractions in denervated muscle. AC is a continuous two-directional flow of ions, which is commonly used for pain control (e.g., transcutaneous electrical neurostimulation, interferential, premodulated) and for muscle contraction (e.g., neuromuscular electrical stimulation). PC is a flow of ions in direct or alternating current that is briefly interrupted (e.g., Russian current). Like AC, PC is used in many applications, including pain control, tissue healing, and muscle contraction. In clinical use, each current can be manipulated by altering the amplitude, frequency, intensity, and duration of the wave or pulse.

b) Amplitude

The amplitude is the magnitude of the current or voltage and is often also called the "intensity" of the current. Amplitude is controlled by the therapist and can affect how intense the stimulation feels, as well as what types of nerves are activated by the current. The amplitude of ES is usually set "to effect." For instance, when treating pain, the amplitude is slowly increased until the patient feels tingling sensation, but not so high as to be uncomfortable.

c) Frequency

Frequency, commonly known as pulse rate, is referred to the number of pulses delivered to the tissue per second and is measured in Hertz (Hz) or pulses per second (pps). Different frequencies are chosen by the therapist depending on the goal of the treatment. In general, low-frequency stimulation causes the muscle to twitch with each pulse, cycle, or burst. As frequency increases, the stimulation generates a sustained, maximal contraction (tetany). Clinically, frequency affects fatigue of muscle, quality of muscle contraction (twitch of tetanic), and activation of fiber types.

d) Pulse Duration and Phase duration

Pulse duration, measured in microseconds (μsec), is the length of a single pulse of monophasic or biphasic current (how long each pulse lasts). Phase duration refers to the length of time that current is flowing (duration of one phase of the pulse). Clinically, shorter pulse durations (50 to 150 μsec) are usually used for pain control, whereas

Integrative Veterinary Medicine, First Edition. Edited by Mushtaq A. Memon and Huisheng Xie.
© 2023 John Wiley & Sons, Inc. Published 2023 by John Wiley & Sons, Inc.
Companion Website: www.wiley.com/go/memon/veterinary

longer pulse durations (200 to 400 μsec) generate powerful muscle contractions.

e) Duty Cycle

Duty cycle represents the on-and-off time of an electrical stimulation unit, and are measured in seconds (s). "On" time is the period of time the current is delivered to the tissue. "Off" time is the period current flow stops. Duty cycle is usually used only when ES is used to produce muscle contractions. During "on" time, the muscle contracts, and during "off" time, it relaxes (to reduce muscle fatigue).

f) Treatment Duration

Duration of treatment is the total time the patient receiving ES, and the length of treatment depends on the individual tolerable to ES, condition being treated, injured site, and the goal of treatment. When ES is used for pain control with transcutaneous electrical neurostimulation (TENS), the stimulation may be applied for 20 to 40 minutes once or twice daily or as needed. When using neuromuscular electrical stimulation (NMES) for preventing muscle atrophy or muscle re-education, it should only be used for about 10 minutes. Prolonged stimulation of muscle contractions can cause muscle fatigue or delayed-onset muscle soreness.

Adverse Effects of Electrical Stimulation

Adverse effects resulting from the clinical application of ES is uncommon in animals when it is performed by trained therapist or personnel. Common adverse effects include pain, muscle spasm, skin irritation or redness, muscle fatigue, and delayed onset muscle soreness [1]. To minimize the likelihood of any adverse effects, firstly, the therapist should carefully evaluate the patient and review its pertinent medical history and current medical status. During the session, the therapist should increase the current amplitude slowly over a few minutes so that the patient could tolerate the stimulation, and the patient should be monitored throughout the session with electrical therapy. If clients are provided with an ES unit for home use on their pets, they should be clearly instructed on its use and monitor for any potential adverse effect. In patients who could not tolerate all forms of ES, other treatment approaches should be used.

Precautions and Contraindications of

Electrical Stimulation

Electrical stimulation should be used cautiously on patient with pain of unknown origin or cause. It should be used cautiously in areas of poor or absent sensation. Peripheral neuropathies or areas of denervation may not generate muscle contractions at stimulation levels that are comfortable and safe [3]. Electrical stimulation should be used

cautiously in the presence of obesity. Fat is an electrical insulator and greater current amplitude or intensity is often required to achieve the desired physiological effect [3]. However, higher intensity may cause pain to the animal. Electrical currents may exacerbate dermatitis and can spread infections [2]. In the presence of metal, either internal implants or external fixation devices, electrodes should be positioned away from the metal and the pathway of current should not crossing the metal.

The contraindications of include electrical stimulation should not be used over (current flows across) the heart (normal or diseased), pacemaker, neoplasm, infected or hemorrhagic lesion, and active osteomyelitis. Pregnancy should be considered a contraindication even when applied to an area distant from the abdomen. Electrical stimulation should not be used over the carotid sinus or in the presence of fever or systemic infection [2].

Electrical Stimulation Units

There are several different types of electrical units, and each type has its characteristics, parameters, and clinical indications, such as Transcutaneous electrical nerve stimulation (TENS) and interferential current stimulation (IFS) are used for pain control; Neuromuscular electrical stimulation (NMES) is use for muscle contractions or re-educating muscles.

Transcutaneous Electrical Nerve Stimulation

Transcutaneous electrical nerve stimulation (TENS) is the use of electrical stimulators to deliver pulsed or continuous currents to induce analgesia by stimulating (depolarizing) peripheral nerve fibers through the skin (hence the term transcutaneous) using surface electrodes. TENS is noninvasive with minimal side effects and is commonly used as an adjunct therapy in rehabilitation for managing symptomatic acute and chronic pain of nociceptive, neuropathic, and musculoskeletal origin [4]. TENS techniques include conventional TENS (high frequency/low intensity), acupuncture-like TENS (low frequency/high intensity), and intense TENS (high frequency/high intensity). In animal rehabilitation practice, the conventional TENS is most used in animal rehabilitation. It can be administered easily at clinic or by the client at home.

Interferential current stimulation (IFS) or interferential current therapy (IFC) is another common technique of TENS for pain control. IFC is also claimed to reduce inflammation and edema, heal chronic wounds, strengthen weakened muscles, and relieve abdominal organ dysfunction, and assist tissue repair (including bone fractures) [5]. IFS uses paired electrodes of two independent circuits carrying high-frequency (also known as carrier frequency; usually

4,000 Hz) and medium-frequency (also known as beat frequency; can be either low or high frequency as in TENS) alternating currents, hence its name – interferential current [6]. It is believed that IFS permeates the tissues more deeply and effectively, with less unwanted stimulation of cutaneous nerves, thus is more comfortable than TENS [2]. Like TENS, IFS may vary according to the frequency of stimulation, the pulse duration, treatment time, and electrode-placement technique [6]. Evidence suggests that TENS and IFS have similar effects on pain and improvements in functional outcome measures [7].

Mechanisms of TENS

The mechanisms of action for TENS appear to be frequency, not intensity, dependent. There are generally two types of frequencies applied clinically, low frequency (<50 Hz) and high frequency (50–100 Hz) [8]. These can be applied at either a sensory intensity that produces a tingling sensation (for pain control) or at motor intensity that produces an additional motor contraction (for muscle contractions). Varying pulse durations (e.g., 50 μs versus 200 μs) also have no effect on the magnitude of anti-hyperalgesia produced [8].

In general, the analgesic mechanisms of TENS is related to the gate control theory, the endogenous opioid system, and the neuropharmacology [4]. According to the gate control theory of pain, conventional TENS with high-frequency and low-intensity selectively activates large-diameter Aβ fibers (non-noxious afferents), which at dorsal horn level inhibit the incoming nociceptive information transmitted via small-diameter, slow-conducting Aδ and C fibers innervating skin areas [9]. With acupuncture-like TENS (low frequency/high intensity), the current stimulates primarily the A delta (Aδ) fibers, which will activate the opioid mechanisms, and provide pain relief by releasing endogenous opiates in the spinal cord [4]. In additional, the neuropharmacology of TENS is complex with many neurotransmitters and neuromodulators implicated. TENS effects are mediated by many neurochemicals including opioids, serotonin, acetylcholine, noradrenaline, and gamma-aminobutyric acid (GABA) [10]. Low frequency (<50 Hz) but not high frequency (50–100 Hz) TENS has been shown to involve mu opioid and 5-HT2 and 5-HT3 receptors. Contrary, high but not low-frequency TENS has been shown to involve delta opioid receptors and reduce aspartate and glutamate levels in the spinal cord [10].

Applications of TENS

Clinically, it is unlikely that there is a single frequency (low or high) that works best for every patient. Therapist should be encouraged to explore the options where possible and

take a trial-and-error approach on each treatment session to establish the most comfortable pattern, frequency, and duration for pain for their patients. Figure 14.3.1 to 14.3.3 show patients received TENS as a multimodal pain management regimen for different pain conditions. The parameters and settings of TENS that the author commonly use as follows:

a) Frequency (Hz or pulse per second, pps):
   - Acute pain: 50–150 Hz; *the pain relief is short-lasting (a few hours).*
   - Chronic pain: < 50 Hz (typically 20 or 35 Hz); *it provides longer lasting pain relief (from a few hours to days).*
b) Pulse Duration (μsec):
   - Acute or chronic pain: 50–100 μsec (typically 50 μsec); *higher pulse duration (>200 μsec) may cause more pain.*
c) Mode: there are three different mode settings.
   - Normal: constant/continuous current stimulation; *most used for pain relief; nerve adaptation is common likely depreciating effect of TENS.*
   - Modulation: the frequency or pulse rate varies between different settings and uses a cyclical (sweep) to help reduce nerve adaptation; *this mode is most commonly used by the author.*
   - Burst: the pulses will be allowed out in bursts or "trains," usually at a rate of 2–3 bursts per second;

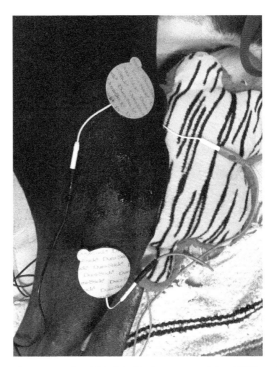

Figure 14.3.1 A Pit Bull Terrier was receiving TENS on his right stifle joint as an adjunct treatment to manage pain following cranial cruciate ligament surgery.

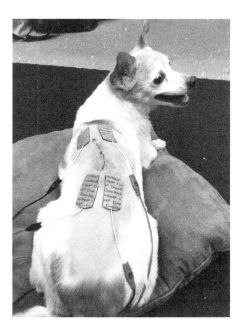

Figure 14.3.2 A Terrier mix was receiving TENS around the incision for managing pain and edema two days after her hemilaminectomy surgery for thoracolumbar intervertebral disc herniation.

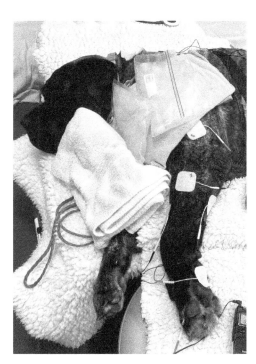

Figure 14.3.3 An English Mastiff was extremely pain in his left shoulder due to osteosarcoma. His left thoracic limb was also swollen. Because TENS is contraindicated over malignancy, it was then applied proximally and distally to the lesion to provide pain relief. Cryotherapy was applied over the lesion to reduce pain and edema. This rehabilitation treatment was performed prior to his radiation.

although it is most useful for chronic pain relief, it is not commonly used on animals because it startles them easily due to its sudden bursts of current.

d) Intensity (Amplitude):
- This is set "to effect." When use for pain control, the amplitude should be high enough for the patient to feel tingling, but not so high as to be uncomfortable. *The author recommends that the operator should try it on themselves to find out the comfort intensity for their patients.*
- It is important to remember that intense stimulation may result in muscle spasm and/or muscle soreness.

e) Duty Cycle:
- This is not important in TENS.

f) Ramp:
- This is not important in TENS.

g) Treatment time:
- Treatment time varies with the conditions. Typical 10 to 30 min for acute pain and 20–45 min for chronic pain on each session, once to twice daily, 2 to 3 times per week or as needed; *prolonged stimulation may result in muscle spasm and/or muscle soreness.*
- It is important to remember that TENS is generally considered as a symptomatic treatment. It may not prevent pain.

h) Placement of electrodes:
- Choose an electrode that is appropriately sized and shaped for the target area – multiple and varied options are available. In general, the larger the electrode, the lower the resistance, thus the more comfortable for the patient. However, larger electrode may stimulate unnecessarily areas.
- The usual practice is to apply the electrodes to where the pain is felt in order to get the maximal benefit.
- Electrodes can be placed over painful areas, trigger points, acupuncture points, peripheral nerves (proximal to the pain), nerve root level/spinal cord segment, and close to the areas of pain ("sandwich" the pain).
- The distance of electrodes placement affects the depth of current penetration:
  - Close placement = superficial current penetration
  - Farther placement = deep current penetration

Neuromuscular Electrical Stimulation

Neuromuscular electrical stimulation (NMES) is a modality designed to elicit a muscle contraction. It utilizes electrodes placed over specific skeletal muscles or motor points with an electric current applied to produce contraction of the muscle in either synchronous or alternating sequence [1]. In animal rehabilitation, NMES has been used for muscle strengthening, prevent or muscle delay atrophy, maintenance of muscle mass, and strength during prolonged periods of immobilization, muscle reeducation, and the control of edema [1]. The type of NMES that is used to retrain and enhance impaired motor functions of spinal cord injury or myelopathy patients is sometimes referred to as functional electrical stimulation (FES).

While voluntary muscle contraction and training remain the best rehabilitation method to enhance muscle and mobility and muscle functions (i.e., strengthening), with patients who are immobilized or unable or perform volitional exercise at adequate intensity and duration to gain benefits, the use of NMES provides therapists with an alternative muscle-strengthening method that mimics muscle contraction trainings. The therapeutic effect of NMES, therefore, helps attenuate the muscle's response to disuse, and accelerate functional recovery [11]. It is successfully used to strengthen skeletal muscles in patients after many types of neurologic injury. In addition, when NMES is used in combination with active exercises, they appear to provide the most optimal functional response, particularly enhance muscle strengthening by improving motor unit activation [11, 12].

Mechanisms of NMES

NMES is thought to strengthen muscles through two mechanisms: overload and specificity [13]. According to the overload principle, the more the load placed on a muscle, the greater force contraction muscle produces, hence the more strength that muscle will gain [14]. This principle applies to contractions produced by physiological exercise or training, which the load can be progressively increased by increasing the resistance, as with weights [15]. NMES utilizes similar principle to electrically stimulate muscle contractions, in which the force is increased primarily by the adjustments of amplitude (intensity), pulse duration, and electrode size [2].

According to the specificity theory, muscle contractions strengthen specific muscle fibers that contract because skeletal muscle contains slow-twitch type I and fast-twitch type II muscle fibers that are distinguished based on specific myosin heavy chain isoforms they express [16]. With voluntary contractions, the slow-twitch type I muscle fibers, are activated before fast-twitch type II muscle fibers [17]. In contrast, with NMES induced contractions, the type II muscle fibers are activated first, and type I muscle fibers are recruited later [18]. Although these type II muscle fibers produce the strongest and quickest contractions, they fatigue rapidly and atrophy rapidly with disuse.

Applications of NMES

NMES for stimulating muscle contractions have proved helpful in a variety of clinical conditions in animals, including strengthening and improving motor control in patients with orthopedic conditions, neurological disorders, and occasionally for other diseases that lead to immobilizations. It is important to remember that NMES should not replace voluntary exercise training whenever

possible if the patient has regained its voluntary motor function and strength. In fact, the combination of both NMES and voluntary exercise produce greater strength gains and optimize functional improvement than either intervention alone [19, 20]. Figures 14.3.4 and 14.3.5 show a tetraplegic patient receiving NMES to maintain muscle mass of his thoracic and pelvic limbs following a ventral slot for cervical intervertebral disk disease. The parameters and settings recommended by the author for NMES are summarized here:

a) Frequency (Hz or pps):
   - It determines the amount of muscle tension; strong muscle contractions are often elicited with frequencies of 35–80 Hz.
     - Low frequency (1–10 Hz): muscle twitch, maybe less comfortable but less fatigue; good for heavily atrophied muscle.
     - Moderate frequency (20–60 Hz): tetanic muscle contraction sufficient for physiological joint movement; good for muscle reeducation and functional tasks training; the author typically starts at 35 Hz; 20 Hz may be more effective on smaller muscles such as the muscles of extremities (carpal extensors and tarsal flexors) and in small size animals.
     - High frequency (>60 Hz): strong tetanic contraction; causes maximal force of contraction and increase risk of muscle fatigue.

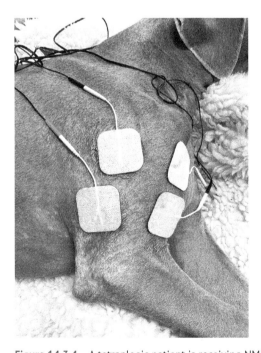

Figure 14.3.4 A tetraplegic patient is receiving NMES to maintain muscle mass of his thoracic limb following a ventral slot for cervical intervertebral disk disease. Note electrodes were placed on muscle belly of triceps brachii and biceps brachii to induce strong muscle contractions.

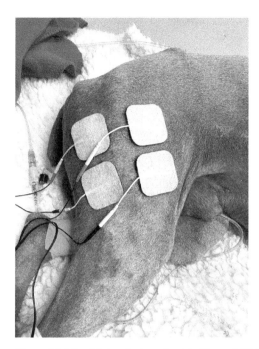

Figure 14.3.5 A tetraplegic patient in Figure 14.3.5 is also receiving NMES to maintain muscle mass of his pelvic limbs following a ventral slot for cervical intervertebral disk disease. Note electrodes were placed on muscle belly of quadriceps brachii and hamstrings to induce strong muscle contractions.

b) Pulse Duration or Pulse Width (μsec):
- When electrical stimulation is used to produce a muscle contraction in an innervated muscle, the pulse duration should be between 100 and 500 μsec to produce contractions while minimizing the likelihood of recruiting many pain fibers; > 600 *μsec causes muscle pain*.
  - Low (50–200 μsec): weak and superficial contraction but will feel less intense; good for smaller muscle groups.
  - Medium (200–350 μsec): stronger contraction recruiting more motor fibers but may begin to overflow in smaller muscles.
  - High (350–500 μsec): powerful, deeper, and more intense contraction; good for larger muscle groups.
- Shorter pulse duration is generally more comfortable to animals. However, as the pulse duration is shortened, higher amplitude current will be needed to achieve the same strength of contraction produced by a longer pulse duration.

c) Duty Cycle (on:off time):
- The ratio of on and off time to total cycle time (expressed in seconds) to allow the muscles to contract and then relax during treatment. The relaxation time is needed to prevent fatigue.
- As a general rule, longer on-time will increase muscle fatigue; weak muscles will require longer off-time.

- When NMES is used for muscle strengthening, the recommended on-time is in the range of 6 to 10 seconds, and the recommended off time is in the range of 30 to 60 seconds, with an initial on:off ratio of 1:5. A patient with severe atrophy or long-term immobilization may require a longer off-time to minimize muscle fatigue and to recover between contractions.
- With subsequent treatments, as the patient gets stronger, the on:off ratio may be decreased to 1:4, or even 1:3 (e.g., 6–10s on: 18–30s off).
- When treatment is intended to relieve a muscle spasm, the on:off ratio is set at 1:1, to produce muscle fatigue and relax the spasm.

d) Ramp up:
- The ramp time allows for a gradual increase and decrease of force rather than a sudden increase when switching from off time to on time, and a sudden decrease when switching from on time to off time.
- When NMES is used for gait training, where muscles should contract and then relax rapidly, a ramp time should not be used.

e) Amplitude (Intensity):
- The strength of contraction produced depends the most on the current amplitude.
- The amplitude should be increased to achieve the best possible contraction within tolerable levels.
- During recovery from injury or surgery, an amplitude that produces contractions of a strength equal to or greater than 10% of the maximal isometric contraction of the uninjured limb is recommended.
- When the goal is to strengthen muscles in paralyzed animals, the amplitude should be high enough to produce a contraction that is at least 50% of the maximal isometric contraction of the uninvolved side.

f) Mode: Most NMES units offer three treatment modes:
- Constant: the current is delivered without breaks; *it is not recommended on any muscle*.
- Simultaneous or co-contraction: the current is delivered according to the on:off settings for both channels concurrently, e.g., when treating bilateral quadriceps concurrently.
- Alternating or Reciprocal: the current delivery is still based on on:off settings but the timing between channels can be adjusted, e.g., when treating quadriceps and hamstrings on the same limb.

g) Treatment Time and Frequency:
- When NMES is used for muscle strengthening, it is generally recommended that treatment allows for 10 to 20 contractions, which usually take about 10 minutes. This treatment session should be repeated multiple times throughout the day.

- When NMES is used for muscle reeducation, treatment time will vary based on the functional activity being addressed, but generally it takes no longer than 20 minutes at a single session – less if a patient shows signs of inattentiveness or fatigue.
- Treatment frequency will vary from 1 to 3 times daily, over a period of 3 to 5 weeks based on the functional activity being addressed.

h) Placement of Electrode:
- Choose an electrode that is appropriately sized and shaped for the target area – multiple and varied options are available. More coverage of the chosen muscle will activate more of the muscle (gaining a better contraction), however too large and the electrical stimulation will outflow into other muscle groups affecting the quality of the muscle action/contraction.
- One electrode should be placed over the motor point of the muscle (usually located over the middle of the muscle belly), and the other electrode should be placed on the muscle to be stimulated so that the two electrodes are aligned parallel to the direction of the muscle fibers, allowing the current to travel parallel to the direction of the muscle fibers. The motor point of the muscle produces the greatest contraction with the least amount of electricity.
- The electrodes should be at least two inches apart to keep them from becoming too close.
- In general, the larger the electrode, the greater the comfort, but too large may stimulate unwanted muscles.

Conclusion

Electrical stimulation is a very useful physical agent for the treatment of pain and the reeducation of muscle in veterinary patients. Any modification of parameters is based on treatment outcome. TENS and IFS modulate pain via electrically stimulation of sensory or motor nerves. There is moderate to strong scientific evidence in human showing that TENS can induce significant pain modulation for pain conditions, including post-surgical, musculoskeletal, and neurological conditions. Currents of IFS encounter a low electrical resistance and can thus penetrate deeply without causing undue discomfort to the patient. NMES is the delivery of electrical current through the skin causing motor nerve depolarization, which in turn evokes muscle contraction. It is commonly used in immobilized or paralyzed patients to prevent muscle atrophy, reeducate muscle, and maintain or regain muscle strength. NMES stimulated contractions preferentially recruit type II muscle fibers, and it is not more effective than voluntary exercise, therefore it cannot be considered as an alternate exercise training method, but as an adjunct to muscle training.

References

1 Levine, D. and Bockstahler, B. (2014). Electrical stimulation. In: *Canine Rehabilitation and Physical Therapy*, 2e (ed. D.L. Millis and D. Levine), 342–358. Elsevier.

2 Sara Shapiro, S. and Ocelnik, M. (2013). Part IV Electrical currents. In: *Physical Agents in Rehabilitation: From Research to Practice*, 4e (ed. M.H. Cameron), 223–282. St. Louis Mo: Elsevier/Saunders.

3 Benton, L. et al. (1981). *Functional Electrical Stimulation: A Practical Guide*, 2e. Downy, CA: Ranchos Los Amigos Rehabilitation Engineering Center.

4 Johnson, M. (2007 August). Transcutaneous electrical nerve stimulation: mechanisms, clinical application and evidence. *Rev Pain* 1 (1): 7–1.

5 Noble, G.J., Lowe, A.S., and Walsh, D.M. (2001). Interferential therapy review part 2: experimental pain models and neurophysiological effects of electrical stimulation. *Physical Therapy Reviews* 6 (1): 17–37.

6 Kitchen, S. (ed.) (2001). *Electrotherapy E-Book: Evidence-based Practice*, 11e. Elsevier Health Sciences.

7 Almeida, C.C., Silva, V.Z.M.D., Júnior, G.C. et al. (2018 September–October). Transcutaneous electrical nerve stimulation and interferential current demonstrate similar effects in relieving acute and chronic pain: a systematic review with meta-analysis. *Braz J Phys Ther* 22 (5): 347–354.

8 Sluka, K. (2007). TENS, mechanisms of action. In: *Encyclopedia of Pain* (ed. R. Schmidt and W. Willis). Berlin, Heidelberg: Springer. doi: 10.1007/978-3-540-29805-2_4409.

9 Melzack, R. and Wall, P.D. (1965 November 19). Pain mechanisms: a new theory. *Science* 150 (3699): 971–979.

10 Sluka, K.A. and Walsh, D. (2003 April). Transcutaneous electrical nerve stimulation: basic science mechanisms and clinical effectiveness. *J Pain* 4 (3): 109–121.

11 Bickel, C.S., Gregory, C.M., and Dean, J.C. (2011 October). Motor unit recruitment during neuromuscular electrical stimulation: a critical appraisal. *Eur J Appl Physiol* 111 (10): 2399–2407.

12 Knutson, J.S., Fu, M.J., Sheffler, L.R., and Chae, J. (2015 November). Neuromuscular electrical stimulation for motor restoration in hemiplegia. *Phys Med Rehabil Clin N Am* 26 (4): 729–745.

13 Delitto, A. and Snyder-Mackler, L. (1990 March). Two theories of muscle strength augmentation using percutaneous electrical stimulation. *Phys Ther* 70 (3): 158–164.

14 Miller, C. and Thépaut-Mathieu, C. (1993 Janaury). Strength training by electrostimulation conditions for efficacy. *Int J Sports Med* 14 (1): 20–28.

15 De Luca, C.J., LeFever, R.S., McCue, M.P., and Xenakis, A.P. (1982 August). Behaviour of human motor units in different muscles during linearly varying contractions. *J Physiol* 329: 113–128.

16 Jostarndt-Fogen, K., Puntschart, A., Hoppeler, H., and Billeter, R. (1998). Fibre-type specific expression of fast and slow essential myosin light chain mRNAs in trained human skeletal muscles. *Acta Physiol Scand* 164: 299–308.

17 Millard, R. (2014). Exercise physiology of the canine athlete. In: *Canine Rehabilitation and Physical Therapy*, 2e (ed. D.L. Millis and D. Levine), 162–179. Elsevier.

18 Hennings, K., Kamavuako, E.N., and Farina, D. (2007 February). The recruitment order of electrically activated motor neurons investigated with a novel collision technique. *Clin Neurophysiol* 118 (2): 283–291.

19 Herrero, A.J., Martín, J., Martín, T. et al. (2010 June). Short-term effect of strength training with and without superimposed electrical stimulation on muscle strength and anaerobic performance. A randomized controlled trial. Part I. *J Strength Cond Res* 24 (6): 1609–1615.

20 Paillard, T. (2008). Combined application of neuromuscular electrical stimulation and voluntary muscular contractions. *Sports Med* 38 (2): 161–177.

15

Modalities Used in Rehabilitation—Land and Aquatic Exercises

*Ronald B. Koh and Janice Huntingford**

* *Corresponding author*

Introduction

Therapeutic exercises are the cornerstone of veterinary rehabilitation. Therapeutic exercises, whether land or aquatic, are a crucial component of any patient's rehabilitation program regardless of problem or diagnosis. The purpose of this chapter is to introduce the integrative practitioner to both land and water exercises that may be applied to post-surgical, post injury, geriatric or athletic patients. Rehabilitation is a holistic specialty as it encompasses pain management, improvement of functional impairments, nutrition and supplements, and improvement in overall health.

Exercise Physiology

Unless the therapist understands how exercise impacts the body, it is impossible to design an appropriate exercise program [1]. Exercise physiology is a complex topic and the reader should be referred to further textbooks of exercise physiology, however a brief outline is included here.

Skeletal muscle performance is dependent on muscle fiber type. Traditionally, muscles are classified as type I (oxidative or slow twitch) or type II (glycolytic or fast twitch) with subclassifications of these two types [2]. However, all muscles consist of a mix of different fiber types, in different ratios depending on the individual muscle and on training. Postural muscles (stabilizer muscles) such as the quadriceps femoris are capable of slow and sustained contraction and contain about 50 % more type I fibers [3] than muscles like the gracilis, which contain more type II and are speed and power (mobilizing) muscles [4]. Type I muscle fibers have been thought of as the endurance muscle fibers and type II as the sprinting muscle fibers. However, when compared to humans, all dogs have a high oxidative capacity in all their muscles and are adapted for endurance activities [5]. Certain breeds, for example Greyhounds, do have more fast twitch muscle fibers than others [6].

When muscles are immobilized, such as in casts or splints, muscle strength decreases rapidly, with as much as 50% of strength lost within the first week [7]. With disuse, postural muscles that contain a predominance of type I fibers, atrophy more than the mobilizing muscles containing type II fibers. In dogs with geriatric sarcopenia, the epaxial muscles atrophy early in the process. One study compared epaxial, quadriceps, and temporalis muscle size in aged dogs to young dogs that were matched in size and body condition. The results showed that epaxial muscles were smaller in aged dogs but quadriceps and temporal muscles did not differ significantly [8]. Fiber type lost, however, appears preferential for the large type II fibers [9, 10]. This is an important consideration in designing an exercise program for an athlete with muscle loss due to injury, versus a geriatric patient with age-related sarcopenia [11].

Muscle contractions can be described as having two variables: force and length. The force is either tension or load. Load is the force exerted on the muscle by an object and muscle tension is the force the muscle exerts on an object. Isometric contractions occur when muscle tension changes with no change in muscle length. This is a static exercise, for example lifting a front leg so that more weight/load is on the muscles of the contralateral front limb and the rear limbs; these limb muscles are undergoing isometric contractions to support more body weight. Tension bands applied to the standing patient rely on the instinct to lean into pressure. As a patient maintains the same body position under an increased load (whether push or pull), the muscle work has increased without a change in muscle length [12].

Isotonic contractions occur when the muscle tension remains the same, but the muscle length changes. Isotonic contractions occur as either concentric or eccentric contraction. Concentric contraction occurs when tensions in the

Integrative Veterinary Medicine, First Edition. Edited by Mushtaq A. Memon and Huisheng Xie.
Companion Website: www.wiley.com/go/memon/veterinary

muscle increase along with shortening. An example of this would be a human weightlifter performing a biceps curl. Eccentric contraction occurs when the muscle contracts but lengthens because the tension generated in the muscle is insufficient to overcome the load pulling down on the muscle. An example of this would be a slowly released biceps curl and with the weightlifter extending the elbow to put down the weight [12]. The eccentric contraction controls the movement – it is the natural braking force that occurs during motion [13]. Eccentric contractions can predispose to injury in untrained individuals [14]. Resistive exercise of all forms leads to the preferential hypertrophy of type II fibers and eccentric contractions render type II fibers more susceptible to damage when compared to type I fibers in humans, rabbits, and rodents [15]. In an exercise program, generally, concentric exercises are performed first to help accustom the muscle to movement. Eccentric exercises are added later as these have the potential to cause damage to the muscle and delayed-onset muscle soreness, but they help develop greater strength. A balanced program between concentric and eccentric muscle contractions is desired.

Designing an Exercise Program

Before designing an exercise program, the practitioner must consider any underlying pathology or pre-existing conditions that may affect muscular performance. As an example, a dog with geriatric onset laryngeal paralysis/polyneuropathy will have some respiratory compromise that should be considered when exercising. The experience of the client or handler and the willingness of the patient to perform exercises must also be considered. An agility dog with an experience handler will have a very different exercise program from that of a geriatric companion dog with an inexperienced owner [12].

Exercise improves physical function and reduces pain [16]. Balance and proprioception exercises are indicated for patients with neurological disease. Post-operative and geriatric patients benefit from strengthening exercises and exercises to increase ROM of affected joints. According to Fry et al. obese patients who combined a restricted calorie diet with an exercise program, lost more weight and had improved fitness [17]. All dogs can benefit from regular controlled exercise.

After evaluating the patient and assessing tissue integrity, it is important to set long- and short-term goals. For success, the client and the therapist should have the same goals for the patient. Regular reassessment throughout therapy can insure that goals are met and changed as the patient progresses through therapy. Goals should be SMART – Specific, Measurable, Achievable, Relevant, and Time-Bound. Care plans can be based on functional progression [16].

According to McCauley and Van Dyke (2018), there are five variable parameters for each therapeutic exercise [18]:

1) Frequency of work done (multiple times per day, daily or weekly)
2) Speed/intensity
3) Duration of work (time or number of reps)
4) Environment (terrain, footing, substrate)
5) Impact (low, high or no impact).

The frequency, intensity, and duration of each exercise is increased as the patient heals and progresses through rehabilitation, however this is based on improvement in functional abilities and tissue healing [19]. Patients should be assessed based on passive and active assessments as outlined in Chapter 13.

Canine Rehabilitation Exercise Equipment

Physioballs/Peanuts/BOSU® Balls

Exercise balls come in many shapes and sizes and have many different uses. Peanut balls look exactly like a peanut shell, with an indent in the middle providing two separate points of ground contact for added stability over an oval ball. A physio roll is like a peanut ball but lacks the middle indent. Egg-shaped balls have less stability, which makes exercises on these more challenging. Round balls are the most challenging as they allow movement in all directions. A BOSU® ball is flat on one side and has a half ball attached, allowing the patient to balance on the half ball side or when flipped over to balance on the flat side. The patient may stand on the ball or stand with front feet on the ball and roll the ball forward or backward depending on which muscle groups are being strengthened. Most ball work will start with an under-inflated peanut for the most stability. As the patient progresses, more air is added for an additional challenge; later, more challenging ball shapes, along with more challenging postures, are used [12, 16]. See Figure 15.1 for another use of a physioball.

Cavaletti Poles

Although these ground poles have been used for exercising horses for many years, in the small animal patient they are used to train gait, improve proprioception, and strengthen front and hind limb flexor muscles. They are also used to improve active ROM – specifically they increase flexion and extension of stifle and flexion of the carpus and elbow along with flexion of the tarsus [16, 20]. Figure 15.2 shows a cat walking over cavaletti poles. Cavalettis are placed in a series and are adjustable in height. They are placed low or on the ground when the patient begins the exercise or has significant muscle weakness. The height can be adjusted as the patient progresses through rehabilitation. Spacing is patient-dependent; it depends roughly on height and body

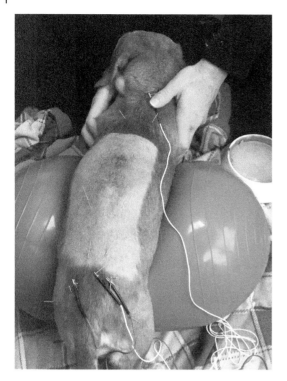

Figure 15.1 A dog receiving acupuncture while strengthening on a physioball.

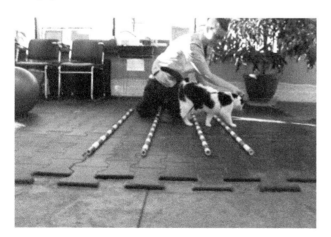

Figure 15.2 A cat walking over cavaletti poles.

length, but most importantly on stride length. Cavalettis are easily made from pylons with holes and PVC pipe. The cones can then be used for weaving exercises [16].

Weave Cones

These poles and cones are used for circling, walking in a figure eight, and weaving (in a serpentine). Weaving in and out of cones creates lateral flexion of the spine, aims to strengthen the adductor and abductor muscles and to improve balance and proprioception. Six to eight cones can be used to make up an obstacle course for the patient to weave in and out of. Alternatively, multiple objects such as bowling pins, water bottles, or a line of trees, for large dogs, can be used if they are

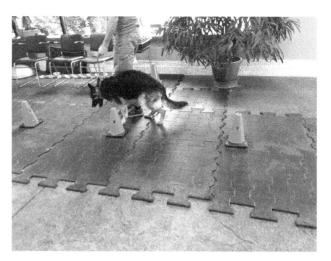

Figure 15.3 A dog weaving through cones during an assessment.

evenly spaced so the dog can weave in and out of the objects. Vertical weave pole agility sets, or safety cones can be used. The distance between the poles needs to be adjusted so that sufficient lateral bending occurs. Weaves are used to help build core strength and improve proprioception [16]. Figure 15.3 shows a dog weaving through cones.

Planks/Blocks/Stairs

All of these exercises improve balance and proprioception and build core strength [12].Planks are 2.5–3.0 m (8–10 feet) long pieces of wood that are either 5 × 20 cm or 5 × 25 cm (2 × 8–10 inches) in length. The dog walks along the planks which are initially placed on the floor. As the dog progresses, he is further challenged by elevating the planks or placing obstacles on the plank.

Blocks are smaller and thicker pieces of wood generally 10 × 15 cm with a grip tape added to create a non-skid surface. The blocks can be made in heights of 5, 10, and 15 cm (2, 4, and 6 inches). The dog stands with one foot on each block or any combination of diagonals or front or back paws. Strengthening of the stabilizer muscles of the trunk is emphasized by this exercise [16].

Stairs can be made of any material and many different types of stairs exist in a home or clinical setting. Climbing stairs is good for proprioceptive training, core muscle strengthening, improved hind-limb weight bearing, and improving ROM of pelvic limb joints (improved extension of hip and hock and improved/increased flexion of stifle and hock) [21]. Descending stairs is also good for balance and proprioception and should increase forelimb weight bearing [16]. Figure 15.4 shows a dog doing stair training.

Uneven Surface Training

Rehabilitation therapists use many different surfaces to improve balance and strength particularly in the stabilizer muscles. Balance discs such as BOSU balls, or textured surface balls are particularly good for neurological rehabilitation. See Figure 15.5. Balance boards can be made be acquired commercially or made by gluing a half tennis ball to a piece of plywood which can be covered in a non-slip surface. For small dogs recovering from back surgery, mini trampolines can be used to helps activate multiple muscles and increase core strength. They can also be used to build core strength in dogs at risk of back problems [12, 16]

Elastic Resistance Bands

Resistance bands are 15 cm (6 in) wide latex bands that are color coded by the thickness of the material providing

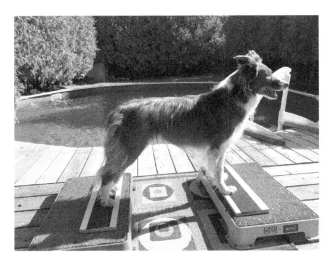

Figure 15.4 A dog doing stair training.

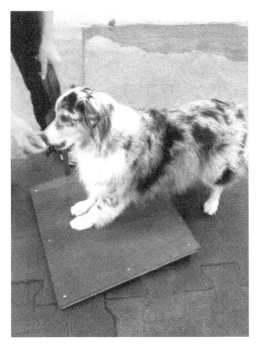

Figure 15.5 A dog doing uneven surface training on a rocker board.

different resistance levels. They can be used in both beginner and advanced therapy as a means of pulling a paralyzed leg forward, mimicking regular gait. They can also be used to increase tension and resistance to facilitate muscle development [12].

Land Treadmills

Land treadmills can be used in dogs and cats to provide a cardiovascular workout, increase limb strength particularly in the pelvic limbs, and to aid in rebalancing gait during ambulation. Laurer et al. reported a 5 % incline increased hamstring activity in dogs walking on a treadmill [22]. It can also be used in neurological patients for gait retraining during recovery from paralysis. See Figure 15.6.

The integrative practitioner needs to evaluate each patient's performance on the treadmill to determine the optimal speed and incline to maintain a normal gait without overexertion. Neurological patients should be started at 0.1–0.5 mph (0.2–0.8 km/h) whereas most medium to large dogs will comfortably walk at a rate of approximately 2 mph (3.2 km/h). Some important things to consider when purchasing a treadmill are belt size, incline/decline capacity, speed variability with a low starting speed, side rails and easy on/off switch or button. Specific dog treadmills can be used or a human treadmill if the belt is a minimum of 6 feet/2 m [23]. See Box 15.1 for treadmill safety.

Dogs that are leash trained can be treadmill trained with the use of treats and positive re-enforcement.

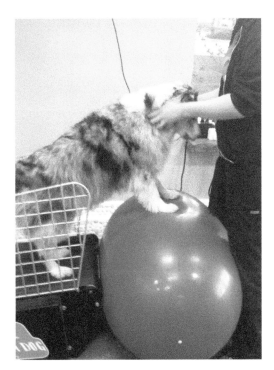

Figure 15.6 A dog strengthening on a land treadmill.

Box 15.1 Treadmill safety [12]. Huntingford JL, Bale J. 2017 / John Wiley & Sons

- Always use a leash and harness with the patient. Collars can be dangerous.
- Never tie the patient to the treadmill or leave the patient unattended. Stand next to the dog throughout the entire workout.
- Do not face the treadmill into a wall – the dog will resist walking "into" the wall.
- Lead the patient onto the treadmill using an incentive such as a treat or toy, and then the treadmill can be slowly turned on.
- If your treadmill does not have safety walls you may need assistance to keep the pet's attention looking and walking forward. Place one side against the wall so the patient does not fall off the side.
- Short intervals are important until the patient gets accustomed to the treadmill. Go slow and let the patient get acclimatized to the routine.
- Always monitor the amount of panting, the pet's gait, body language, and signs of fatigue (excess or rapid panting, glazed eyes, change to gait (wobbling, staggering), and drooping tongue) the entire time.
- Allow rest periods where stretching, massage, and ROM can be performed.
- A water dish can be offered during intermission time as well.
- Remember that each session should be positive and time on the treadmill should be dictated by the patient's condition and response.

Special Considerations during Exercise

There are some special considerations when adding exercise therapy into integrative practice. These considerations have to do with facility, patient, client, and staff. These are summarized in Box 15.2:

Box 15.2 Special Consideration for Exercises [18]. McCauley L, Van Dyke JB. 2018 / John Wiley & Sons

- Good footing and good flooring are paramount to avoid slipping. Ensure nails and paw fur are trimmed.
- Adequate space to perform exercises with as little distraction as possible.
- Use harnesses (rather than collars) for better control of the patients.
- Consider patient's condition and stage of wound healing and tissue strength when progressing exercise.
- The most appropriate exercise depends on specific goals and factors that were identified during the initial evaluation.

- Exercise sessions should always be positive. Treats and/or praises should always be used for rewarding. Exercise sessions should always be like a game rather than treatment session.
- An exercise program should be started slowly, usually begin with 3–5 exercises per session to avoid fatigue, weakness, lameness, and pain.
- The rate of progression of the rehabilitation program is based on the patient's response and outcomes (i.e. limb circumference, joint angles (ROM), pain level, strength level).
- The number, duration, and intensity of exercise should be increased gradually (no more than 20% per week), depending on patient tolerance.
- Recognition of fatigue is very important. Do not overstress the patient.
- It is best for the patient to get exercise (at home) on a regular basis throughout the week, in addition to one or two days at rehab facility.

Therapeutic Exercises

Table 15.1 lists therapeutic exercises by category. This list is not exhaustive, but it should give the practitioner a place to start. Neurological exercises and gait patterning are very important for paralyzed patients to encourage recovery. Pattern training (mimicking walking, running, scratching, or any normal movement) takes advantage of neuroplasticity and is very complementary to acupuncture for neurological stimulation. Feline exercises are included here as well. When dealing with cats, it is important to be patient and tailor exercises to include things the cat likes to do and will do. For more information on specific therapeutic exercises, please consult a good rehabilitation resource or consider further training in rehabilitation.

Aquatic Therapy

Any exercise or therapy performed in water can be considered aquatic therapy. Swimming and underwater treadmill (UWTM) therapy are the two most used forms of aquatic therapy in small animal rehabilitation. One of the major benefits of aquatic therapy is the ability of the patient to exercise without pain. Swim therapy improves cardiorespiratory and muscular endurance, and ROM whereas the UWTM is important for strengthening, improved weight bearing, proprioceptive gait training, improved balance and improved active ROM while decreasing joint stress. Both pool and UWTM therapy take advantage of the properties of water that make it an ideal therapeutic environment [25]. See Table 15.2.

Table 15.1 Therapeutic exercises by category [24].

Goal	Exercises
Encourage Weight-bearing	• Standing/walking exercises (harness, slings, carts, water) • Weight shifting and various other weight shifting activities • Cookie stretching • Cavaletti course • Three-leg standing – pick up opposite leg • Foreign object on opposite foot or leg (syringe cap, therapy band, scrunchies) • Therapy ball activity – front or rear limbs on ball
Improve joint ROM	• Incline and decline walking • Stair climbing • Sit-to-stand exercises • Cavaletti rails • Underwater treadmill activities • Swimming • Tunnel and limbo walking
Improve balance and proprioception	• Assisted standing or walking (slings, carts, water) • Balance board/disc activity • Cookie stretching • Circling, figure-of-eight walking • Wobble board • Therapy ball activity (FL/HL on ball or entire body stand on ball) • Cavaletti rails • Three-leg standing – pick up opposite or diagonal leg • Stand or walk on uneven surfaces (carpet, grass, sand, foam, mattresses, trampoline) • Step-ups (may begin at low and work up to 6" or more) • Side stepping • Incline ramp • Climbing stairs • Zigzag walking on a hill
Muscle strengthening	• Sit-to-stand – HL strengthening • Sit-to-down – FL strengthening • Three- or two-leg standing • Cavaletti rails • Weave poles • Figure-of-eights • Circles • Declines (ramps, hills, stairs, steps) – FL strengthening • Inclines (ramps, hills, stairs, steps) – HL strengthening • Backward walking – hamstring, gluteal, and triceps strengthening • Aquatic therapy (underwater treadmill walking or swimming) • Therapy band resistance on leg • Treadmill activity with resistance • Tunnel/crawling/Limbo walking
Core strengthening	• Sit-to-stands or down-to-stands (on ground or ball) • Physioball or trampoline • Walking with a rolling object/cart • Rolling over • Rolling slowly to pause in each direction • Begging • Bowing • Plank on Physioroll or narrow board • Crawling • Standing on a BOSU • Pulling or carrying weight.

(Continued)

Table 15.1 (Continued)

Goal	Exercises
Cardiopulmonary conditioning	• Incline and decline walking • Stair climbing • Treadmill activity • Jogging • Running controlled • Aquatic therapy (underwater treadmill or swimming)Sport-specific activities
Endurance	• Walking, running, and swimming are used to condition patients whose jobs require long duration running and/or trotting. • Increase the duration and intensity of training as the patient's fitness improves.
Feline exercises	• Proprioceptive exercises (e.g., weight-shifting activities, balance board, wobble board, and standing on a therapy ball or roll). • Walking with a harness. • Ground treadmill walking with support and assistance. • Treadmill walking with small leg weights or therapy bands. • Playing with feathers or toys tied on the end of the string. • Scratching post. • Put cat in box (shallow/deep) and allow it to jump out of it • Can opener. • Low cavaletti rails. • Chasing a flashlight beam or laser light (use caution to avoid obsessive-compulsive light chasing). • Aquatic therapy.
Neurological rehabilitation	• Brushing • Tapping • Tickling • Quick stretch • Tail stimulation • Withdrawal reflex • Joint compression • Sphinx lying • Standing • Transitions • Weight shifting for balance • Wobble board • Patterning

Table 15.2 Important properties of water as they affect rehabilitation [25]. Mucha M, 2019 / VBS GmbH.

Property of water	Action on the body
Buoyancy	Decreases stress on joints – water depth at greater trochanter = 38% of normal weight bearing
Hydrostatic pressure	Reduces edema
Viscosity	Strengthening, proprioception
Surface tension	Strengthening
Warm water temperature	Promotes circulation

UWTM Speed and Duration

The speed for the initial UWTM session often slower than subsequent sessions as the patient needs to become accustomed to the treadmill. Slower speeds generally encourage weight bearing whereas faster speeds are better for muscular and cardiovascular conditioning. It is important to monitor the patient's gait and adjust as needed. Common speeds used for initial UWTM sessions are between 0.3 and 0.5 m/s (0.7 and 1.1 mph) for medium to large dogs. Dachshunds most often need to begin between 0.18 and 0.25 m/s (0.4 and 0.6 mph), given their chondrodystrophic stature. Other small and toy breeds often walk comfortably between 0.2 and 0.3 m/s (0.5 and 0.7 mph) [26].

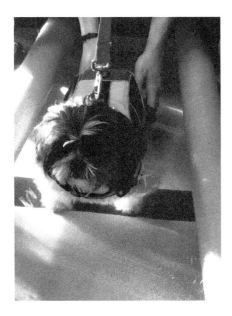

Figure 15.7 A dog in the underwater treadmill.

There is no perfect duration of time for every patient and the authors use intervals for the first several sessions particularly in deconditioned animals. For example, a standard cruciate repair would begin with the water level at the level of the flank, a speed of 0.36 and 0.45 m/s (0.8–1.0 mph) and duration of two minutes, repeated three times with two-minute rest intervals. Massage and ROM exercises are often done during the rest interval. Ending the sessions with a vigorous massage is often enjoyed by the patients [24]. Figure 15.7 shows a dog undergoing underwater treadmill therapy.

Swim Therapy

In swimming, dog and cats use different muscles than those used on land and have increased ROM of the front limbs [25]. Swimming can be used for rehabilitation after surgery or injury or for athletic conditioning or weight loss. Figure 15.8 shows a dog enjoying swim therapy. Therapeutic swimming exercises can be performed on a set of stairs in the water or a series of exercises in the water. A floating board can be used to improve balance and core strength in patients under 40 lbs.

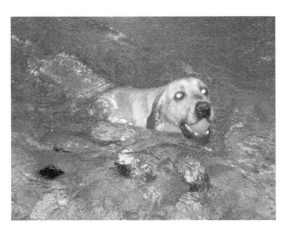

Figure 15.8 A dog enjoying swim therapy.

Swimming helps with co-ordination, postural awareness, endurance and overall fitness [25]. Life vests and harnesses are essential for safety, control of the patient and to improve confidence in swimming. Assistive devices such as water wings can be used on the patient's legs to improve ROM. Bunge cord leashes can be attached to harnesses while swimming for extra resistance. If the pool has jets, then resistance swimming is also an option. Figure 15.9 shows a dog in the underwater treadmill receiving treatment.

Case Study: Hydrotherapy for Brachial Plexus Injury

Signalment: Three-year old F/S Labrador Retriever.

History: Hit by car one week prior to presentation. Diagnosed with brachial plexus injury by emergency clinic and was presented for therapy.

Examination: Left foreleg paresis with some areas of pain sensation present on the dorsum of paw but none on ventrum. Able to move shoulder and elbow but lower limb had CP deficits and paresis.

TCVM Examination: Earth dog, tongue is pale and purple, pulse is wiry and deep.

Main TCVM Pattern: Front limb Qi/Blood Stagnation with local Qi Deficiency.

Goals: Improve function of front limb, improve weight bearing.

Treatments and Outcome:

Treated three times weekly initially with Acupuncture/Laser/UWTM.

Home with home exercises and recommended swimming at home.

After two weeks, went to twice weekly acupuncture and UWTM for two weeks then once weekly acupuncture and twice weekly UWTM. Twice weekly UWTM was continued for one month after which dog was treated only with home exercises and swimming at home.

Electroacupuncture
- Lui-feng to Lui-feng 4 points
- LI-4 to LI 15 on affected side
- GB21 to GB21
- SI9 to SI9
- Jing Ja jie points

Dry Needle
- LI-10, ST-36, GB-34

UWTM sessions: Initially 0.9 mph for 3 minutes x 3 sessions. Gait patterning was done by technician to insure proper foot placement. Rest for 2 minutes occurred between sessions in which the technician did massage and ROM. As she progressed sessions increased to 6 minutes x 3 sessions and eventually to 10 minute sessions.

Herbal therapy: Double P II and Cervical Formula (both Jing Tang Products).

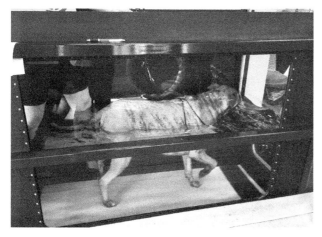

Figure 15.9 A dog receiving UWTM therapy for brachial plexus injury.

References

1 Bockstahler, B., Millis, D.L., and Egner, B. (2019). Exercise physiology. In: *Essential Facts of Physical Medicine, Rehabilitation and Sports Medicine in Companion Animals*, 1e (ed. B. Bockstahler, K. Wittek, D. Levine, J. Maieri, and D. Millis), 47–61. VBS GmbH.

2 Armstrong, R.B., Sauber, C.W.T., Seeherman, H.J., and Taylor, C.R. (1982 January). Distribution of fiber types in locomotory muscles of dogs. *Am J Anat* 163 (1): 87–98.

3 Lieber, R.L., McKee-Woodburn, T., and Gershuni, D.H. (1989 May). Recovery of the dog quadriceps after 10 weeks of immobilization followed by 4 weeks of remobilization. *J Orthop Res* 7 (3): 408–412.

4 Amann, J.F., Wharton, R.E., Madsen, R.W., and Laughlin, M.H. (1993 August). Comparison of muscle cell fiber types and oxidative capacity in gracilis, rectus femoris, and triceps brachii muscles in the ferret (Mustela putorius furo) and the domestic dog (Canis familiaris). *Anat Rec* 236 (4): 611–618.

5 Wakshlag, J.J., Cooper, B.J., Wakshlag, R.R. et al. (April 1, 2004). Biochemical evaluation of mitochondrial respiratory chain enzymes in canine skeletal muscle. *Am J Vet Res* 65 (4): 480–484.

6 Guy, P.S. and Snow, D.H. (September 1, 1981). Skeletal muscle fibre composition in the dog and its relationship to athletic ability. *Res Vet Sci* 31 (2): 244–248.

7 Boyd, A.S., Benjamin, H.J., and Asplund, C.A. (September 1, 2009). Splints and casts: indications and methods. *Am Fam Phys* 80 (5): 491–499.

8 Hutchinson, D., Sutherland-Smith, J., Watson, A.L., and Freeman, L.M. (November 1, 2012). Assessment of methods of evaluating sarcopenia in old dogs. *Am J Vet Res* 73 (11): 1794–1800.

9 Deschenes, M.R., Gaertner, J.R., and O'Reilly, S. (December 1, 2013). The effects of sarcopenia on muscles with different recruitment patterns and myofiber profiles. *Curr Aging Sci* 6 (3): 266–272.

10 Pagano, T.B., Wojcik, S., Costagliola, A. et al. (October 1, 2015). Age related skeletal muscle atrophy and upregulation of autophagy in dogs. *Vet J* 206 (1): 54–60.

11 Appell, H.J. (1990 July). Muscular atrophy following immobilisation. *Sports Med* 10 (1): 42–58.

12 Huntingford, J.L. and Bale, J. (September 14, 2017). Therapeutic exercises part 1: land exercises. In: *Physical Rehabilitation for Veterinary Technicians and Nurses* (ed. M.E. Goldberg and J.E. Tomlinson), 286–307.

13 Gillette, R. and Dale, R.B. (January 1, 2014). Basics of exercise physiology. In: *Canine Rehabilitation and Physical Therapy* (ed. D. Levine and D. Millis), 155–161.

14 Whitehead, N.P., Morgan, D.L., Gregory, J.E., and Proske, U. (2003 September). Rises in whole muscle passive tension of mammalian muscle after eccentric contractions at different lengths. *J Appl Physiol* 95 (3): 1224–1234.

15 Quindry, J., Miller, L., McGinnis, G. et al. (December 1, 2011). Muscle-fiber type and blood oxidative stress after eccentric exercise. *Int J Sport Nutr Exerc Metab* 21 (6): 462–470.

16 Wittek, K. and Bockstahler, B. (2019). Active therapeutic exercise. In: *Essential Facts of Physical Medicine, Rehabilitation and Sports Medicine in Companion Animals*, 1e (ed. B. Bockstahler, K. Wittek, D. Levine, J. Maieri, and D. Millis), 119–164. VBS GmbH.

17 Frye, C., Carr, B.J., Lenfest, M., and Miller, A. (2022). Canine geriatric rehabilitation: considerations and strategies for assessment, functional scoring, and follow up. *Front Vet Sci* 9.

18 McCauley, L. and Van Dyke, J.B. (April 23, 2018). Therapeutic exercise. In: *Canine Sports Medicine and Rehabilitation* (ed. C. Zink and J.B. Van Dyke), 177–207.

19 Kirkby Shaw, K., Alvarez, L., Foster, S.A. et al. (2020 January). Fundamental principles of rehabilitation and musculoskeletal tissue healing. *Vet Surg* 49 (1): 22–32.

20 Holler, P.J., Brazda, V., Dal-Bianco, B. et al. (July 1, 2010). Kinematic motion analysis of the joints of the forelimbs and hind limbs of dogs during walking exercise regimens. *Am J Vet Res* 71 (7): 734–740.

21 Durant, A.M., Millis, D.L., and Headrick, J.F. (2011). Kinematics of stair ascent in healthy dogs. *Vet Comp Orthop Traumatol* 24 (02): 99–105.

22 Lauer, S.K., Hillman, R.B., Li, L., and Hosgood, G.L. (May 1, 2009). Effects of treadmill inclination on electromyographic activity and hind limb kinematics in healthy hounds at a walk. *Am J Vet Res* 70 (5): 658–664.

23 Ciuperca, I. and Wittek, K. (2019). Land treadmill. In: *Essential Facts of Physical Medicine, Rehabilitation and Sports Medicine in Companion Animals*, 1e (ed. B. Bockstahler, K. Wittek, D. Levine, J. Maieri, and D. Millis), 167–172. VBS GmbH.

24 Koh, R. and Huntingford, J.L. (2022). *Certified Canine Rehabilitation Veterinarian Lab Notes, Session 2. Exercise Therapy*. Chi University.

25 Mucha, M. (2019). Aquatic therapy. In: *Essential Facts of Physical Medicine, Rehabilitation and Sports Medicine in Companion Animals*, 1e (ed. B. Bockstahler, K. Wittek, D. Levine, J. Maieri, and D. Millis), 175–188. VBS GmbH.

26 Chiquoine, J., Martens, E., McCauley, L., and Van Dyke, J.B. (April 23, 2018). Aquatic therapy. In: *Canine Sports Medicine and Rehabilitation* (ed. C. Zink and J.B. Van Dyke), 208–226.

16

Integrative Treatment of Common Musculoskeletal and Neurological Conditions

Ronald B. Koh* and Janice Huntingford*

* Corresponding authors

Introduction

Integrative practitioners are frequently asked to evaluate patients with musculoskeletal or neurologic diseases. Most of these patients can benefit from a multi-modal approach integrating pharmaceutical and non-pharmaceutical therapy. Treatment of orthopedic and neurologic disease form the basis of what most rehabilitation practitioners do. Integrating these therapies with TCVM acupuncture, food therapy, manual therapy, and modalities improves outcomes for patients with these issues.

Orthopedic Conditions

Degenerative Joint Disease (Osteoarthritis)

From a TCVM standpoint, conditions such as degenerative joint disease, osteochondritis dissecans, and hip and elbow dysplasia are considered Bi syndrome [1, 2]. Bi syndrome simply refers to pain and stiffness (stagnation) in bones, joints, tendons, ligaments and muscles, and the resultant aberration of gait or deformities associated with the stagnation [2, 3]. Integrative treatment can improve the quality of life (QOL) of patients with Bi syndrome by improving circulation, strengthening muscles and tendons, and decreasing pain. Each treatment is individual and must fit the TCVM pattern as well as the Western diagnosis.

Bi syndrome is a disorder resulting from the obstruction of meridians, sluggishness of Qi and blood circulation after the invasion of pathogenic wind, cold, dampness or heat, and is characterized by pain, numbness and heaviness of muscles, tendons, and joints, or swelling, hotness, and limitation of movement of joints [1, 2]. Invasion of pathogenic factors and deficiency of healthy Qi are the two underlying causes of this disorder. Six types of Bi syndrome have been identified owing to difference in body constitutions and pathogenic factors [1–3].

1) Wind or Wandering Bi Syndrome

This occurs when wind-cold-damp, predominantly wind, invades the body causing Qi and dlood stagnation and wandering pain (difficult to localized painful area).

2) Cold or Painful Bi Syndrome

This occurs when wind-cold-damp invades the body with cold predominating. Cold cause Qi and blood stagnation and severe pain. Cold Bi is worse in cold wet weather.

3) Damp or Fixed Bi Syndrome

This occurs when wind-cold-damp invades the body with damp predominating. Dampness creates heavy and stiff movements and impairs the flow of Qi. It is worse in damp weather.

4) Heat or Re Bi Syndrome

Either wind-cold-damp Bi syndrome or deficient heat from Yin deficiency Bi syndrome can turn into heat Bi syndrome resulting in inflamed and swollen joint. It is aggravated by warmth or pressure.

5) Kidney Qi/Yang Deficiency Bi Syndrome

This is a chronic Bi syndrome, and when bony degeneration is involved it is called bony Bi.

6) Kidney Qi/Yin Deficiency Bi Syndrome

This is another form of bony Bi but occurs when the Yin is depleted in chronic disease. This is a very common pattern in geriatrics with arthritis.

Integrative Veterinary Medicine, First Edition. Edited by Mushtaq A. Memon and Huisheng Xie.
© 2023 John Wiley & Sons, Inc. Published 2023 by John Wiley & Sons, Inc.
Companion Website: www.wiley.com/go/memon/veterinary

Degenerative joint disease (DJD) occurs most commonly in weight bearing joints and joints which are overused [4]. The main symptoms of DJD are pain and stiffness in the affected joint. Pain is aggravated by movement, but stiffness generally follows a short period of inactivity. The affected joint may be swollen, and crepitus may be palpated on movement. Rehabilitation of DJD is multimodal utilizing pharmaceuticals (such as non-steroidal anti-inflammatories (NSAIDS), gabapentin, amantadine, tricyclic anti-depressants, or opioids) and non-pharmaceutical supplements and modalities [5–7]. A discussion of pharmaceuticals for use in DJD is beyond the scope of this chapter but more information on integrative pain management appears in Chapter 18.

Treatment for DJD may be different from joint to joint depending on the Bi syndrome being treated. Hip dysplasia, elbow dysplasia and osteochondritis dissecans are all classified as DJD from a conventional perspective. From a TCVM perspective, they all have underlying components of kidney deficiency and need to be treated as such [2]. Dogs and cats with DJD may show a myriad of different signs related to the severity of the pathologic change in the joint. Degree of lameness may be inconsistent with radiographic signs of disease particularly in cats. The wide range of factors affecting this disease make it difficult to provide recommended blanket treatments thus underscoring the need for multimodal individual treatment.

Integrative treatment of DJD focuses on pain relief. Weight loss has been shown to decrease the severity of pain in dogs with DJD [6]. A combination of weight loss and PT was demonstrated to improve patient mobility by Mlacnik Purina study. These studies show that restricted diet or weight loss alone may be an important aspect of managing dogs with OA [8].

Rehabilitation modalities such as cryotherapy, thermotherapy, physical exercises, hydrotherapy (pool or treadmill), laser, ultrasound, shockwave, and massage therapy are all valuable in treating patients with DJD [5–10]. These modalities increase circulation of blood and lymph, decrease inflammation, improve joint range of motion, improve strength, balance and proprioception, and help restore normal joint function. A discussion of common therapeutic modalities appears in Chapter 14. Frequently acupuncture, Tui-na and food therapy are employed for pain relief and to help relieve Qi stagnation and bring the DJD patient back into balance [2]. DJD is a lifelong management issue for the client and the veterinarian alike. See Figure 16.1.

TCVM treatments for DJD and other common orthopedic conditions are summarized in Table 16.1. Rehabilitation modalities for common orthopedic conditions are summarized in Table 16.2. Table 16.3 summarizes herbal treatments for Bi syndrome.

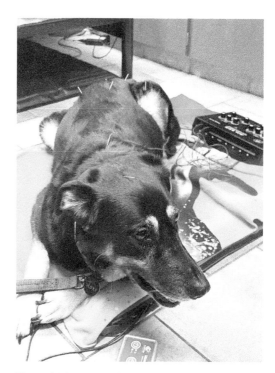

Figure 16.1 A dog with DJD receiving acupuncture.

Shoulder Conditions

Shoulder injuries can include medial shoulder instability, supraspinatus, or biceps tenosynovitis or contractures. Meridians that run through the shoulder area are associated with the lung (LU), large intestine (LI), bladder (BL) and Triple Heater (TH) channels and meet at the acromion. Qi and blood stagnation with underlying liver Yin or blood deficiency are common patterns. In TCVM, the liver governs the sinews (tendons and ligaments) [13]. Common injuries in the shoulder are generally related to tendon or ligament pathology such as medial shoulder instability and tenosynovitis of the supraspinatus or biceps. TCVM treatments for these are summarized in Table 16.1. Modalities, pharmaceuticals, and herbals are all used for these conditions. Exercise therapy and the use of hobbles or supports may be suggested. Some of these conditions require surgery. Table 16.2 summarizes the treatment of these conditions.

Elbow Conditions

Elbow problems include elbow dysplasia and traumatic fragmented medial coronoid process. Elbow dysplasia is a term use to describe inherited elbow disease that includes fragmented medial coronoid process (FCP) or medial compartment disease (MCD), osteochondritis dissecans (OCD), ununited anconeal process (UAP), and joint incongruity [11]. The dog may have one or all of these syndromes. Traumatic Fragmented Medial Coronoid process or Jump Down Syndrome is a repetitive stress injury found in performance dogs [12]. Dogs with elbow

Table 16.1 TCVM diagnosis and treatment of common orthopedic conditions [1]. Zhang, EQ, 2010; [2]. Preast V, Xie H, 2007; [3]. Hu, J., 2003.

Condition	TCVM patterns	TCVM treatments
Degenerative joint disease or Osteoarthritis	Excess patterns: wind, cold, damp, heat Bi Deficiency patterns: kidney Qi, Yin or Yang deficiency bone Bi	**Wind Bi**: GB-20, BL-17, SP-10; *Juan Bi Tang* **Cold Bi**: GV-4, CV-4, Bai-hui, moxibustion; *Du Huo Ji Sheng Tang* **Damp Bi**: ST-40, BL-20, SP-9; *Yi Yi Ren Tang* **Heat Bi**: GV-14, LI-11, LIV-2; *Bai Hu Tang* **Kidney Qi-Yin Deficiency**: SP-6, KID-3, KID-7; *Di Gu Pi San* **Kidney Yang Deficiency**: BL-23, GV-4, Bai-hui, Moxibustion; *Sang Ji Sheng San**
Osteochondritis dissecans/hip or elbow dysplasia	Kidney Jing deficiency with Qi blood stagnation	**Kidney Jing Deficiency**: BL-23, BL-26, KID-3; *Sheng Jing San** **Qi Blood Stagnation**: LIV-3, ST-36, BL-60; *Shen Tong Zhu Yu Tang*
Bicipital/ supraspinatus tendinopathy	Liver Yin or blood deficiency with Qi- blood stagnation	**Liver Yin or Blood Deficiency**: BL-18, LIV-3, GB-34; *Bu Gan Qiang Jin San** **Qi Blood Stagnation**: LIV-3, ST-36, BL-60; *Shen Tong Zhu Yu Tang*
Medial shoulder instability	Liver Yin or blood deficiency with Qi- blood stagnation	**Liver Yin or Blood Deficiency**: BL-18, LIV-3, GB-34; *Bu Gan Qiang Jin San** **Qi Blood Stagnation**: LIV-3, ST-36, BL-60; *Shen Tong Zhu Yu Tang*
Contractures	Qi or blood stagnation with or without spleen Qi deficiency	**Qi Blood Stagnation**: LIV-3, ST-36, BL-60; *Shen Tong Zhu Yu Tang* **Spleen Qi Deficiency**: BL-20, ST-36, SP-9; *Si Jun Zi Tang*
Carpal hyperextension	Liver Yin or blood deficiency	**Liver Yin or Blood Deficiency**: BL-18, LIV-3, GB-34; *Bu Gan Qiang Jin San**
Cranial cruciate rupture	Liver Yin or blood deficiency with Qi blood stagnation	**Liver Yin or Blood Deficiency**: BL-18, LIV-3, GB-34; *Bu Gan Qiang Jin San** **Qi Blood Stagnation**: LIV-3, ST-36, BL-60; *Shen Tong Zhu Yu Tang*
Patellar luxation	Kidney Jing deficiency with or without liver Yin deficiency	**Kidney Jing Deficiency**: BL-23, BL-26, KID-3; *Sheng Jing San** **Liver Yin or Blood Deficiency**: BL-18, LIV-3, GB-34; *Bu Gan Qiang Jin San**
Calcaneal tendon/ Achilles injury	Liver Yin or blood deficiency with Qi blood stagnation	**Liver Yin or Blood Deficiency**: BL-18, LIV-3, GB-34; *Bu Gan Qiang Jin San** **Qi-Blood Stagnation**: LIV-3, ST-36, BL-60; *Shen Tong Zhu Yu Tang*
Iliopsoas and other muscle injuries	Qi or blood stagnation	**Qi-Blood Stagnation**: LIV-3, ST-36, BL-60; *Shen Tong Zhu Yu Tang*

Sang Ji Sheng San: Loranthus Formula (Dr Xie's Jing Tang Herbal)*
Sheng Jing San: Epimedium Formula (Dr Xie's Jing Tang Herbal)*
Bu Gan Qiang Jin San: Tendon Ligament Formula (Dr Xie's Jing Tang Herbal)*

Table 16.2 Rehabilitation treatments for common orthopedic conditions [5]. Millis DL, Levine D., 1997; [7]. Mosley C, et al., 2022; [11]. Vezzoni A, Benjamino K, 2021; [12].Tan DK, et al., 2016.

Condition	Rehabilitation modalities	Rehabilitation exercises	Supplements/injections
Degenerative Joint Disease – can occur in any joint secondary to injury, genetic predisposition, congenital deformity, or growth aberration (osteochondritis dissecans or hip or elbow dysplasia) or surgery	Pain Control: Pharmaceuticals, herbs, modalities Photobiomodulation EWST Acupuncture UWTM PEMF Hot and cold therapy Manual therapy – Massage, Chiropractic, Joint mobilization, Stretching TENS Weight loss if needed	Depends on location and condition of patient but could include Sit to Stand, Cavalettis, Backwards walking, Swimming, Ball work, Obstacle course, Hill walking. Goals include pain relief, weight loss, increased joint movement, and strengthening adjacent muscles.	Joint injections with platelet rich plasma (PRP), stem cells, hyaluronic acid (HA), steroids, Synovetin*; Injectable monoclonal antibody (MAB) or polysulfated glycosaminoglycan (PSGAG); Dietary supplements with undenatured collagen type II (UCII), green lipped mussel (GLM), omega (ω)-3 polyunsaturated fatty acids (ω3-PUFAs), glucosamine and chondroitin, egg shell membrane, cannabidiol (CBD)

Table 16.2 (Continued)

Condition	Rehabilitation modalities	Rehabilitation exercises	Supplements/injections
Osteochondritis dissecans/Hip or elbow dysplasia	See DJD above OCD is most often a surgical problem that requires follow up rehabilitation and therapies to minimize future DJD. Surgery may be indicated for hip and elbow dysplasia if recognized early enough. If no surgery is performed it is treated in the same manner as DJD	As for DJD above For elbows can add Commando crawling and rocker board work	Joint injections with PRP, stem cells, HA, steroids, Synovetin[*]; Injectable MAB or PSGAG; Dietary supplements with UCII, GLM, ω3-PUFAs, glucosamine and chondroitin, egg shell membrane, CBD
Medial shoulder instability	Treatment depends on severity but may include: Hobbles, EWST, laser, acupuncture UWTM, PEMF, stretching and mobilization Surgery may be needed for severe cases or canine athletes	Sit to Stand, Cavalettis, swimming, ball work, hill walking Avoid exercises that require lateral movement	Joint injections with PRP, stem cells, HA, steroids; dietary supplements with UCII, GLM, ω3-PUFAs, glucosamine and chondroitin, egg shell membrane, CBD, Fortetrophin
Bicipital/Supraspinatus Tendinopathy	Treatment depends on severity but may include: rest, NSAIDs, EWST, laser, acupuncture, weight control UWTM, PEMF, stretching and mobilization, cross friction massage, therapeutic ultrasound surgery may be needed for chronic cases or canine athletes	Note: acute injuries should not be stretched PROM (flexion/extension of limb while not weight bearing) In acute phase exercises increase strength of muscles Controlled leash walking, therapy ball work, rocker board balancing, cavletti, weaves (slow), figure 8s and hill walking	Joint injections with PRP, stem cells, HA, steroids; Tendon injections with PRP or stem cells; Dietary supplements with UCII, ω3-PUFAs, CBD
Contractures	Ultrasound, cross friction massage Mature contractures usually require surgery UWTM and general conditioning, leash walking also appropriate	Depends on location but heating with therapeutic ultrasound and then stretching is recommended. PROM	Regenerative medicine with PRP or stem cells may help some patients
Jump Down Syndrome (Traumatic Fragmented medial coronoid process)	Arthroscopic removal of fragments followed by rehabilitation therapy, pharmaceuticals, herbs modalities UWTM, massage	Cavalettis, high fives, weaves, backward walking, zig zag hill walking – timing of exercises depends on healing	Injectable PSGAGs; Dietary supplements with UCII, GLM, ω3-PUFAs, glucosamine and chondroitin, egg shell membrane, CBD, other supplements as per DJD
Carpal Hyperextension	Acupuncture treatment, braces, UWTM	Exercises on textured surfaces, rocker board, ball work, cavaletti, backwards walking, zigzag hill walking	Joint injections with PRP or stem cells; Injectable PSGAGs; Dietary supplements with UCII, ω3-PUFAs
Cranial Cruciate Rupture	If complete rupture and unstable, surgery is indicated Post surgery or for medical treatment use acupuncture, laser therapy, EWST, UWTM, massage NOTE: according to tissue healing principles complete healing of CCL injury may take 6 to 12 months even post surgery	Sit to stand, Controlled leash walks, cavaletti, paws up on ball, backward walking, Weaves, progress to zig zag hill walking, cross legged standing,	Joint injections with PRP or stem cells; Injectable PSGAGs; Dietary supplements with UCII, GLM, ω3-PUFAs, glucosamine and chondroitin, egg shell membrane, avocado soybean unsaponifiables (ASU), CBD

(Continued)

Table 16.2 (Continued)

Condition	Rehabilitation modalities	Rehabilitation exercises	Supplements/injections
Patellar luxation	Medical therapy indicated for Grade 1–2 luxation, chronic or Grade 3 or 4 often have surgery Treatments include pharmaceutical, herbs and modalities acupuncture, laser therapy, EWST	Sit to stand, backward walking, cavaletti, weaves, circles, zigzag hill walking, cross legged standing	Injections with PRP or stem cells; Injectable PSGAGs; Dietary supplements with UCII, GLM, ω3-PUFAs, glucosamine and chondroitin, egg shell membrane, CBD, other supplements as per DJD
Calcaneal tendon/achilles injury	Chronic conditions may not require surgery. Acute traumatic conditions do require surgery Treatments include pharmaceutical, herbs and modalities. Post surgery rehabilitation often involves a brace and gradual return to flexion. After tendon has healed then exercises commence Laser, EWST, acupuncture, UWTM are common modalities used.	Sit to stand, backward walking, cavaletti, weaves, circles, zigzag hill walking Can Progress to backward walking up hill when tendon is sufficiently healed	Injections with PRP or stem cells; Injectable PSGAGs; Dietary supplements with UCII, GLM, ω3-PUFAs, Fortetrophin
Iliopsoas and other muscle injuries	Treatments include pharmaceutical, herbs and modalities Trigger point therapy Laser, massage, stretching, UWTM	Sit to stand, cookie stretches, cross legged standing	Injections with PRP or stem cells; Dietary supplements with UCII, GLM, ω3-PUFAs, Fortetrophin

Table 16.3 Common Chinese herbals used for Bi Syndrome [1]. Zhang, EQ, 2010; [2]. Preast V, Xie H, 2007; [3]. Hu, J., 2003.

Chinese herbal name	Western indication	TCVM indication
Xiao Chai Hu Tang (Minor Bupleurum Combination)	Hip Dysplasia, IVDD, CCL injury, OA, DM, collapsing trachea – particularly good post disc surgery and for sacroiliac joint pain *Can be modified by adding *Qin Jiao* to improve anti-inflammatory action	*Shao Yang* disharmony, dampness obstructing the spleen and stomach and *Qi* deficiency.
Chai Ge Jie Ji Tang (Bupleurum and Kudzu Combination)	Acute IVDD, acute neck and back pain, meningitis, and spinal cord tumors *Can be modified by adding *Du Huo* for more disc pain relief	*Shao Yang* disharmony (Bupleurum) and sudden wind invasion that obstructs the normal flow of blood and *Qi*
Du Huo Ji Shen Tang	Severe acute neck pain especially in Dachshunds, DJD, back issues, hind limb lameness, and muscle spasms, upper and lower motor neuron disorders	Boney *Bi* formula. Invigorates blood, expels wind-cold-damp Used for liver blood deficiency, kidney and liver *Yin* deficiency and *Qi* deficiency
Xiao Huo Luo Dan (Minor Invigorate the Collaterals Combination)	Iliopsoas muscle tears, IVDD, DJD, partial cruciate tears, soft tissue injuries, OA that is worse with cold weather. Helpful when NSAIDS no longer work well – Important geriatric formula	For treating blood stasis, *Yang* deficiency and stagnation in the channels
Da Huo Luo Dan (Major Invigorate the Collaterals)	Acute IVDD and neck pain (with caution) *Caution for long-term use as some forms use contains Aconite	Dispels wind, tonifies *Qi* and blood, invigorates the blood, disperses cold, clears heat, opens the channels and collaterals, and relieves pain
Yi Yi Ren Tang (Coix Combination)	Polyarthritis, OCD, chronic elbow osteoarthritis, back pain and IVDD. This is an important formula for large breed dogs with severe back pain.	Wind cold damp invasion, *Qi* deficiency, blood deficiency and Blood stasis. It is used for acute invasion of wind in the dorsum, extremities and joints. The underlying deficiency that allows wind invasion is blood stasis or decreased circulation. Contraindicated with *Yin* deficiency

Table 16.3 (Continued)

Chinese herbal name	Western indication	TCVM indication
Shen Tong Zhu Yu Tang	Muscle and generalized body soreness	Pain in joints due to *Qi*-blood stagnation
San Ren Tang	Lumbosacral disease with less pain and more ataxia, concurrent neurogenic bladder	Damp heat, dampness obstructing the spleen and stomach, and wind damp dnvasion
Si Miao San	Severe lumbosacral pain with toneless, full pulse	Damp heat *Bi* syndrome

dysplasia have an underlying Jing deficiency. As well as treating the elbow issues, the integrative medical practitioner should address the Jing deficiency through the use of acupuncture, herbs, Tui-na and food therapy. TCVM treatments for this are summarized in Table 16.1. Treatments with rehabilitation for this condition are summarized in Table 16.2.

Carpal Hyperextension

This condition is common is older performance dogs and often affects the collie breeds. Ligaments in carpal joint become lax as the dog ages and repetitive stress from landing on hard surfaces when jumping, fall from heights, osteoarthritis, trauma, and inflammatory diseases affect the carpal joint [14]. See Figure 16.2. Treatment of carpal hyperestension is summarized in the tables that follow.

Stifle Issues

The two most common problems seen in the stifle are patellar luxation and ruptured cranial cruciate ligaments (CCL). CCL injuries are the most common cause of hind limb lameness and may need to be treated surgically or medically [15]. A complete tear that also involves the meniscus may best be treated with surgical joint stabilization [16]. Partial tears and strains may be treated conservatively with a combination of rehabilitation, acupuncture, and herbal therapy. See Figure 16.3. Treatments are summarized in the following tables.

Hock Issues

Achilles tendon (more frequently defined as the common calcaneal tendon) ruptures and strains are common hock problems. These injuries are most often the result of direct force, leading to the tendon's tearing or complete rupture [17]. Surgery, regenerative medicine, acupuncture, and

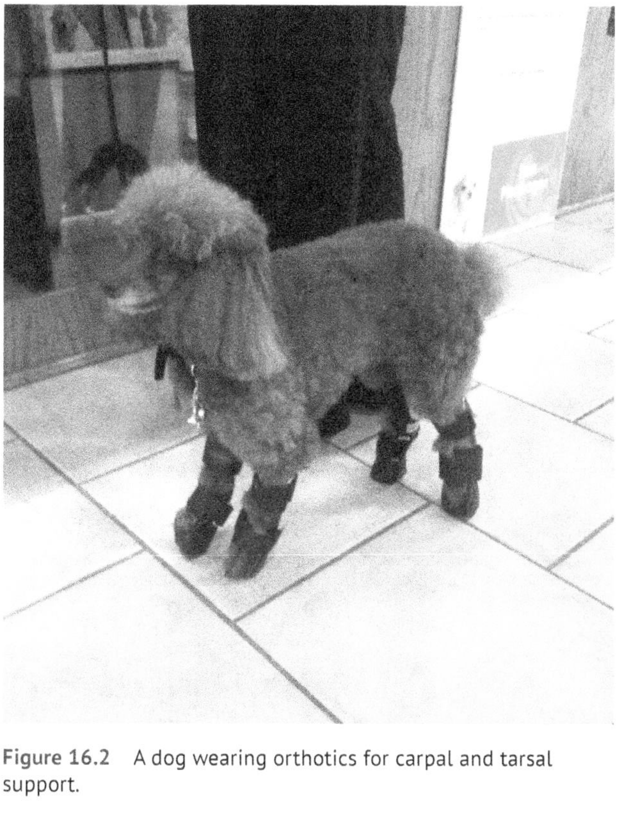

Figure 16.2 A dog wearing orthotics for carpal and tarsal support.

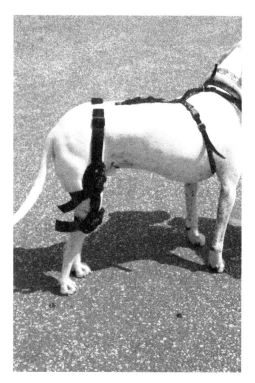

Figure 16.3 A dog with a CCL partial tear wearing a custom cruciate orthotics.

herbals are commonly used to treat these conditions. Treatments are summarized here.

Muscle Injuries

These are common and are best treated with a combination of pharmaceuticals, herbs, acupuncture, and other modalities. Chinese herbals such as Xiao Huo Luo Dan and Shen Tong Zhu Yu tang have been very helpful for many patients. Muscle injuries do not respond well to treatment with NSAIDs but instead need rehabilitation and modalities.See Figure 16.4.

Neurological Conditions

TCVM and conventional medicine differ in their diagnosis and treatment of neurological diseases. However, an integration of these two systems provides the best treatment for patients particularly those with paresis and paralysis. A Western neurological exam as well as a TCVM pattern diagnosis contribute to the treatment of these patients.

Intervertebral Disc Disease

Canine Intervertebral Disc Disease involves "the degeneration and protrusion or extrusion of disc material into the vertebral canal causing a variety of clinical signs ranging from pain to paralysis." [18] Disc disease is divided into two categories based on extrusion (Hansen Type I and Type III) and protrusion (Hansen type II) [18]. See Table 16.4.

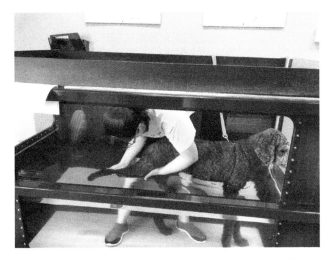

Figure 16.4 A dog receiving hydrotherapy for a muscle injury.

We further classify these cases based on the severity of clinical signs from I to IV. Please see Table 16.5.

From a conventional standpoint, the IVDD patient needs to be treated for pain, paresis, ataxia, muscle atrophy, weakness, and perhaps incontinence. The mitigation of pain needs to be the practitioner's primary concern. Pain is most frequently treated with NSAIDs or steroids and other adjuncts such as gabapentin or tramadol or perhaps surgery. Once the pain is under control, the practitioner can focus on restoring the dog to normal neurological function if possible [19].

Table 16.4 IVDD summary after Dewey [18]. Dewey, CW and Da Costa RC, 2016.

	Hansen Type I	Hansen Type II	Hansen Type III
Pathophysiology	Chondroid degeneration (Extrusion)	Fibroid degeneration (Protrusion)	Acute Non-compressive Nucleus Pulposus Extrusion (ANNPE) Explosive disc herniation – low volume, high velocity
Etiology			Strenuous exercise, trauma
Breeds	Chondrodystrophic breeds with Dachshund most common	Non-chondrodystrophic larger breed dogs	Any breed of dogs, cats as well but mid size to larger dogs are over represented
Age	>2 years usually 3 to 6 years	> 5 years	>1 year
Onset	Peracute to acute	Chronic	Acute
Anatomic location	Thoracolumbar with T12-L1 most common in small dogs, L1-L3 for larger dogs and L4-L5 in cats	Cervical most common, L7-S1	Any
Clinical signs	Acute pain that may rapidly progress to paresis and paralysis. Severe neck pain can result. Nerve root signature pain is seen	Slowly developing paresis over weeks, months, or years. Often a component of cervical spondylomyelopathy (Wobblers)	Acute spinal bruising but not compressive
Treatment	See Table 16.5	If not associated with L/S disease or Wobblers, medical management usually works. Surgery frequently makes this condition worse	Only treatment is physical therapy and acupuncture

Table 16.5 IVDD classes or stages after Dewey [18]. Dewey, CW and Da Costa RC, 2016.

Stage or class	Clinical signs
Stage 1	Mild back pain no neurological deficits, usually self corrects in a few days
Stage 2	Moderate to severe neck or lumbar pain
Stage 3 * surgery preferred treatment	Partial Paralysis (Paresis) resulting in ataxia, but has intact pain sensations
Stage 4 * surgery preferred treatment	Paralysis but with deep pain present
Stage 5 * surgery preferred treatment ASAP before 72 hours	Paralysis with no deep pain sensation

Intervertebral Disc Disease from a TCVM Standpoint

Disc disease affects nerves, the discs, and muscles as well as the vertebrae themselves. Nerves are considered marrow and disc extrusion or protrusion creates an obstruction which could be blood, Qi, or phlegm [2, 20]. The discs themselves are under the influence of blood. Often the dog has a deficiency of kidney Jing, Qi, Yin, or Yang [21]. In TCVM, pain is recognised as an obstruction of Qi and or Blood [2]. Qi Stagnation is categorized as a dull intermittent and shifting pain whereas blood stagnation is sharp, fixed, and constant. When the disk degenerates, it dehydrates and loses its elasticity. This is a failure of the disc to be nourished by blood and blood stagnation occurs. It is possible for the patient to have an overall kidney Qi deficiency with a local blood stagnation (local excess) which is the most commonly diagnosed TCVM pattern. However, the final TCVM diagnosis is made based on the pattern observed by the practitioner at the time of examination. This stagnation may be around the disc, or it can radiate down the channel or meridian and cause Qi stagnation within the channel. For most thoraco-lumbar disc issues, both the bladder meridian and the governing vessel meridian will be affected. The gall bladder, small intestine and Triple Heater meridians may be affected with cervical disc issues.

Integrative treatment of IVDD has the same goals as conventional treatment – relieve pain, improve paresis, ataxia, muscle atrophy, weakness, and perhaps incontinence and return the patient to full function. Pain relief can be accomplished by acupuncture and herbals, and therapeutic modalities such as laser, PEMF therapy, exercise therapy, manual therapy, and hydrotherapy. Rehabilitation therapies have been proven to be effective to help patients with IVDD to return to normal function [22–25]. Acupuncture has also been recognized to be an effective therapy for IVDD [23, 26–31]. See Figure 16.5. Summary of IVDD treatment based on pattern diagnosis appears in Table 16.6.

Rehabilitation Modalities

Pulsed Electromagnetic Field Therapy (PEMF)

Pulsed electromagnetic field (PEMF) therapy has been shown to reduce postoperative pain, inflammation, and narcotic usage in both human and animal studies [32].

Photobiomodulation (LASER) Therapy

One use of laser therapy is in spinal cord injuries. PBMT has been shown to modulate oxidate stress, reduce inflammation, promote axonal regeneration, and accelerate functional recovery [33, 34]. Draper performed a prospective study to determine if low-level laser therapy and surgery for intervertebral disk herniation encouraged ambulation faster than surgery alone [35]. A 5×200 mW, 810 nm, cluster array laser was used to deliver 25 W/cm2 to the skin. All dogs were scored daily by the investigators using the modified Frankel scoring system. The time to achieve a modified Frankel score of 4 was significantly lower ($p = 0.0016$) in the low-level laser therapy group (median 3.5 days) than the control group (median 14 days). They concluded that low-level laser therapy in combination with surgery decreases the time to ambulation in dogs with T3-L3 myelopathy secondary to intervertebral disc herniation [35].

Proprioceptive Neuromuscular Facilitation

After stretching and PROM, it is important to re-educate the muscles that are unresponsive. Generally, these are muscles that are antagonistic to those shortened through contracture or by spasticity. This re-education process takes place through Proprioceptive Neuromuscular Facilitation patterning (PNF). PNF is used to simulate movement patterns that are ingrained and functional [36]. Common patterns are

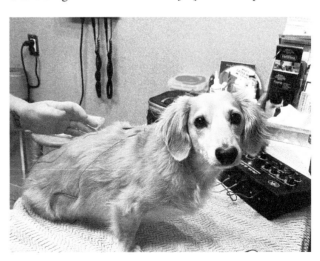

Figure 16.5 Acupuncture is frequently used post IVDD surgery or for conservative treatment.

Table 16.6 Summary of IVDD treatment based on pattern and Western Diagnosis.

Problem/TCVM pattern	Acupuncture points	Common Chinese herbals
Lower motor neuron Flaccidity (Could be L/S disease, cauda equina injury or DM) Qi/blood stagnation with local Qi stagnation, or could involve spleen *Qi*, kidney *Qi* or *Yang* or *Jing* if DM	**DN:** BL-40, BL-36, ST-36,KID-1, KID-3 through to BL-60, LIV-3, BL-62, BL-23 **EAP:** GV-1-GV-3, CV-1-CV-3, BL-39-BL-39, BL-54 -BL-54, BL-36-BL36, GV-14-*Bai-hui* For DM add BL-20/21, *Shen-shu, Shen-peng, Shen-jiao*	*Bu Yang Huan Wu* (weakness), *Da Huo Luo Dan* if painful, *Ba Zhen Tang* to Tonify *Qi* and blood and move blood and relieve pain
Upper motor neuron lesion Hypertonicity – cervical Qi/blood stagnation with local Qi stagnation or could involve kidney *Qi* or *Yang* deficiency	**DN:** LU-7, BL-23, KID-3, SI-3, BL-60, BL-62, LI-11, LI-4, ST-36, GB-39, ST-36 **EAP:** GB-20-GB-21 (same side), SI-16-SI-9, *Jing-jia-jji* bilaterally, GV-14-*Bai-hui*, BL-17-Bl-17, BL-40-BL-54, KID-1-BL-11	Cervical formula (JT) or *Jing Tong Fang* *Bu Yang Huan Wu* may be added for kidney *Qi* deficiency and weakness
Upper motor neuron lesion Hypertonicity-thoracolumbar Qi/blood stagnation with local Qi stagnation or could involve kidney *Qi* or *Yang* deficiency	**DN:** LIV-3, LI-4, BL-60 (KID-3),BL-62,LI-10, ST-36, GV-1, KID-10, GB-39, PC-8, *Hua-tuo-jia-ji, Shen-shu, Shen-peng, Shen-jiao* **EAP:** GV-14-*Bai-hui*, BL-17-Bl-17, BL-40-BL-54, KID-1-BL-11, *Liu-feng*	*Da Huo Luo Dan, Du Huo Ji Sheng Tang* (for Dachshunds) *Shen Tong Fang* *Xiao Chai Hu Tang*
Pain	LI-4, GV-14, LI-11 GV-20, ST-36, SP-6, LIV-3, BL-60, GB-34, TH-5, PC-6 *Hua-tuo Jia Ji, Bai-Hui, Shen-shu, Shen-Peng*, BL-40	*Shen Tong Fang, Si Miao San* if damp, *Xiao Chai Hu Tang*
Muscle weakness/atrophy Kidney Qi/Yang deficiency Qi and Yin deficiency Spleen Qi deficiency	DN: BL-20, BL-21, ST-36, LI-10, GV-3, GV-4, Shen -shu, KID-7 **EAP:** GV-14-*Baihui, Shen-shu-Shen-shu*,	*Bu Yang Huan Wu* (Yang deficiency) *Di Gu Pi* (Yin signs)
Decreased proprioception Qi stagnation and deficiency	**DN:** TH-21/20/17, GB-3, ST-36, SI-3, LI-4, LI-10, LU-7 **EAP:** BL54-BL-60, GV14-*Bai-hui*, BL-17-*Shen-shu*, BL-23-BL-23	

walking, running, scratching, sit to stand, movement from lateral to sternal recumbency, kicking back, turning, and many others. See Figure 16.6. PNF patterns can be done in any position depending on the disability [37]. One example of PNF patterning is rhythmic stabilization. This involves placing dog in normal standing position or sternal recumbency and applying a resistance in one direction that is gradually decreased and then applied in the opposite direction. This movement strengthens the patient's isometric contractions. Passive running is another PNF pattern that is easily performed [36–38].

Tips for Neurological Patients [36–38]

1) Try a small vibrator or an electric toothbrush to stimulate weak muscles.
2) Tapping over muscle bellies stimulates the muscles to contract.
3) Postural reflexes such as wheelbarrowing or hopping are useful.
4) Wrap a tensor around the patient from the front to the back to create awareness and connect front and back end. Alternatively use a Thunder shirt or Snuggly.

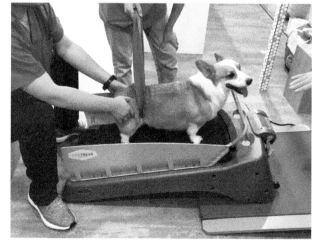

Figure 16.6 PNF patterning a patient with neurological disease.

5) Any sensory stimulation you can provide will stimulate the superficial receptors.
6) Do not forget to counsel clients about lifestyle changes. Non-slip flooring, raised bowls, no stairs are jumping are imperative.

Therapeutic Exercises

Therapeutic exercises are used for pain reduction, strengthening of muscles and joints, to mitigate muscle atrophy and improve proprioception and balance. Hydrotherapy is extensively used for patients with neurological disease as often these patients walk on the treadmill before they walk on land.

One common exercise used in non-ambulatory patients is assisted standing. This can be use for patients with either front or hind limb paresis. The patient can be draped over a therapy roll to assist with support of the limbs. To further increase sensory input and improve proprioception, the ball can be rocked back and forth gently with the dog over it. With a very small patient, the patient can be placed on the ball and bounced slightly. NMES can also be utilized at this time to facilitate and increase the force of contraction. Standing exercises utilizing balls, rocker boards and slings may be incorporated into the exercise regime also. See Figure 16.7.

Ambulatory patients can be assisted with harness or sling walking. Harnesses are available to assist front and back-end mobility. These harnesses are easy to use and ergonomically designed for the patient and the owner. They provide support for early ambulation and joint stability (Help -em-up Harnesses available through Helpemup.com and in this authors opinion are a superior harness). When the patient is ambulatory, assisted incline walking, figure 8s, walking in circles, cavalettis, varied terrain walking, and stepping over obstacles can be added. Backwards walking can be incorporated to strengthen hamstring and gluteal muscles. Good footing is essential for these exercises and enhances proprioception and proper limb placement [38].

Table 16.7 gives approximate time scale for recovery for an IVDD patient.

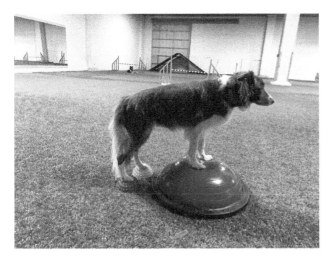

Figure 16.7 A patient on a Bosu ball working on proprioceptive training.

Table 16.7 Approximate time scale for recovery for an IVDD patient [19]. Campbell MT and Huntingford JL, 2016; [39]. Huntingford JL, Fossum T, 2019.

Timescale	Physiotherapy aims	Treatment options
0–4 weeks	Reduce inflammation	Laser, Assisi Loop
	Reduce muscle guarding	Laser
	Improve core strength/stability	Massage
		Heat
	Increase sensation	Acupuncture
	Management at home	Home Ex Program (HEP)
		NMES
		Hydrotherapy
		PNF patterns
		Acupuncture
		Exercise restriction
		Mobility Aids–Harness
		Advice re flooring
4–6 weeks	Continue as above	HEP increasing challenges
		Other modalities as needed
6–12 weeks	Increase exercise tolerance	Increase exercise level
	Improve proprioception and balance	Acupuncture
		HEP
12 weeks	Return to full function	Continue as needed

Other Neurological Diseases

A complete discussion of the integrative diagnosis and treatment of other neurological diseases is beyond the scope of this chapter, but the following table summarizes most the common integrative diagnosis, TCVM pattern and treatment for other common neurological diseases. Of particular note is treatment of Degenerative Myelopathy as recent publications outline the use of high dose photobiomodulation (PBMT) combined with physiotherapy for the treatment of these dogs [40, 41]. Table 16.8 outlines common neurological diseases and their integrative treatment.

Conclusions

Integrative practitioners can treat many musculoskeletal and neurological conditions by integrating rehabilitation with TCVM pattern treatment. Combinations of western medicine, acupuncture, and rehabilitation modalities facilitate recovery and improve mobility faster more quickly than any single treatment. Improving function and quality of life should be paramount when treating any of these patients.

Table 16.8 Integrative treatment of common neurological diseases except IVDD [2]. Preast V, Xie H, 2007; [37]. Wang RY, 1994; [38]. Huntingford JL and Bale J, 2017; [39]. Huntingford JL, Fossum T, 2019; [40]. Kathmann I, et al, 2006; [41]. Miller LA, et al. 2020.

Diagnosis	TCVM pattern	TCVM treatment	Rehabilitation modalities	Comments
Degenerative myelopathy	Kidney Qi, Yin, or Yang deficiency with spleen Qi deficiency (muscle atrophy)	**Kidney Qi-Yin deficiency**: SP-6, KID-3, KID-7; *Hu Qian Wan* **Kidney Yang Deficiency**: BL-23, GV-4, Bai-hui, Moxibustion; *Di Huang Yin Zi*	High dose laser therapy, Intensive rehabilitation therapy including exercise therapy and UWTM	Patients treated with Rehab therapy live considerably longer than those who are not [40]
Vestibular disease	Kidney Qi, Yin, or Yang deficiency with internal wind	GV-20, GV-26, GB-20, LI-4, PC-6, BL-23, ST-36, KID-3, LIV-3, Er-jian; *Bu Yang Huan Wu*	Stand the dog on its four feet for 5 minutes per hour initially to provide input into the nervous system, UWTM, exercise, home modification, PEMF, PNF patterns	Home modification with non skid floors, raised food, and water bowls
Peripheral neuropathies	Kidney Qi, Yin, or Yang deficiency	TH-5, LI-4, LI-10, BL-23, ST-36, KID-3, LIV-3, GB-39, Liu-feng (forelimb); *Bu Yang Huan Wu or Di Huang Yin Zi*	UWTM, exercise therapy, acupuncture, PNF, PROM, PEMF	
Brachial plexus injuries	Kidney Qi or Yin deficiency	SI-9, TH-5, TH-14, LI-4, LI-10, PC-8, BL-23, ST-36, KID-3, Liu-feng (forelimb); *Di Huang Yin Zi*	UWTM, exercise therapy, acupuncture PNF, PROM, PEMF	Remember to add Gabapentin as these patient will experience tingling in the affected foot as recovery progresses

References

1 Zhang, E.Q. (2010). Bi Syndrome (arthralgia syndrome). *J Tradit Chin Med = Chung I Tsa Chih Ying Wen Pan* 30 (2): 145–152.

2 Preast, V. and Xie, H. (2007). Acupuncture for treatment of musculoskeletal and neurological disorders. In: *Xie's Veterinary Acupuncture* (ed. V. Preast and H. Xie), 247–250. Iowa: Blackwell Pub.

3 Hu, J. (2002). How to differentiate and treat Bi-syndrome by acupuncture and moxibustion? *J Tradit Chin Med = Chung I Tsa Chih Ying Wen Pan* 22 (1): 73–76.

4 Johnston, S.A. (1997 July). Osteoarthritis. Joint anatomy, physiology, and pathobiology. *Vet Clin North Am Small Anim Pract* 27 (4): 699–723. doi: 10.1016/s0195-5616(97)50076-3. PMID: 9243777.

5 Millis, D.L. and Levine, D. (1997 July). The role of exercise and physical modalities in the treatment of osteoarthritis. *Vet Clin North Am Small Anim Pract* 27 (4): 913–930. doi: 10.1016/s0195-5616(97)50086-6. PMID: 9243787.

6 Johnston, S.A., McLaughlin, R.M., and Budsberg, S.C. (2008 November). Nonsurgical management of osteoarthritis in dogs. *Vet Clin North Am Small Anim Pract* 38 (6): 1449–70, viii. doi: 10.1016/j.cvsm.2008.08.001. PMID: 18954692.

7 Mosley, C., Edwards, T., Romano, L. et al. (April 26, 2022). Proposed Canadian consensus guidelines on osteoarthritis treatment based on OA-COAST stages 1-4. *Front Vet Sci* 9: 830098. doi: 10.3389/fvets.2022.830098. PMID: 35558892; PMCID: PMC9088681.

8 Mlacnik, E., Bockstahler, B.A., Müller, M. et al. (December 1, 2006). Effects of caloric restriction and a moderate or intense physiotherapy program for treatment of lameness in overweight dogs with osteoarthritis. *J Am Vet Med Assoc* 229 (11): 1756–1760. doi: 10.2460/javma.229.11.1756. PMID: 17144822.

9 Corti, L. (2014 June). Massage therapy for dogs and cats. *Top Companion Anim Med* 29 (2): 54–57. doi: 10.1053/j.tcam.2014.02.001. Epub 2014 Feb 14. PMID: 25454377.

10 Alvarez, L. (2022 July). Extracorporeal shockwave therapy for musculoskeletal pathologies. *Vet Clin North Am Small Anim Pract* 52 (4): 1033–1042. doi: 10.1016/j.cvsm.2022.03.007. PMID: 35715112.

11 Vezzoni, A. and Benjamino, K. (2021 March). Canine elbow dysplasia: ununited anconeal process, osteochondritis dissecans, and medial coronoid process disease. *Vet Clin North Am Small Anim Pract* 51 (2): 439–474. doi: 10.1016/j.cvsm.2020.12.007. PMID: 33558015.

12 Tan, D.K., Canapp, S.O., Jr, Leasure, C.S. et al. (July 19, 2016). Traumatic fracture of the medial coronoid process in 24 dogs. *Vet Comp Orthop Traumatol* 29 (4): 325–329. doi: 10.3415/VCOT-15-09-0154. Epub 2016 Apr 22. PMID: 27102430.

13 Xie, H.S. and Vanessa, P. (2013). *Traditional Chinese Veterinary Medicine: Fundamental Principles*, 2e. Chi Institute, 85–107.

14 Beierer, L.H. (2021 March). Canine carpal injuries: from fractures to hyperextension injuries. *Vet Clin North Am Small Anim Pract* 51 (2): 285–303. doi: 10.1016/j.cvsm.2020.12.002. Epub 2021 Jan 13. PMID: 33451806.

15 Kowaleski, M.P., Boudrieau, R.J., and Pozzi, A. (2012). Stifle joint. In: *Veterinary Surgery Small Animal*, vol. 1 (ed. K.M. Tobias and S.A. Johnston), 906–988. St. Louis, MO: Elsevier.

16 Vasseur, P.B. (2003). Stifle joint. In: *Textbook of Small Animal Surgery*, 3e, vol. 2 (ed. D. Slatter), 2090–2116. Philadelphia, PA: Elsevier Science Saunders.

17 Carmichael, S. and Marshall, W.G. (2012). Tarsus and metatarsus. In: *Veterinary Surgery Small Animal*, vol. 1 (ed. K.M. Tobias and S.A. Johnston), 1014-1028. St. Louis, MO: Elsevier.

18 Dewey, C.W. and da Costa, R.C. (2016). Myelopathies: disorders of the spinal cord. In: *Practical Guide to Canine and Feline Neurology* (ed. C.W. Dewey and R.C. da Costa), 329–403. Ames: Wiley Blackwell.

19 Campbell, M.T. and Huntingford, J.L. (2016). Nursing care and rehabilitation therapy for patients with neurologic disease. In: *Practical Guide to Canine and Feline Neurology* (ed. C.W. Dewey and R.C. da Costa), 559–585. Ames: Wiley Blackwell.

20 Choi, K.H. and Hill, S.A. (2009 August). Acupuncture treatment for feline multifocal intervertebral disc disease. *J Feline Med Surg* 11 (8): 706–710. doi: 10.1016/j.jfms.2008.11.013. Epub 2009 Jan 31. PMID: 19186087.

21 Xie, H. (2008). *Chinese Veterinary Herbal Handbook*, 2e. Chi Institute of Chinese Medicine, 6.

22 Lewis, M.J., Granger, N., and Jeffery, N.D. (October 15, 2020). Canine Spinal Cord Injury Consortium (CANSORT-SCI). Emerging and adjunctive therapies for spinal cord injury following acute canine intervertebral disc herniation. *Front Vet Sci* 7: 579933. doi: 10.3389/fvets.2020.579933. PMID: 33195591; PMCID: PMC7593405.

23 Frank, L.R. and Roynard, P.F.P. (2018 June). Veterinary neurologic rehabilitation: the Rationale for a comprehensive approach. *Top Companion Anim Med* 33 (2): 49–57. doi: 10.1053/j.tcam.2018.04.002. Epub 2018 May 16. PMID: 30236409.

24 Spinella, G., Bettella, P., Riccio, B., and Okonji, S. (August 13, 2022). Overview of the current literature on the most common neurological diseases in dogs with a particular focus on rehabilitation. *Vet Sci* 9 (8): 429. doi: 10.3390/vetsci9080429. PMID: 36006344; PMCID: PMC9414583.

25 Sims, C., Waldron, R., and Marcellin-Little, D.J. (2015 January). Rehabilitation and physical therapy for the neurologic veterinary patient. *Vet Clin North Am Small Anim Pract* 45 (1): 123–143. doi: 10.1016/j.cvsm.2014.09.007. Epub 2014 Oct 14. PMID: 25440754.

26 Roynard, P., Frank, L., Xie, H., and Fowler, M. (2018 January). Acupuncture for small animal neurologic disorders. *Vet Clin North Am Small Anim Pract* 48 (1): 201–219. doi: 10.1016/j.cvsm.2017.08.003. Epub 2017 Oct 14. PMID: 29037432.

27 Joaquim, J.G. et al. (June 1, 2010). Comparison of decompression surgery. Electroacupuncture, and decompressive surgery followed by electroacupuncture for the treatment of dogs with intervetebral disc disease with long-standing neurologic deficits. *JAVMA* 236: 1225–1229.

28 Hayashi, A.M., Matera, J.M., and Fonseca Pinto, A.C. (2007). Evaluation of electroacupuncture treatment for thoracolumbar intervertebral disc disease in dogs. *J Am Vet Med Assoc* 231: 913–918.

29 Hayashi, A.M., Matera, J.M., da Silva, T.S. et al. (2007). Electro-acupuncture and Chinese herbs for treatment of cervical intervertebral disc disease in a dog. *J Vet Sci* 8: 95–98.

30 Janssens, L.A. and Rogers, P.A. (1989). Acupuncture versus surgery in canine thoracolumbar disc disease. *Vet Rec* 124: 283.

31 Janssens, L.A. (1992). Acupuncture for the treatment of thoracolumbar and cervical disc disease in the dog. *Probl Vet Med* 4: 107–116.

32 Alvarez, L.X., McCue, J., Lam, N.K. et al. (2019). Effect of targeted pulsed electromagnetic field therapy on canine postoperative hemilaminectomy: a double-blind, randomized, placebo-controlled clinical trial. *J Am Anim Hosp Assoc* 55 (2): 83–91.

33 da Cruz Tobelem, D., Silva, T., Araujo, T. et al. (2022 August). Effects of photobiomodulation in experimental spinal cord injury models: a systematic review. *J Biophotonics* 15 (8): e202200059. doi: 10.1002/jbio.202200059. Epub 2022 May 19. PMID: 35484784.

34 Ayar, Z., Gholami, B., Piri, S.M. et al. (2022 February). The effect of low-level laser therapy on pathophysiology and locomotor recovery after traumatic spinal cord injuries: a systematic review and meta-analysis. *Lasers Med Sci* 37 (1): 61–75. doi: 10.1007/s10103-021-03301-5. Epub 2021 Mar 31. PMID: 33791887.

35 Draper, W.E., Schubert, T.A., Clemmons, R.M. et al. (2012). Low-level laser therapy reduces time to ambulation in dogs after hemilaminectomy: a preliminary study. *J Small Anim Pract* 53: 465–469.

36 Gardiner, M.D. (2005). *The Principles of Exercise Therapy: Proprioceptive Neuromuscular Facilitation*, 4e, vol. 9. New Delhi: CBS Publishers, 78–90.

37 Wang, R.Y. (1994 December). Effect of proprioceptive neuromuscular facilitation on the gait of patients with hemiplegia of long and short duration. *Phys Ther* 74 (12): 1108–1115. doi: 10.1093/ptj/74.12.1108. PMID: 7991652.

38 Huntingford, J.L. and Bale, J. (2017). Therapeutic exercises. In: *Physical Rehabilitation for Veterinary Technicians and Nurses* (ed. M.E. Goldberg and J.E. Tomlison), 238–307. Ames: Wiley.

39 Huntingford, J.L. and Fossum, T. (2019). Fundamentals of physical rehabilitation. In: *Small Animal Surgery*, 5e (T.W. Fossum and L.P. Duprey), 105–109. Philadelphia PA: Elsevier.

40 Kathmann, I., Cizinauskas, S., Doherr, M.G. et al. (2006 July). Daily controlled physiotherapy increases survival time in dogs with suspected degenerative myelopathy. *J Vet Intern Med* 20 (4): 927–932.

41 Miller, L.A., Torraca, D., and De Taboada, L. (April 1, 2020). Retrospective observational study and analysis of two different photobiomodulation therapy protocols combined with rehabilitation therapy as therapeutic interventions for canine degenerative myelopathy. *Photobiomodul Photomed Laser Surg* 38 (4): 195–205.

Section VII

Additional Complementary Therapies
(Section Editor – Mushtaq A. Memon)

17

Ayurveda
Tejinder Sodhi* and Rupali Sodhi*

* Corresponding authors

Introduction

Ayurveda is a holistic science of balance and health. It not only deals with the prevention of diseases, promotion of health and longevity, but also cures disease. This system of medicine determines the quality and power of herbs according to the laws of nature; thus herbs can collectively or individually be used to match individual diseases or conditions. It should be noted that a majority of Ayurvedic herbs are well-researched and backed by research and clinical trials [1]. Ayurveda in veterinary medicine focuses on animal welfare, treatment, therapies, management, and surgery. Salihotra was the first to be credited as an animal healer and he wrote the Ayurvedic materia medica in veterinary medicine [2]. He also wrote *Mrig* (animal) and *Hasti* (elephant) Ayurvedic texts dedicated to animal welfare and treatment. The first recorded veterinary hospital was opened by King Ashoka in 1463 BC and used Ayurvedic botanicals [3]. Knowledge of basic philosophy and principles of Ayurveda is an essential tool that goes hand in hand with using Ayurvedic products. However, due to the abundance of scientific data on clinical research about Ayurvedic herbs, any clinician should be able to utilize the benefits for their animal patients.

Theory of Tridoshas

Body typing is a unique concept in Ayurvedic medicine, based on three primary constitutions known as Vata, Pitta, and Kapha. These three are collectively referred to as the *Doshas*. Determining the constitution is a vital tool to uniquely approach patients, allowing the clinician to best tailor recommendations. It is believed that balancing the dosha doesn't just improve the health of the individual being, but also the whole world that interacts with that being. Therefore, healing according to dosha is thought to heal not only the patient, but contributes to healing the world itself.

Kapha types tend to be calm, slower moving, and more relaxed compared to others in their species. They have a mesomorph body type. A breed it can be likened to would be an old, loyal, golden retriever.

Pitta types tend to be competitive, fast acting, and will take the lead in social settings most often. They tend toward endomorphic body types. They are also the type that are fastest toward dominant and protective aggression, not to be confused with fear-based aggression, which is considered more Vata. A pit bull or rottweiler is a good example.

Vata types tend to be outgoing albeit nervous types that have an ectomorph body type and tend toward fear and nervousness in new situations. Greyhounds, Afghans, and Whippets are all breeds that symbolize the Vata type.

Functions of the Tridosha

Maintaining balance within the tridosha is fundamental for optimal health. Together, the doshas govern all metabolic activities; anabolism (Kapha), catabolism (Vata), and metabolism (Pitta) [4]. Each dosha is enhanced by anything that is similar to it, be it food, emotions, or the season. Similarly, each dosha is decreased by things that are its opposite. For example, Vata is dry, light, and cold; so, any food, lifestyle, or behavior that increases these qualities will increase the activity of Vata within the body. Conversely, factors that are oily, heavy or hot will decrease Vata influence.

There can be up to ten different constitutions, depending on the combinations of Vata, Pitta, and Kapha. Doshas can be manifested in an individual in various combinations like Vata-Pitta, Pitta-Kapha, Kapha-Vata and so on, with one predominant Dosha governing it. The combination of the three dosha remains unchanged throughout an individual's lifetime and can indicate lifelong inherent strengths and susceptibilities.

I) Disease and Classification of Disease

To understand disease, we must understand health. Health is constantly challenged by the external environment as well as the internal environment of the body. When these two are not in equilibrium, disease process starts. A state of health occurs where digestion is well balanced, and body types "Vata, Pitta, and Kapha" are in equilibrium and waste products (urine, feces, and sweat) are produced and eliminated at normal levels. Along with these processes, sensory organs work normally, and mind and consciousness are harmoniously working as a unit.

Along with other classifications, diseases are also classified according to the doshas Vata, Pitta or Kapha.

Kapha body types have tendency toward Kapha disease. Most Kapha diseases are related to recurring tonsillitis, sinusitis, and bronchitis and lung congestion. Kapha disorders originate at stomach.

Pitta types will have pitta type disease like bile and liver disorders, gall bladder diseases, GI ulcers and acid reflux as well as inflammatory bowel disease. Pitta disease originates in the small intestine.

Vata types are susceptible to gas, colic, lower back pain, arthritis, scratches and paralysis. These diseases of Vata originate at large intestine.

Any imbalance in the disease process affecting body will ultimately reflect on one's mind and behavior as well. Vata imbalance creates fear, depression, and nervousness. Pitta imbalance will create anger, heat, and jealousy. Kapha produces greed, passiveness, and lassitude.

II) Diet

In veterinary medicine, dietary strategies are exceptionally useful. By assessing the constitution of the animal and understanding the impacts different foods have on the dosha, one can tailor their dietary recommendations to help achieve balance and thus cure disease. Dietary advice is tailored to balance the dosha of the patient, while also reducing the dosha of the disease manifesting, which is usually the same Dosha, though not always.

Vata promoting foods are dry and light such as dried fruits, apples, melons, potatoes, tomatoes, eggplant, ice cream, beef, peas and green salad. Those predominantly Vata should limit these foods, as there is already enough Vata activity in their natural being that foods which promote more Vata, will surely lead to imbalance and therefore disease. However, sweet fruits, avocadoes, coconut, brown rice, red cabbage, bananas, grapes, cherries, and oranges are good for Vata types.

Pitta promoting foods are spicy foods, peanut butter, sour fruits, bananas, papayas, tomatoes and garlic. Foods that inhibit Pitta are mangoes, oranges, pears, plums, sprouts, green salad, sunflower seeds, asparagus, and mushrooms.

Kapha promoting foods tend to be moist and cool such as bananas, melons, coconut, dates, papayas, pineapple, and dairy products. However, pomegranate, cranberry, basmati rice, sprouts, and chicken are also beneficial for Kapha constitution.

Seasonal variations should also be considered as well. In summer avoiding pitta aggravating foods like spices or pungent foods are beneficial. In autumn vata food should be avoided, e.g. dry fruits, high protein foods. In winter, avoid cold drinks, ice cream, cheese and yogurt. Certain foods are incompatible such as milk and fish, meat, milk, beef and yogurt as well as sour fruits and milk. So they should not be taken together.

III) Seasonal Variations of Vata, Pitta, and Kapha

The seasons are also considered in Ayurvedic treatments as each season naturally encourages a particular dosha. When in balance, you can see this play out naturally when a Pitta type, who runs warm, has a preference for fall and winter, which are Vata and Kapha times of year. The coolness of Vata and Kapha complement the individual's hot tendency. Whereas, in the summer, this same individual may become irritable and agitated. This is true for animals as well, most notably in behavior changes and the occurrences of common cyclical conditions, such as rashes or otherwise inexplicable diarrhea for instance.

IV) Ayurvedic Materia Medica

Ayurvedic herbs are classified by energetics and effects on the dosha which are determined by a plant's flavor, and its effects on, during, and after digestion. Today, research continues to elucidate the mechanisms and the value these traditional plants have as potential treatments and adjunct therapies.

Amla (*Emblica officinalis*)

Amla fruit (*Emblica officinalis*), also known as Indian gooseberry, is revered for its anti-aging and immune system enhancing properties. This plum-sized fruit contains up to 700 mg of vitamin C per berry [5]. The natural ascorbate is also synergistically enhanced by the bioflavonoids and polyphenols contained in each fruit. In traditional Ayurvedic medicine, amla has been particularly indicated for anemia, asthma, bleeding gums, diabetes [6], respiratory viruses [7], hyperlipidemia [8], and hypertension [9].

Ashwagandha (*Withania somnifera*)

Ashwagandha literally means "to impart the strength of a horse" and is used in Ayurveda as a daily rasayana, or anti-aging therapy. It is one of the most highly regarded and widely used Ayurvedic herbs and is believed to increase energy and overall health and longevity. Ashwagandha can be used on a long-term daily basis without the risk of side effects. Some select uses include that it supports the activity of lymphocyte and macrophages [10]. Ashwagandha has potent anti-inflammatory properties and is used in osteoarthritis and other inflammatory conditions and is considered neuro-protective in nervous tissue injury and inflammation [11]. It also has anti-carcinogenic activity and is used in patients undergoing chemotherapy and radiation [12]. It is used for anemia due to its higher iron content and steroidal lactone which affects bone marrow. Ashwagandha is also used in thyroid problems [13]. I have successfully used Ashwagandha liquid in chronic renal failure in cats and in inappropriate urination (behavioral) in cats as well. I have also used it in stress-related issues such as travel, addition of a new pet or family member, etc.

Bacopa (*Bacopa monnieri*)

Bacopa (also known as Brahmi which in Sanskrit means Creator) is a potent herb for supporting the mind and has been shown also decrease signs of stress in animals in a dose-related activity that was similar to lorazepam [14]. It has also been shown to support T4 concentrations in hypothyroid mice [15].

Boswellia (*Boswellia Serrata*)

This is one of the most potent anti-inflammatory herbs in the Ayurvedic materia medica. Used alone or in combination with other herbs, it can be taken externally and internally to treat various arthritic and inflammatory conditions. As an anti-arthritic and anti-inflammatory agent, Boswellia is a promising alternative to conventional NSAIDS with the added effect of sparing the GI lining, unlike NSAIDS. It is most commonly used for osteoarthritis, degenerative disc disease, and any inflammatory condition of bones, joints, and spine [16]. Additionally, inflammatory bowel disease [17], antitumor [18], anti-asthma activity [19], and neuroprotective activities have been reported [20]. Lastly, dermatological actions [21] and cholesterol lowering [22] effects have been documented.

Ginger (*Zingiber officinalis*)

The rhizomes are highly valued as a spice for their characteristic odor and warm pungent taste. Ginger possesses antioxidant properties [23] and is known to act as a systemic anti-inflammatory [24]. It is also used as an antiemetic and digestive aid [25], supports fertility [26], neuroprotective [27], and analgesic [28].

Guggal (*Commiphora Mukul*)

Guggal is a plant native to India that has been successfully used for centuries to treat a wide variety of ailments. Not only has it effectively remedied lipid disorders [29] and thyroid problems [30] but it has also been used against cancer [31], skin lesions, and wounds [32].

Neem (*Azadirachta Indica*)

Neem has attracted worldwide attention in the medical community due to its wide range of medicinal properties. It has been used to treat skin wounds including wound myiases from bug bites [33]. Similarly, it is known to be insecticidal [34] and fungicidal [35] as well as an insect repellent [36]. It also has been used in sheep as an anthelminthic [37].

Phyllanthus Niruri

Phyllanthus niruri is a perennial herb found in Central and Southern India and Ceylon. This plant, also known as *Phyllanthus amarus*, is one of a variety of Phyllanthus species that is used medicinally. Traditionally, *Phyllanthus niruri* has a wide variety of applications, with use of all parts of the plant. A decoction of the whole plant may be given in cases of jaundice [38]. Other indications for use of the whole plant include certain other genitourinary infections [39].

Triphala

Triphala is a combination of three herbs – *Terminalia chebula* (Haritaki), *Terminalia belerica* (Bahera), and *Emblica officinalis* (Amla). This long revered herbal blend has been used for thousands of years and is referred to in almost every Ayurvedic textbook. It is considered a powerful antioxidant [40] and has digestive and bowel regulating properties [41]. It has also been shown to support dental health [42] and visual acuity [43].

Turmeric (Curcuma longa)

Turmeric is a famous culinary spice from India that is an essential staple of Indian food and culture. It has been used medicinally since antiquity. Today, the phenolic pigment curcumin is largely credited many of its anti-inflammatory effects. In canines, it has been studied for osteoarthritis favorably [44]. Additionally, it has been shown to improve immune function [45], improve liver health [46], and support cardiovascular health [47].

Tylophora Indica (Anantamul)

Tylophora indica, also known as anantamul in Sanskrit, has been used for respiratory conditions such as asthma, bronchitis, and whooping cough [48]. It has also been used for dysentery, and diarrhea. It is recommended for rheumatic ailments and gout pains. The leaves and roots are used as a substitute of lpecacuanha. The leaves contain alkaloids tylophorine and tylophorinine which help cure dermatitis [48].

References

1 Yurdakok-Dikmen, B., Turgut, Y., and Filazi, A. (2018). Herbal bioenhancers in veterinary phytomedicine. *Front Vet Sci* 5: 249.

2 Jamanadas, K. (2004). *Decline and Fall of Buddhism: A Tragedy in Ancient India*, 1e. 235.

3 Somvanshi, R. (2006). Veterinary medicine and animal keeping in ancient India. *AAHF* 10 (2): 1–12.

4 Konjengbam, H., Leona Devi, Y., and Meitei, S.Y. (2021). Correlation of body composition parameters and anthropometric somatotypes with Prakriti body types among the Meitei adults of Manipur, India. *Ann Hum Biol* 48 (2): 160–165.

5 Abeysuriya, H.I., Bulugahapitiya, V.P., and Loku Pulukkuttige, J. (2020). Total vitamin c, ascorbic acid, dehydroascorbic acid, antioxidant properties, and iron content of underutilized and commonly consumed fruits in Sri Lanka. *Int J Food Sci* 2020: 4783029.

6 Patel, S.S. and Goyal, R.K. (2011). Prevention of diabetes-induced myocardial dysfunction in rats using the juice of the Emblica officinalis fruit. *Exp Clin Cardiol* 16 (3): 87–91.

7 Lv, J.J., Yu, S., Xin, Y. et al. (2015). Anti-viral and cytotoxic norbisabolane sesquiterpenoid glycosides from Phyllanthus emblica and their absolute configurations. *Phytochemistry* 117: 123–134. 1.

8 Koshy, S.M., Bobby, Z., Jacob, S.E. et al. (2015). Amla prevents fructose-induced hepatic steatosis in ovariectomized rats: role of liver FXR and LXRα. *J Int Menopause Society* 18 (2): 299–310.

9 Ojha, S., Golechha, M., Kumari, S., and Arya, D.S. (2012). Protective effect of Emblica officinalis (amla) on isoproterenol-induced cardiotoxicity in rats. *Toxicol Ind Health* 28 (5): 399–411.

10 Priyanka, G., Anil Kumar, B., Lakshman, M. et al. (2020). Adaptogenic and immunomodulatory activity of ashwagandha root extract: an experimental study in an equine model. *Front Vet Sci* 7: 541112.

11 Gupta, M. and Kaur, G. (2019). Withania somnifera (L.) Dunal ameliorates neurodegeneration and cognitive impairments associated with systemic inflammation. *BMC Complement Altern Med* 19 (1): 217.

12 Malik, F., Kumar, A., Bhushan, S. et al. (2009). Immune modulation and apoptosis induction: two sides of antitumoural activity of a standardized herbal formulation of Withania somnifera. *Eur J Cancer* (Oxford, England: 1990) 45 (8): 1494–1509.

13 Abdel-Wahhab, K.G., Mourad, H.H., Mannaa, F.A. et al. (2019). Role of ashwagandha methanolic extract in the regulation of thyroid profile in hypothyroidism modeled rats. *Mol Biol Rep* 46 (4): 3637–3649.

14 Wynn, S.G. and Fougère, B.J. (2007). Veterinary herbal medicine: a systems-based approach. *Vet Herb Med* 291–409.

15 Kar, A., Panda, S., and Bharti, S. (2002). Relative efficacy of three medicinal plant extracts in the alteration of thyroid hormone concentrations in male mice. *J Ethnopharmacol* 81: 281–285.

16 Majeed, M., Nagabhushanam, K., Lawrence, L. et al. (2021). Boswellia serrata extract containing 30% 3-acetyl-11-keto-boswellic acid attenuates inflammatory mediators and preserves extracellular matrix in collagen-induced arthritis. *Front Physiol* 12: 735247.

17 Abdel-Tawab, M., Werz, O., and Schubert-Zsilavecz, M. (2011). Boswellia serrata: an overall assessment of in vitro, preclinical, pharmacokinetic and clinical data. *Clin Pharmacokinet* 50 (6): 349–369.

18 Khan, M.A., Ali, R., Parveen, R. et al. (2016). Pharmacological evidences for cytotoxic and antitumor properties of Boswellic acids from Boswellia serrata. *J Ethnopharmacol* 191: 315–323.

19 Soni, K.K., Meshram, D., Lawal, T.O. et al. (2021). Fractions of boswellia serrata suppress LTA4, LTC4, cyclooxygenase-2 activities and mRNA in HL-60 cells and reduce lung inflammation in BALB/c mice. *Curr Drug Discov Technol* 18 (1): 95–104.

20 Gomaa, A.A., Farghaly, H.A., Abdel-Wadood, Y.A., and Gomaa, G.A. (2021). Potential therapeutic effects of boswellic acids/Boswellia serrata extract in the prevention and therapy of type 2 diabetes and

Alzheimer's disease. *Naunyn-Schmiedeberg's Arch Pharmacol* 394 (11): 2167–2185.

21 Singh, S., Khajuria, A., Taneja, S.C. et al. (2008). Boswellic acids: A leukotriene inhibitor also effective through topical application in inflammatory disorders. *Phytomedicine: Int J of Phytotherapy and Phytopharmacology* 15 (6-7): 400–407.

22 Kiczorowska, B., Samolińska, W., Al-Yasiry, A., and Zając, M. (2020). Immunomodulant feed supplement Boswellia serrata to support broiler chickens' health and dietary and technological meat quality. *Poult Sci* 99 (2): 1052–1061.

23 Ali, B.H., Blunden, G., Tanira, M.O., and Nemmar, A. (2008). Some phytochemical, pharmacological and toxicological properties of ginger (Zingiber officinale Roscoe): a review of recent research. *Food and Chemical Tox: Int J = for the British Industrial Biological Research Association* 46 (2): 409–420.

24 Öz, B., Orhan, C., Tuzcu, M. et al. (2021). Ginger extract suppresses the activations of NF-κB and Wnt pathways and protects inflammatory arthritis. *Eur J Rheumatol* 8 (4): 196–201.

25 Amber, K., Badawy, N.A., El-Sayd, A. et al. (2021). Ginger root powder enhanced the growth productivity, digestibility, and antioxidative capacity to cope with the impacts of heat stress in rabbits. *J Therm Biol* 100: 103075.

26 Gholami-Ahangaran, M., Karimi-Dehkordi, M., Akbari Javar, A. et al. (2021). A systematic review on the effect of Ginger (Zingiber officinale) on improvement of biological and fertility indices of sperm in laboratory animals, poultry and humans. *Vet Med Sci* 7 (5): 1959–1969.

27 Hussein, U.K., Hassan, N., Elhalwagy, M. et al. (2017). Ginger and propolis exert neuroprotective effects against monosodium glutamate-induced neurotoxicity in rats. *Molecules (Basel, Switzerland)* 22 (11): 1928.

28 Wilson, P.B. (2015). Ginger (Zingiber officinale) as an analgesic and ergogenic aid in sport: a systemic review. *J Strength Cond Res* 29 (10): 2980–2995.

29 Bellamkonda, R., Karuna, R., Sasi Bhusana Rao, B. et al. (2017). Beneficiary effect of Commiphora mukul ethanolic extract against high fructose diet induced abnormalities in carbohydrate and lipid metabolism in wistar rats. *J Tradit Complement Med* 8 (1): 203–211.

30 Panda, S. and Kar, A. (2005). Guggulu (Commiphora mukul) potentially ameliorates hypothyroidism in female mice. *Phytother Res PTR* 19 (1): 78–80.

31 Anwar, H.M., Moghazy, A.M., Osman, A., and Abdel Rahman, A. (2021). The Therapeutic Effect of Myrrh (Commiphora molmol) and Doxorubicin on Diethylnitrosamine Induced Hepatocarcinogenesis in Male Albino Rats. *Asian Pac J Cancer Prev APJCP* 22 (7): 2153–2163.

32 Gebrehiwot, M., Asres, K., Bisrat, D. et al. (2015). Evaluation of the wound healing property of Commiphora guidottii Chiov. ex. Guid. *BMC Complement Altern Med* 15: 282.

33 Carnevali, F., Franchini, D., Otranto, D. et al. (2019). A formulation of neem and hypericum oily extract for the treatment of the wound myiasis by Wohlfahrtia magnifica in domestic animals. *Parasitol Res* 118 (8): 2361–2367.

34 Mulla, M.S. and Su, T. (1999). Activity and biological effects of neem products against arthropods of medical and veterinary importance. *J Am Mosq Control Assoc* 15 (2): 133–152.

35 de Rezende Ramos, A., Lüdke Falcão, L., Salviano Barbosa, G. et al. (2007). Neem (Azadirachta indica a. Juss) components: candidates for the control of Crinipellis perniciosa and Phytophthora ssp. *Microbiol Res* 162 (3): 238–243.

36 Aidoo, O., Kuntworbe, N., Owusu, F., and Nii Okantey Kuevi, D. (2021). Chemical composition and in vitro Evaluation of the mosquito (anopheles) repellent property of neem (Azadirachta indica) seed oil. *J Trop Med* 2021: 5567063.

37 Chagas, A.C., Vieira, L.S., Freitas, A.R. et al. (2008). Anthelmintic efficacy of neem (Azadirachta indica A. Juss) and the homeopathic product Fator Vermes in Morada Nova sheep. *Vet Parasitol* 151 (1): 68–73.

38 Maity, S., Nag, N., Chatterjee, S. et al. (2013). Bilirubin clearance and antioxidant activities of ethanol extract of Phyllanthus amarus root in phenylhydrazine-induced neonatal jaundice in mice. *J Physiol Biochem* 69 (3): 467–476.

39 Sarin, B., Verma, N., Martín, J.P., and Mohanty, A. (2014). An overview of important ethnomedicinal herbs of Phyllanthus species: present status and future prospects. *Sci World J* 2014: 839172.

40 Peterson, C.T., Denniston, K., and Chopra, D. (2017). Therapeutic uses of triphala in ayurvedic medicine. *J Altern Complement Med* (New York, N.Y.) 23 (8): 607–614.

41 Tarasiuk, A., Mosińska, P., and Fichna, J. (2018). Triphala: current applications and new perspectives on the treatment of functional gastrointestinal disorders. *Chin Med* 13: 39.

42 Shanbhag, V.K. (2015). Triphala in prevention of dental caries and as an antimicrobial in oral cavity – a review. *Infect Disord Drug Targets* 15 (2): 89–97.

43 Gangamma, M.P. and Rajagopala, M. (2010). A clinical study on "Computer vision syndrome" and its management with Triphala eye drops and Saptamrita Lauha. *Ayu* 31 (2): 236–239.

44 Sanderson, R.O., Beata, C., Flipo, R.M. et al. (2009). Systematic review of the management of canine osteoarthritis. *Vet Rec* 164 (14): 418–424.

45 Khodadadi, M., Sheikhi, N., Haghbin Nazarpak, H., and Nikbakht Brujeni, G. (2021). Effects of dietary turmeric

(Curcuma longa) on innate and acquired immune responses in broiler chicken. *Vet Anim Sci* 14: 100213.

46 Moghadam, A.R., Tutunchi, S., Namvaran-Abbas-Abad, A. et al. (2015). Pre-administration of turmeric prevents methotrexate-induced liver toxicity and oxidative stress. *BMC Complement Altern Med* 15: 246.

47 Kumar, F., Tyagi, P.K., Mir, N.A. et al. (2020). Dietary flaxseed and turmeric is a novel strategy to enrich chicken meat with long chain ω-3 polyunsaturated fatty acids with better oxidative stability and functional properties. *Food Chem* 305: 125458.

48 Gururani, R., Patel, S., Yaduvanshi, N. et al. (2020). Tylophora indica (Burm. f.) merr: an insight into phytochemistry and pharmacology. *J Ethnopharmacol* 262: 113122.

18

Veterinary Ozone and Prolotherapy

Signe Beebe

Veterinary Ozone

Introduction

Ozone (O_3) is a blue, gaseous molecule, composed of three atoms of oxygen with a cyclical structure; ozone is O_3 oxygen is O_2. O_3 occurs naturally in the stratosphere and acts as a filter to protect the earth from harmful ultraviolet radiation. It has a distinctive pungent acrid odor and is explosive in its liquid or solid form. O_3 can also be formed from electrical discharges that catalyze the formation of ozone from atmospheric oxygen during lightning strikes and can often be smelled after a storm. O_3 is a highly reactive, unstable form of oxygen that cannot be stored; and due to its instability, the half-life of ozone is temperature-dependent and quite short (at 20°C, O_3 concentration will be reduced by half within 40 min) upon which it reverts back to the more stable form of oxygen [1–3]. The word "ozone" comes from the Greek word "ozein," which means "smell" and was first isolated by the German-Swiss chemist Christian Friedrich Schönbein in the mid-nineteenth century [4].

The effects of O_3 have been studied and recorded for over 150 years, and the medical use of O_3 for water treatment, disinfection, and its antimicrobial properties have been well documented [1–3]. However, the use and application of O_3 in veterinary medicine is still in the developmental stage. O_3 was initially used as a microbicidal molecule in 1856 and subsequently used as an operating room disinfectant and in water treatment. The first medical use of O_3 is said to have been during World War I for the treatment of gangrene in German soldiers, and to follow, a Swiss dentist began to use O_3 in endodontic treatments [1]. Since this time, the medical use of O_3 has been expanded and its use today is based on its anti-oxidant, immunostimulant, anti-microbial, and anti-protozoal properties. In addition, current research shows the potential use of O_3 to treat HIV and cancer [5–7]. Although O_3 is well known as a toxic gas, its medical use in low concentrations has been well-established as a promising medical modality for many different conditions because of its broad mechanism of actions [8–11]. Medical O_3 (also known as oxygen-ozone therapy) is produced by a medical generator that uses high voltage electrical discharge as the source of energy to produce a standardized medical oxygen-ozone gas. Medical O_3 concentration should be composed of no less than 95% O_2 and no more than 5% O_3 [2, 8]. In this process, oxygen molecules are pulled apart and reorganized in the form of O_3. The first ozone generator was developed in 1857 by the French chemist Marius Paul Otto and the first O_3 generator in the US was patented by Nikola Tesla in 1896, later forming the "Tesla Ozone Company," in the late nineteenth century [12].

Ozone Paradoxical Mechanism of Action

Chronic inflammatory processes are characterized by high oxidative stress, reactive oxygen species, suppression of anti-oxidant capacity, and immunologic dysregulation, each of which in turn creates a perpetual cycle of promotion and maintenance of the inflammatory process. In these cases, medical O_3 therapy is thought to act as a bioregulator to help control and stop these chronic processes. O_3 is one of the most powerful known oxidizing agents, surpassed only by flourine and persulphate [1, 12–14]. O_3 as an oxidant, shows a paradoxical activity when it encounters organic molecules, causing a powerful antioxidant response. Antioxidants are critical for the maintenance of cellular integrity and cytoprotection. Once O_3 contacts body fluids and tissues it rapidly reacts with all macromolecules (lipids, proteins, carbohydrates, and DNA) of the cellular membranes [15] to create hydrogen peroxide (ROS-reactive oxygen species) and a mixture of lipid ozonation products (LOP), mainly composed of 4-hydroxynonenal (4-HNE), one of the major end products of lipid peroxidation and an inducer of oxidative stress, and trans-4 hydroxy-2-hexenal (4-HHE) from

Integrative Veterinary Medicine, First Edition. Edited by Mushtaq A. Memon and Huisheng Xie.
© 2023 John Wiley & Sons, Inc. Published 2023 by John Wiley & Sons, Inc.
Companion Website: www.wiley.com/go/memon/veterinary

polyunsaturated fatty acids (PUFA). These two important groups of by-products, ROSs that rapidly stimulate important biochemical processes in the early phase and LOPs, in the later phase, act as secondary messengers to promote and modulate the nuclear factor-erythroid-derived 2-related factor 2 (Nrf2) pathway. Nrf2 is a key transcription factor that coordinates expression of genes encoding antioxidant and detoxifying enzymes and stimulates the synthesis of several substances such as: γ-glutamyl transferase, γ-glutamyl transpeptidase, HSP-70, HO-1, and antioxidant enzymes such as such as super-oxide dismutase (SOD), glutathione peroxidase (GSH-Px), catalase, and glucose-6-phosphate dehydrogenase (G6PDH). This process represents the basis of the paradoxical phenomenon, for which an oxidizing molecule, such as O_3, triggers a potent anti-oxidant reaction [9, 15] (Figure 18.1). At a therapeutic dose, O_3 acts as a modulator or pro-drug and by inducing secondary messengers, facilitates the ensuing adaptive responses by the body. The main goal behind the use of repeated O_3 treatments is to create resistance against oxidative stress (oxidative preconditioning) through the stimulation of the antioxidant system to produce cytoprotective effects in order to help treat and control different pathological conditions [16–19].

O_3 Antimicrobial Effects

The antimicrobial effects are one of the most important properties of O_3. The oxidant activity of O_3 has long been used to disinfect and kill bacteria, viruses, fungi, yeast, and protozoa. In bacterial, infections O_3 therapy disrupts the bacterial cell wall through oxidation of the phospholipids and lipoproteins. This action is non-specific and selective to microbial cells; it does not damage human body cells because of their major antioxidative ability [20, 21]. After the membrane is damaged by oxidation, its permeability increases, and O_3 molecules can enter the cells [19–21]. In viral infections, O_3 damages the viral capsid and disrupts the reproductive cycle via peroxidation [19, 22–25], and destroys fungi via the same oxidative mechanism. In its gaseous and oiled forms, O_3 has been successfully used in the treatment of epidermophyton, microsporum, and trichophyton dermatophyte infections, showing inhibitory effects on sporulation via inhibition of enzymes required for multiplication [25, 26]. A study on yeasts evaluated the fungicidal effects of O_3 on different forms of Candida albicans that showed O_3 was highly effective in killing C. albicans in yeast form and inhibited germ tube formation [27]. O_3 has demonstrated activity to destroy protozoa (leishmania giardia, cryptosporidia, and microsporidia) in vitro, using ozonated oil and ozonated water [19, 28, 29].

O_3 Immunomodulation Effects

O_3 can stimulate cells of the immune system due to its reaction with polyunsaturated fatty acids (PUFA) in cellular membranes. When in contact with biological fluids, it forms reactive oxygen species as well as lipid oxidation products. After the peroxidation compounds are formed, H_2O_2 can then diffuse into immune cells and regulate signal transduction, stimulate cellular/humoral

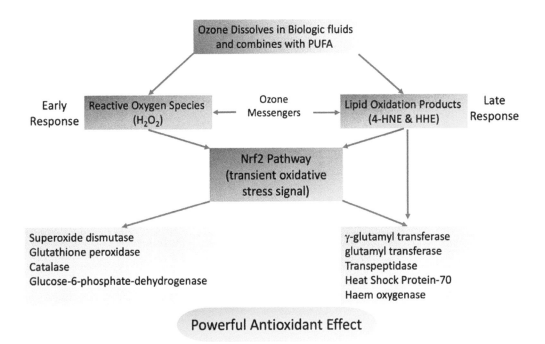

Figure 18.1 Ozone therapy: Paradoxical mechanism of action.

immunity/phagocytic function and immune responses such as reduction of cytokines (interleukin-1, interleukin-6, tumor necrosis factor-α, and interleukin-10 etc.), induction of interferon-γ, and others. O_3 also has a promoting effect on vascular endothelial growth factor (VEGF), platelet-derived growth factor (PDGF), and TGF-β [30–34].

O_3 Anti-inflammatory and Analgesic Effects

Many studies have suggested O_3 therapy as an effective therapeutic option in the management of musculoskeletal disorders [11, 35–38]. The activation of Nrf2-antioxidant signaling pathway is thought to attenuate NF-$\kappa\beta$, a key regulator of the inflammatory response and prevent muscle atrophy, as discussed in several in vivo studies [39–41]. Other studies have assessed the effects of O_3 on musculoskeletal pain. It is well known that pain is a common clinical sign related to the inflammatory process, and O_3 therapy might play a key role in the modulation of nociceptive pain perception [11, 42].

Ozone Method of Administration and Veterinary Applications

O_3 has a broad range of action, making it an effective therapy for many types, conditions, and diseases in veterinary medicine (Table 18.1). O_3 generators today can generate a precise volume and oxygen-ozone concentration where ozone constitutes 3–5% of the total. The therapeutic effects of O_3 are dose-dependent, and safe when given by the recommended route. The same type of precautions for systemic administration of any medication should be taken when using medical O_3. The use of the appropriate product or concentration of O_3 for the condition is essential to avoid toxicity [1, 2, 12]. Rapid administration is to be avoided and breathing in O_3 directly can be toxic to the lungs. Adverse effects occur when ozonation products overwhelm the body's anti-oxidant system, and can lead to toxicity that includes the formation of free radicals and reactive intermediates, induction of lipid peroxidation chain reaction, destruction of biomolecules and enzymes, and alteration of cellular membranes with tissue destruction [19, 43]. O_3 can be administered via the systemic [44] and local routes and the volume of ozone will be different depending on the route of administration.

Ozone Studies/Research in Veterinary Medicine

There are few research studies available on medical O_3 therapy in veterinary medicine, and most of the current literature is specific for its use in humans. The author

Table 18.1 Medical ozone therapy by species.

Species	Application
Canine	Stifle/hip/elbow arthritis
	Intervertebral disk disease
	Back and neck pain
	Conjunctivitis
	Dentistry/tooth infection
	Wound healing
	Bacterial infection
	IBD
	Anal fistula
	Ulcerative colitis/proctitis
	Adjunct for cancer
	Dermatitis
	Otitis
Feline	Dentistry/tooth infection
	Dermatitis
	Adjunct for cancer
Equine	Laminitis
	Back pain
	Osteoarthritis
	Dentistry
	Wound healing
Bovine	Clinical and subclinical mastitis
	Metritis
	Retained of fetal membranes
	Urovagina
	Wound healing
	Podermatitis
Lagomorph	Dermatitis
	Tooth infection
Ovine/Caprine	Acute foot infection
	Retained fetal membranes
	Wound healing
Porcine	Herniated disk
	Wound healing

recommends reading the reviews that have been recently published [10, 19] in the last three years, which indicate an increasing interest in O_3 as a treatment modality. Two excellent systematic reviews of the current literature on the use of O_3 therapy in veterinary medicine were published in 2020 and 2021 [45, 46]. Both of these reviews discussed the application of O_3 therapy in multiple species. The results of one review [46] showed that two-thirds of the articles selected on the use of O_3 in veterinary medicine were published in the past decade, and the remainder from

2000–2010. The majority of the articles on the use of O_3 as a healing agent referred to experimental studies. Fifty of the 117 papers documented clinical research on laboratory animals or in vitro. The best results were seen on the use of O_3 in cattle and small ruminants where the therapeutic effects of O_3 were confirmed by a large number of articles [10]. In these studies' a large number of animals were treated, and the clinical studies used standardized, reproducible protocols. Some equine medicine O_3 studies also showed good results for several conditions. Several studies indicated beneficial effects of O_3 for musculoskeletal disorders, urinary tract disease, or as adjuvant therapy in oncological patients. However, most of the papers did not use standardized methods or analyzed objective, quantifiable parameters to determine the efficacy of O_3 therapy. Some did not have a high enough number of subjects, to provide statistical significance. Both papers indicated a need for more clinical studies from empirical O_3 administration to standardized methods, in order to develop O_3 therapy protocols that are reproducible in similar circumstances [45, 46].

Major Autohemotherapy (MAHT)-this term is used to describe O_3 therapy as applied to the blood. It is considered to have immunomodulatory, anti-inflammatory, and analgesic effects. A small amount of blood is taken from the patient, mixed with a specific concentration of ozone and then intravenously infused back into the patient. The ozonized blood is typically a much brighter red than the drawn blood. MAHT has been used to treat antibiotic resistant skin infections in the dog, chronic active hepatitis, chronic antibiotic resistant UTI, and cancer.

O_3UV also known as Ultra-Immunotherapy or Ultraviolet Blood Irradiation is the same as MAHT, except that the ozone-blood mixture is then passed through UV light before it is re-infused back to the patient. The use of this application is similar to MAHT and is more effective in cases with immune deficiency and dysregulation and is the choice for immune-mediated diseases.

Minor Autohemotherapy (mAHT) is the intramuscular injection of ozonized blood, using equal parts ozone and blood. The mixture is shaken to obtain a homogenous blend of ozone and blood and then injected into a large muscle group, typically the rear leg. This method is often used to treat dermatitis, wounds, allergies, and local pain.

Ozone Infiltration refers to the administration of ozone gas directly into different tissues of the body. It can be given subcutaneously, intra-muscularly, intra-articular, peri-articular, intra-discal, and intra-lesional. This technique is used to treat disorders of the musculoskeletal system such as herniated disk, osteoarthritis, tendinitis, back and neck pain.

Rectal/Vaginal/Uterus Insufflation involves introducing ozone gas into the colon, vagina, or uterus via catheter. This technique is used for treating metritis, retained fetal membranes and urovagina in large animals and for ulcerative colitis/proctitis, IBD, anal fistula, and gastrointestinal cancer.

Local or Topical therapy includes the use of ozonated creams, oils, water, or saline. Topical oils and creams can be applied to the surface of the body for skin disorders or for wound healing.

O_3 water or saline can be used to flush out the ears, the mammary glands, fistulas, and in dentistry [47]. The use of ozone bagging is especially helpful for non-healing wounds of the extremities, its application is in the form of a transcutaneous O_3 gas bath in a closed system so there is no escape of O_3 into the surroundings, breathing in the gas is to be strictly avoided.

Summary

O_3 therapy in veterinary medicine is in the early stages of development, and the information presented here in terms of the administration and application of O_3 in veterinary medicine can be expected to change as more information becomes available. With the increase in antimicrobial resistance and rising veterinary costs, ozone could be a cost-effective valuable addition to the veterinarian's armentarium.

Veterinary Prolotherapy

Introduction

Prolotherapy is an injection-based treatment for weak and/or damaged tendons and ligaments and for the treatment of chronic musculoskeletal pain [48–51]. This technique is analogous to the historical use of firing and blistering for the treatment of tendon-ligament injuries in the horse.

Modern prolotherapy was developed in the 1930's by George Hackett, a general surgeon that published one of the first textbooks on prolotherapy in 1956 [52, 53]. Dr Hackett coined the phrase prolotherapy because his technique caused the "proliferation" of new healthy connective tissue and a permanent increase in tensile strength of previously weak and/or damaged tendons and ligaments.

Prolotherapy Mechanism of Action

Conventional prolotherapy technique involves injection of a proliferant solution directly into weak or damaged tendon-ligaments; ligament and tendon weakness or laxity can be thought of as connective tissue pathology with insufficient tensile strength or tightness [53]. Prolotherapy is thought to work by creating local inflammation that results in the production and release of growth factors to the area of injection that turns on the body's acute injury healing system [49–54] In essence, prolotherapy solution and injection technique mimics acute injury. The body then produces growth factors that stimulate fibroblast proliferation that in turn produces collagen that is essential to rebuild the weak or injured tendons and ligaments. Over time, tissue strengthening, remodeling and contraction of new collagen deposition occur that tightens the soft tissues injected and reduces joint laxity and subsequently relieves pain. In general, the minimum time between prolotherapy treatments is 4–6 weeks with this time frame being modified depending on the individual case. Anti-inflammatory medications or treatments are contraindicated during treatment as prolotherapy relies on the production of local inflammation to produce its beneficial effects [50, 52, 53, 55].

Prolotherapy Technique

There are numerous types of prolotherapy solutions, however the most commonly used solutions contain hypertonic dextrose, sterile water, and a local anesthetic such as lidocaine or procaine. Other additives include, B12, homeopathics such as Zeel and polysulfated glycosaminoglycan (Adequan^R) [56]. The choice of solution and number of injections depend on the animal's age, breed, weight, condition, and existing cormorbidities. Regenerative injection therapy (RIT) using platelet rich plasma (PRP) [57, 58] as well as intraarticular ozone (prolozone) [59–61] may also be included in prolotherapy protocols particularly in severe conditions. Prolotherapy can be painful depending on the solution used, and many animals require sedation to achieve the needed level of restraint to perform it. The use of a short acting, reversible sedation (e.g. low dose dexmedetomidine) to minimize anesthetic risk is advisable in these cases. The affected joints and surrounding areas are clipped, cleaned, and an antiseptic solution (alcohol or chlorhexadine) and then intra-articular and peri-articular injections are done. Post-procedure pain is variable, and if pain is significant, a narcotic analgesic (tramadol) or a calming neurotransmitter (gabapentin) may be prescribed. No anti-inflammatory drugs may be given as it will interfere with the inflammatory response required for successful prolotherapy results.

Conditions Treated with Prolotherapy

There are many different types of musculoskeletal conditions (Table 18.2.) that can be treated with prolotherapy.

Proper application of prolotherapy technique requires a thorough knowledge of anatomy in order to avoid iatrogenic trauma to the joint and surrounding tissues. Adverse effects seen following prolotherapy are local bruising around the injection sites as well as mild transient pain and stiffness (2–3 days) in some animals. Prolotherapy should be used with caution in animals with any underlying condition that could interfere with healing such as cancer, active infection (e.g., dermatitis, UTI), or immune deficiency.

Prolotherapy Studies

Since the 1930's, studies and reports have demonstrated the effectiveness of prolotherapy for musculoskeletal problems, including case reports, pilot, retrospective, open face prospective, and double-blind placebo-controlled studies. There are several noteworthy studies documenting the effects of prolotherapy to improve tendon-ligament strength. Liu et al. [62, 63] conducted a double blind prolotherapy study in 1983 designed to evaluate the effects of prolotherapy using a solution containing 5% sodium morrhuate on the medial collateral ligament in rabbits. Following the prolotherapy treatments, histopathology was performed on the ligaments and it was shown that repeated injections of 5% sodium morrhuate produced a significant increase in ligament thickness of 28%, mass increase of 47%, and ligament-bone junction strength increase of 27% when compared to saline controls. In a human study of patients undergoing prolotherapy treatment for chronic low back pain, a biopsy of sacroiliac ligaments taken three months after treatment demonstrated a 60% increase in collagen fibril diameter with patients reporting a significant decrease in pain and increased range of motion. Another study in 1985 by Maynard et al. confirmed the findings of the 1982 study, and showed increases in the diameter of the patellar and Achilles tendons of rabbits after injection with sodium morrhuate as compared with saline-injected control [64]. The mechanism of how prolotherapy

Table 18.2   Conditions treated with prolotherapy.

Cranial cruciate ligament tears or rupture

Canine hip dysplasia and hip laxity

Osteoarthritis/DJD

Medial patella luxation

Elbow dysplasia

Neck pain, back pain, lumbo-sacral stenosis

Intervertebral disc disease

Bicipital tendonitis

Ligament-tendon sprain/sprain

Temporomandibular joint dysplasia

Angular limb deformity

is thought to exert its therapeutic effects has been discussed and evaluated in several studies. In 1995, Schmidt et al. evaluated the effect of growth factors on the proliferation of fibroblasts from the medial collateral and anterior cruciate ligaments in humans. It was shown that stimulation of growth factors can induce fibroblast cell division in ligaments which enhances fibroblast proliferation and plays a critical role in ligament repair [65] Another study done in 2005, evaluated the effect of multiple growth factors on canine flexor tendon fibroblast proliferation and collagen synthesis in vitro. Results showed that growth factors significantly increased flexor tendon fibroblast proliferation and matrix synthesis [66].

Summary

Prolotherapy is a cost-effective, safe, low-risk procedure for pain especially when compared to conventional surgical treatment of weak tendon-ligaments and angular limb deformity. It can be used in animals where existing comorbidities preclude surgery, it decreases the need for chronic non-steroidal anti-inflammatory (NSAID) or steroidal drug administration, prevents early euthanasia, and improves the quality of life and longevity of the animals treated.

References

1 Bocci, V. (2010). *Ozone. A New Medical Drug*, 2e. 101 Philip Drive, Norwell, MA: Springer.

2 Bocci, V.A. (May 1, 2006). Scientific and medical aspects of ozone therapy. State of the art. *Arch Med Res* 37 (4): 425–435.

3 Elvis, A.M. and Ekta, J.S. (2011). Ozone therapy: a clinical review. *J Nat Sci Biol Med* 2 (1): 66–70.

4 Schonbein, C.F. (1843). Uber Die Natur des Eigenthumlichen Geruches, Welcher Sich Sowohl Am Positiven Pole Einer Saule Wahrend der Wasserelektrolyse, wie auch Beim Ausstromen der Gewohnlichen Elektrizitat aus Spitzen Entwickelt. *Ann Phys* 1: 1.

5 Qi, H. and Wang, M. (2021). Mechanism of medical ozone and its clinical application in HIV/AIDS patients. *J Chinese Phys* 1588–1591.

6 Gil-del Valle, L., Suarez, M.A., Rabeiro-Martinez, C.L. et al. (2019). Facial biostimulation with PRP activated with ozone resound on cellular redox balance, improves lipoatrophy and quality of life in HIV patients. *J Pharm Pharmacognosy Res* 7 (4): 273–287.

7 Bocci, V. (January 1, 1994). A reasonable approach for the treatment of HIV infection in the early phase with ozonetherapy (autohaemotherapy). How 'inflammatory' cytokines may have a therapeutic role. *Med Inflamm* 3 (5): 315–321.

8 Bocci, V., Zanardi, I., and Travagli, V. (2011). Oxygen/ozone as a medical gas mixture. A critical evaluation of the various methods clarifies positive and negative aspects. *Med Gas Res* 1 (1): 1–9.

9 Sagai, M. and Bocci, V. (2011). Mechanisms of action involved in ozone therapy: is healing induced via a mild oxidative stress? *Med Gas Res* 1 (1): 1–8.

10 de Souza, A.K., Colares, R.R., and de Souza, A.C. (May 1, 2021). The main uses of ozone therapy in diseases of large animals: a review. *Res Vet Sci* 136: 51–56.

11 de Sire, A., Agostini, F., Lippi, L. et al. (2021). Oxygen-ozone therapy in the rehabilitation field: state of the art on mechanisms of action, safety and effectiveness in patients with musculoskeletal disorders. *Biomolecules* 11 (3): 356.

12 Bocci, V. (1996). Ozone as a bioregulator. Pharmacology and toxicology of ozonetherapy today. *J Biol Reg Homeostatic Agents* 10 (2–3): 31–53.

13 Bocci, V., Borrelli, E., Travagli, V., and Zanardi, I. (2009). The ozone paradox: ozone is a strong oxidant as well as a medical drug. *Med Res Rev* 29: 646–682.

14 Viebahn-Haensler, R. and León Fernández, O.S. (2021). Ozone in medicine. The low-dose ozone concept and its basic biochemical mechanisms of action in chronic inflammatory diseases. *Int J Mol Sci* 22 (15): 7890.

15 Clavo, B., Rodríguez-Esparrago´, N.F., Rodríguez-Abreu, D. et al. (2019). Modulation of oxidative stress by ozone therapy in the prevention and treatment of chemotherapy-induced toxicity. *Rev Prospect* 8: 1–20.

16 Inal, M., Dokumacioglu, A., O´zcelik, E., and Ucar, O. (2011). The effects of ozone therapy and coenzyme Q10 combination on oxidative stress markers in healthy subjects. *Ir J Med Sci* 180: 703–707.

17 Bocci, V. (1999). Biological and clinical effects of ozone. Has ozone therapy a future in medicine? *Brit J Biomed Sci* 56 (4): 270.

18 Kozat, S. and Okman, E.N. (2019). Has ozone therapy a future in veterinary medicine. *J Animal Husband Dairy Sci* 3 (3): 25–34.

19 Sciorsci, R.L., Lillo, E., Occhiogrosso, L., and Rizzo, A. (2020). Ozone therapy in veterinary medicine: a review. *Res Vet Sci* 130: 240–246.

20 Bünning, G. and Hempel, D.C. (1996). Vital-fluorochromization of microorganisms using 3′, 6′-diacetylfluorescein to determine damages of cell membranes and loss of metabolic activity by ozonation. *Ozone Sci Eng* 18: 173–181.

21 Seidler, V., Linetskiy, I., Hubálková, H. et al. (2008). Ozone and its usage in general medicine and dentistry. a review article. *Prague Med Rep* 109 (1): 5–13.

22 Bayarri, B., Cruz-Alcalde, A., López-Vinent, N. et al. (2021). Can ozone inactivate SARS-CoV-2? a review of mechanisms and performance on viruses. *J Hazard Mat* 415: 125658.

23 Roy, D., Wong, P.K.Y., Engelbrecht, R.S., and Chian, E.S.K. (1981). Mechanism of enteroviral inactivation by ozone. *Appl Environ Microbiol* 41: 718–723.

24 Akey, D.H. and Walton, T.E. (1985). Liquid-phase study of ozone inactivation of Venezuelan equine encephalomyelitis virus. *Appl Environ Microbiol* 50 (4): 882–886.

25 Ouf, S.A., Moussa, T.A., Abd-Elmegeed, A.M., and Eltahlawy, S.R. (2016). Anti-fungal potential of ozone against some dermatophytes. *Braz J Microbiol* 47: 1–13.

26 Ali, E.M. (2013). Ozone application for preventing fungal infection in diabetic foot ulcers. *Diabetol Croat* 42 (1).

27 Zargaran, M., Fatahinia, M., and Zarei Mahmoudabadi, A. (2017). The efficacy of gaseous ozone against different forms of Candida albicans. *Curr Med Mycol* 3: 26–32.

28 Khalifa, A.M., El Temsahy, M.M., Abou, E., and Naga, I.F. (2001). Effect of ozone on the viability of some protozoa in drinking water. *J Egypt Soc Parasitol* 31: 603–616.

29 Rajabi, O., Sazgarnia, A., Abbasi, F., and Layegh, P. (2015). The activity of ozonated olive oil against Leishmania major promastigotes. *Iran J Basic Med Sci* 18: 915–919.

30 Sánchez, G.M., Re, L., Perez-Davison, G., and Delaporte, R.H. (2012). Las aplicaciones médicas de los aceites ozonizados, actualización. *Rev Esp Ozonoter* 2: 121–139.

31 Yousefi, B., Banihashemian, S.Z., Feyzabadi, Z.K. et al. (2022). Potential therapeutic effect of oxygen-ozone in controlling of COVID-19 disease. *Med Gas Res* 12 (2): 33.

32 Cardoso, C.C., Carvalho, J.C., Ovando, E.C. et al. (2000). Action of ozonized water in preclinical inflammatory models. *Pharmacol Res* 42: 51–54.

33 Seyam, O., Smith, N.L., Reid, I. et al. (2018). Clinical utility of ozone therapy for musculoskeletal disorders. *Med Gas Res* 8 (3): 103.

34 Zhang, J., Guan, M., Xie, C. et al. (2014). Increased growth factors play a role in wound healing promoted by noninvasive oxygen-ozone therapy in diabetic patients with foot ulcers. *Oxid Med Cell Longev* 2014: 1–9.

35 Paoloni, M., Di Sante, L., Cacchio, A. et al. (2009). Intramuscular oxygen-ozone therapy in the treatment of acute back pain with lumbar disc herniation: a multicenter, randomized, double-blind, clinical trial of active and simulated lumbar paravertebral injection. *Spine* 34: 1337–1344.

36 De Sire, A., Baricich, A., Minetto, M.A. et al. (2019). Low back pain related to a sacral insufficiency fracture: role of paravertebral oxygen-ozone therapy in a paradigmatic case of nociplastic pain. *Funct Neurol* 34: 119–122.

37 De Sire, A., Stagno, D., Minetto, M.A. et al. (2020). Long-term effects of intra-articular oxygen-ozone therapy versus hyaluronic acid in older people affected by knee osteoarthritis: a randomized single-blind extension study. *J Back Musculoskelet Rehabil* 33: 347–354.

38 Li, W., Khor, T.O., Xu, C. et al. (2008). Activation of Nrf2-antioxidant signaling attenuates NFkappaβ-inflammatory response and elicits apoptosis. *Biochem Pharmacol* 76: 1485–1489.

39 Mourkioti, F., Kratsios, P., Luedde, T. et al. (2006). Targeted ablation of IKK2 improves skeletal muscle strength, maintains mass, and promotes regeneration. *J Clin Investig* 116: 2945–2954.

40 Buhrmann, C., Mobasheri, A., Busch, F. et al. (2011). Curcumin modulates nuclear factor kappaB (NF-kappaβ)-mediated inflammation in human tenocytes in vitro: role of the phosphatidylinositol 3-kinase/Akt pathway. *J Biol Chem* 286: 28556–28566.

41 Saha, S., Buttari, B., Panieri, E. et al. (2020). An overview of Nrf2 signaling pathway and its role in inflammation. *Molecules* 25: 5474.

42 De Sire, A., Baricich, A., Minetto, M.A. et al. (2019). Low back pain related to a sacral insufficiency fracture: role of paravertebral oxygen-ozone therapy in a paradigmatic case of nociplastic pain. *Funct Neurol* 34: 119–122. [PubMed].

43 Mustafa, M.G. (1990). Biochemical basis of ozone toxicity. *Free Radic Biol Med* 9: 245–265.

44 Viebahn-Hänsler, R., León Fernández, O.S., and Fahmy, Z. (2012). Ozone in medicine: the low-dose ozone concept—guidelines and treatment strategies. *Ozone: Sci Eng* 34 (6): 408–424.

45 Orlandin, J.R., Machado, L.C., Ambrósio, C.E., and Travagli, V. (2021). Ozone and its derivatives in veterinary medicine: a careful appraisal. *Vet Anim Sci* 13: 100191.

46 Peteoacă, A., Istrate, A., Goanță, A.M. et al. (2020). The use of ozone therapy in veterinary medicine: a systematic review. *Agro-Life Sci J* 9 (2): 226–239.

47 Nogales, C.G., Ferrari, P.H., Kantorovich, E.O., and Lage-Marques, J.L. (2008). Ozone therapy in medicine and dentistry. *J Contemp Dent Pract* 9 (4): 75–84.

48 Gladstein, B. (2012). A case for prolotherapy and its place in veterinary medicine. *J Prolother* 4: e870–85.

49 Alderman, D. (2008). *Free Yourself from Chronic Pain and Sports Injuries*. Family Doctor Press.

50 Aldermann, D. (2007). Prolotherapy for musculoskeletal pain. *Pract Pain Manag* 7 (1): 10–15. https://www.practicalpainmanagement.com/pain/other/musculoskeletal/prolotherapy-musculoskeletal-pain.

51 Beebe, S. (February 1, 2018). Chinese herbal medicine and prolotherapy for treatment of forelimb angular deformity in a juvenile bactrian camel. *Am J Trad Chin Vet Med* 13 (1).

52 Hauser, R.A. and Hauser, M.A. (2007). *Prolo Your Pain Away!: Curing Chronic Pain with Prolotherapy*. Beulah Land Press.

53 Hackett, G., Hemwell, G., and Montgomery, G. (1958). *Ligament and Tendon Relaxation (Skeletal Disability) Treated by Prolotherapy (Fibro-osseous Proliferation)*, 3e. Springfield, IL: Charles C Thomas Publishers.

54 Gordin, K. (2011 May). Case for prolotherapy. Patients. 601.

55 Reeves, K. (2000). Prolotherapy: basic science, clinical studies and technique. In: *Pain Procedures in Clinical Practice*, 2e (ed. T. Lennard), 172–190. Hanley and Belfus.

56 Reeves, K. (1996). Prolotherapy: present and future applications in soft-tissue pain and disability. injection techniques: principles and practice. *Phys Med Rehabil Clin N Am* 6 (4): 917–923.

57 Alderman, D.D. and Alexander, R.W. (2011 October). Advances in regenerative medicine: high-density platelet-rich plasma and stem cell prolotherapy for musculoskeletal pain. *Pract Pain Manag* 11 (8): 49–52.

58 Gordin, K. (2011). Comprehensive scientific overview on the use of platelet rich plasma prolotherapy (PRPP). *J Prolotherapy* 3 (4): 813–825.

59 Shallenberger, F., HMD, A. (2011 May). Prolozone™– regenerating joints and eliminating pain. *J Prolotherapy* 3 (2): 630–638.

60 Shallenberger, F. (2018). HMD A. Journal of Prolotherapy Journal of Prolotherapy. Jop 10.

61 Hashemi, M., Jalili, P., Mennati, S. et al. (2015 October). The effects of prolotherapy with hypertonic dextrose versus prolozone (intraarticular ozone) in patients with knee osteoarthritis. *Anesth Pain Med* 5 (5).

62 Liu, Y., Tipton, C., Matthes, R. et al. (1983). An in-situ study of the influence of a sclerosing solution in rabbit medial collateral ligaments and its junction strength. *Connect Tissue Res* 11: 95–102.

63 Klein, R., Dorman, T., and Johnson, C. (1989). Proliferant injections for low back pain: histologic changes of injected ligaments and objective measurements of lumbar spine mobility before and after treatment. *The J Neurol Orthop Med Surg* 10: 2.

64 Maynard, J.A., Pedrini, V.A., Pedrini-Mille, A. et al. (1985). Morphological and biochemical effects of sodium morrhuate on tendons. *J Orthop Res* 3 (2): 236–248.

65 Schmidt, C. (1995). Effect of growth factors on the proliferation of fibroblasts from the medial collateral and anterior cruciate ligaments. *J Orthop Res* 13 (2): 184–190.

66 Thomopoulos, S., Harwood, F., Silva, M. et al. (2005). Effect of several growth factors on canine flexor tendon fibroblast proliferation and collagen synthesis in vitro. *J Hand Surg Am* 30 (3): 441–447.

Section VIII

Integration of Complementary Therapies in Clinical Practice

(Section Editor – Judith E. Saik)

19

Integrative Approach to Cardiovascular Disease
Kristina M. Erwin

Introduction

Congestive Heart Failure (CHF) is commonly seen in veterinary practice. Understanding the pathophysiology from a conventional and Traditional Chinese Veterinary Medicine (TCVM) viewpoint allows the practitioner to identify multiple pathways for intervention to help stabilize the patient and improve quality of life. An integrative, multi-modal approach including conventional drugs, herbal medicine, acupuncture, rehabilitation, nutrition, and husbandry care further helps to address the primary disease as well as other co-morbidities that often occur with CHF. These techniques can benefit CHF patients throughout the course of their illness from initial diagnoses through to hospice and end-of-life care.

Pathophysiology of Congestive Heart Failure (Conventional)

Congestive heart failure (CHF) is a complex clinical syndrome arising from structural or functional impairment of ventricular filling or ejection of blood. Decreased cardiac output (CO) causes lower blood velocity and blood to pool. Left sided heart failure leads to congestion in the lungs with edema while right sided failure leads to systemic venous congestion and peripheral edema or ascites. Decreased CO also causes decreased renal blood flow and GFR, leading to further sodium and fluid retention [1]. These physiological changes lead to neuro-hormonal responses that increase vasoconstriction and peripheral vascular resistance to try to improve circulation. The heart rate increases to compensate for decreased CO and the heart chambers may dilate or the muscle itself may hypertrophy. The result is increased sympathetic nervous system activation [1].

Clinical signs of CHF include dyspnea, cough, exercise intolerance, sarcopenia, and collapse. Affected animals progress through three stages of increasing severity with clinical signs for Class I only apparent during vigorous exercise, Class II seen during minimal exercise and Class III animals affected even at rest [1]. Conventional treatment depends on disease severity with prognosis for these patients greatly improved by the availability of newer pharmaceutical drugs as well as the expertise of veterinary cardiologists (Table 19.1).

Pathophysiology of Congestive Heart Failure (Traditional Chinese Veterinary Medicine)

An understanding of CHF from a TCVM viewpoint can further give the practitioner opportunities for supporting patients and improving quality of life. In TCVM, the Heart is considered the Emperor of the body and it governs Blood circulation, houses the *Shen* (spirit), and controls sweating [1, 2]. Heart *Qi* supplies the power to pump blood through the body, and the Heart, Lung and Liver all play a role in circulating the Blood. The Heart (and Lung) make Blood from nutrients provided by the Spleen. The Blood is the root of the *Shen* and the Heart/Blood complex directly affects the mental activities of memory, thinking, and sleep. In health, the *Shen* will be balanced, peaceful, and joyful. If the *Shen* is deficient, mental activities are weak and anxious [1, 2].

There are six TCVM Heart Patterns involving *Qi*, *Yin*, and *Yang* (Table 19.2) and 2 TCVM Patterns involving *Zang-fu* organ imbalance (Table 19.3).

Integrative Veterinary Medicine, First Edition. Edited by Mushtaq A. Memon and Huisheng Xie.
© 2023 John Wiley & Sons, Inc. Published 2023 by John Wiley & Sons, Inc.
Companion Website: www.wiley.com/go/memon/veterinary

Table 19.1 Common pharmaceuticals for management of CHF (Note: Please check a current veterinary formulary for the most up to date recommendations for dosage and administration).

Pharmaceutical effect	Example
Phosphodiesterase (PDE) III selective inhibitors	Pimobendan Note: Administer tablets at least one hour before feeding as absorption is reduced when administered with food.
ACE inhibitors	Enalapril Benazepril
B-Adrenergic receptor blockers/antagonists	Sotalol Atenolol
Loop diuretics	Furosemide
Aldosterone antagonists	Spironolactone
Pyridine-sulfonyl urea type loop diuretics	Torsemide
Selective phosphodiesterase V inhibitors	Sildenafil
Methylxanthine drugs	Theophylline
Cardiac glycosides	Digoxin
Anti-coagulants	Aspirin Clopidogrel
Na-channel blockers	Mexiletine
Ca-channel blockers	Diltiazem
Nutritional supplements	Taurine Carnitine Potassium

Table 19.2 Heart TCVM pattern differentiation and treatment [1]. Xie, H et al., 2013; [3]. Beebe, S. 2009.

TCVM pattern	Etiology	Clinical signs	Treatment goals	Treatment options
Heart *Qi*-blood stagnation	Excess or deficiency (upper-*Jiao*), causes blood stagnation or sluggish circulation; blocks heart *Qi*	Painful back/chest, restless, deep-slow pulse, tongue-grey/purple with petechia; Class I disease	Eliminate stagnation/pain, activate *Qi*-blood	Compound *Dan Shen*[a]
Heart *Qi* deficiency	Weakened heart (e.g. age, sick, congenital), poor circulation, stagnation with damp accumulation	Shortness of breath, lethargy, pale-tongue, weak-irregular pulse	Tonify Heart *Qi*	Heart *Qi* tonic[a]
Heart *Yang* deficiency	Cold with *Qi* deficiency, stagnation with phlegm obstruction	Shortness of breath, lethargy, loose stool, cool body, pale/purple-tongue, weak-irregular pulse	Tonify Heart *Qi* and warm *Yang*, strengthen Heart, eliminate cold	*Bao Yuan Tang*
Heart and Kidney *Yang* deficiency	Kidney *Yang* deficiency leads to heart *Yang* deficiency; *Shao Yin* pathogens	Ascites, edema rear limbs, cool back/limbs, slow-superficial-toneless pulse, tachycardia	Tonify Kidney and Heart *Yang*, warm the *Yang*	*Zhen Wu Tang*, Epimedium 8 formula[b]
Heart *Yin* and *Qi* deficiency	*Qi-Yin* damaged, weak Kidney *Yin* affects fluid balance = increased blood viscosity, false heat encourages phlegm obstruction/stagnation, *Qi* deficiency weakens heart	Pain in chest exacerbated by moving; dizziness; red tongue; weak-irregular pulse	Tonify Heart *Qi* and *Yin*, activate Blood, regulate pulse	*Sheng Mai San*, *Yi Guan Jian*
Collapse of *Yang Qi*	Extreme progression of Heart *Qi* and *Yang* deficiency with syncope or coma	Coldness limbs/back, urine retention, blue-purple tongue, feeble pulse	Revive *Yang* to resuscitate collapse	*Shen Fu Tang*

[a] Dr Xie's Jing Tang Herbal Inc, Ocala, FL. USA.
[b] Seven Forests Herbal Formulas, Institute for Traditional Medicine (ITM), Portland, OR. USA.

Table 19.3   Heart TCVM patterns involving *Zang-fu* organ imbalance [2].

TCVM pattern	Etiology	Clinical signs	Treatment goals	Treatment options
Wood-Metal imbalance	Cycle of *Qi* not moving into Lung, fluid accumulation, prevents Blood production, creates *Qi* stagnation	Pulmonary edema, harsh chronic cough (worse 3–5 AM); thin-weak pulse, lavender tongue, cool extremities	Move *Qi* and Blood, tonify Blood	*Xue Fu Zhu Yu Tang**
Shao Yang disharmony	Excess: *Yang* trapped internally, *Qi*-blood trapped in Lung, hindering circulation to periphery	Pulse becomes hard, internalized		*Chai Hu Jia Long Gu Mu Li Tang#*
	Deficient: *Yang* trapped in upper-*Jiao* and on body surface; Fluids cannot descend from Lung to Kidney, *Yin* and *Yang* cannot integrate, source *Qi* cannot be made.	Pulses: superficial, slippery to toneless Tongue: red, purple red, or dark red.		

* This formula increases peripheral blood flow, which reduces heart workload; helps clear hilar edema, acts as anti-tussive
# This formula can be added to heart failure patients with severe pulmonary congestion.

Integrative Therapy

Because CHF is a medically complex disease and most patients are clinically fragile, it is helpful for practitioners to approach case management from a broad perspective. Integrative therapies can improve quality-of-life (QOL) and outcomes for CHF patients. Practitioners should work to match treatment recommendations to client goals, patient tolerance, and the patient's overall clinical status. Treatment recommendations should be revisited frequently to ensure they are appropriate as the case evolves and changes.

Botanicals for Cardiovascular Support

Hawthorn (*Crataegus spp.*)

Actions: Mild positive inotrope; anti-arrhythmic; anti-platelet aggregation; vasodilating; endothelial protective; decreases arterial blood pressure; antioxidant [4].

Research: Shown to reduce signs of heart failure, increase functional capacity and improve quality of life in clinical trials, while demonstrating positive safety profiles with concurrent cardiac medications [5].

Dan Shen (*Salvia miltiorrhiza*)

Actions: Hypotensive, anti-platelet, anti-coagulant, hepatoprotective, fibrinolytic, anti-microbial [4].

Research: Chemical constituents of *Dan Shen* have antioxidant, anti-inflammatory, and anti-apoptotic properties that protect the heart from acute ischemic injury. *Dan Shen* has anti-arrhythmic properties that reduces pathological cardiac remodeling that leads to cardiac hypertrophy and fibrosis [5].

Astragalus (*Astragalus membranaceous*)

Actions: Immune enhancing, cardiotonic, diuretic, hypotensive, adaptogen [4].

Research: Demonstrates protective effects on the cardiovascular, immune, digestive, nervous, and renal systems through various mechanisms, including antioxidant, anti-inflammatory, and anti-apoptotic effects [5].

Ginseng (*Panax ginseng, Panax quinquefolius*)

Actions: Adaptogenic, stimulant, tonic, hypoglycemic, immune stimulant, hepatoprotective, cardioprotective, anti-arrhythmic [4].

Research: Ginsenosides can inhibit reactive oxidative species (ROS) production, stimulate nitric oxide (NO) production, increase blood circulation, ameliorate vasomotor tone, and adjust lipid profile. Additionally, ginsenosides have a multitude of activities in both physiological and/or pathologic conditions concerning cardiovascular disease [6]. Ginseng (Panax quinquefolius) can reverse cardiac hypertrophy, myocardial remodeling, and heart failure, which is associated with and likely mediated by reversal of calcineurin activation [7].

Ginkgo (*Ginkgo biloba*)

Actions: Anti-inflammatory, Platelet Activating Factor (PAF) inhibitor, antioxidant, circulatory stimulant, cognitive enhancer [4].

Research: Ginkgo Biloba Extract (GBE) treatment (100 mg/kg/day for 8 days) significantly attenuated the deleterious cardiac actions of sustained β-adrenergic receptor activation in a rodent model study. The pharmacological actions of GBE treatment alone on sympathetic-cholinergic receptors may be involved in a cardioprotective effect.

The antihypertrophic action of GBE occurs via activation of M2 macrophage/NO pathway [8].

Dandelion Leaf (*Taraxacum officinale*)

Actions: Diuretic, cholagogue, nutritive, antioxidant [4].

Research: A human study demonstrated a significant increase in frequency of urination demonstrating dandelion leaf's potential as a diuretic [9]. Additionally, the mineral content of dandelion leaf with potassium at ≈42.5 mg/g and magnesium at ≈2.5 mg/g may mitigate some of the electrolyte imbalance resulting from pharmaceutical diuretic use [9]. The combination of potassium and magnesium in dandelion leaf have been shown to be equally as effective as KCl [9].

Milk Thistle (*Silybum marianum*)

Actions: Hepatoprotective, demulcent, cholagogue, antioxidant, nephroprotective [4].

Research: Cytoprotective due to antioxidant activity and radical scavenging. Mechanisms of action include blockade and adjustment of cell transporters, p- glycoprotein, estrogenic, and nuclear receptors. It also has anti-inflammatory effects through reduction of TNF-α, along with protective effects on erythrocyte lysis and cisplatin-induced acute nephrotoxicity [10].

Cordyceps (*Cordyceps sinensis*)

Actions: Adaptogen, hypocholesterolemic, lipid-lowering, hepatoprotective, nephroprotective, anti-cancer, antioxidant, anti-asthma, hypoglycemic, *Qi*-tonic, anti-arrhythmic, hypotensive [4, 11].

Research: Oral administration of *Cordyceps sinensis* exerted statistically significant rescue effects on the liver and heart by reversely regulating levels of metabolites that are perturbed in chronic kidney disease [12]. It has also been shown that long-term administration of Cordyceps to patients suffering from chronic heart failure, in conjunction with conventional treatments, promoted an increase in the overall quality of life (general physical condition, mental health, sexual drive, cardiac function) compared to the control group [11]. Other research has demonstrated that use of Cordyceps results in cellular ATP increase which drives increased useful energy [11].

Acupuncture

GV-26: This point is used primarily for emergency situations (shock, apnea, coma).

GV-20 and *An-shen*: These points are used to calm the *Shen*.

PC-6: Cardiovascular disease, including arrhythmias; *Qi*-Blood Stagnation in chest; Regulates Heart *Qi*.

HT-7: Cardiovascular disease; Heart *Qi*, *Yang*, *Yin*, or Blood Deficiency.

CV-14: Alarm point for the Heart; cardiac disorders in general; regulates Heart and Lung *Qi*.

CV-17: Alarm point for the Pericardium; Influential Point for *Qi*; Influential Point for the respiratory system; respiratory and thoracic disorders; cough and dyspnea.

BL-14: Association Point for the Pericardium; cough and general respiratory problems; Heart *Qi* Deficiency.

BL-15: Association Point for the Heart; cardiac disorders, arrhythmias; *Qi*-Blood Stagnation of Heart or chest; Heart *Qi*, Blood, *Yin* or *Yang* Deficiency.

ST-36: General *Qi* tonification.

Heart Failure Co-morbidities

Co-morbidities commonly develop secondary to CHF and can create life-limiting states for affected patients. An integrative approach to these cases can benefit and prolong patient QOL.

I) Cachexia

Cachexia arises as inconsistent blood flow to the gastrointestinal tract causes motility changes in the intestines, which may alter nutrient absorption [13]. Additionally, patients have higher caloric needs with increased respiratory rate and effort. In humans, TNF and cytokines increase metabolic rate of tissues creating increased calorie burning [13].

Therapy Options

Fish oil: Anti-inflammatory, anti-arrhythmic, and positive effects on endothelial function. Helps to manage loss of lean muscle mass through improved muscle cell energy metabolism. May have positive effects on myocardial energy metabolism [14].

Dose: EPA and DHA in dogs and cats [14]

- 40 mg/kg EPA
- 25 mg/kg DHA
- Ideally, sourced from small, cold-water fish. Do not use Cod-liver oil [14].

Research: EPA was associated with weight stabilization, gains in lean body mass, and improvements in QOL markers in weight-losing patients with advanced pancreatic cancer [13]. Other effects include: 1) supplementation with EPA downregulates the amount of TNF-α and NF-κB, and 2) it augments the hyperaminoacidemia-hyperinsulinemia induced increase in the rate of muscle protein synthesis [13].

Myostatin Inhibition: Myostatin is a potent negative regulator of muscle growth that triggers muscle breakdown, hinders muscle protein synthesis, and hinders muscle cell differentiation [13, 15]. There is therapeutic potential for antibody-directed inhibition of myostatin for treating sarcopenia by inhibiting protein degradation and/or apoptosis [13, 15].

Dose: 300 mg/kg daily (Fortetropin) [15]

Research: A prospective, double-blinded study by Kansas State University found that the effects of Fortetropin (MYOS Rens Technology) prevented a rise in serum myostatin during periods of exercise restriction in dogs and curtailed disuse atrophy [15].

Ursolic Acid: Ursolic Acid is commonly found in: apple peels, rosemary, persimmon, lavender, sage, oregano, thyme, basil, and hawthorn. Ideally, 0.14% of the human daily diet should be ursolic acid rich foods [16].

Actions: Antioxidant, anti-microbial, anti-inflammatory, anti-apoptotic, anti-carcinogenic, prevents insulin resistance, hepatoprotective, anti-hyperlipidemic, cardioprotective, prevents diabetes/obesity/muscle wasting, supports brain health [16, 17].

Research: Ursolic acid contributed to restoration of normal cardioprotective enzyme activity levels in rats, which suggests it protects against myocardial ischemia. It has an anti-apoptotic effect in cardiac muscle cells [17]. Ursolic acid stimulated skeletal muscle synthesis and increased skeletal muscle strength via signaling pathways, suggesting use for prevention of sarcopenia [17].

Ashwagandha (*Withania somnifera*):

Actions: Adaptogenic, nervine tonic, sedative, anti-inflammatory, anodyne, anti-oxidant [4].

Research: *Withania somnifera* effectively modulated antioxidant activity, inflammatory cytokines and cell death in a cell line study with THP-1 monocyte cells. Results suggested it may alleviate cancer cachexia and excessive leukemic cell growth [18]. Withaferin-A [reduces] NF-κB-dependent pro-inflammatory cytokine production leading to an attenuation of the cachectic phenotype in a xenograft model of ovarian cancer [19].

II) Gastrointestinal Disturbances

Changes in blood flow secondary to CHF can negatively impact the gastrointestinal (GI) tract causing nausea, diarrhea, and constipation. The clinician should consider feeding strategies, acupuncture, essential oils, probiotics, and conventional drugs to improve GI function and promote appetite.

Chinese Herbal Medicine

Liu Jun Zi Tang (Si Jun Zi Tang + Er Chen Tang): This formula is helpful for digestive weakness coupled with secondary production of Dampness and Phlegm (secondary to Spleen or Stomach *Qi* Deficiency). It regulates the *Qi* [2, 20]. Indications include: chronic vomiting, loose stools, low stamina/lethargy, and shortness of breath. This formula contains Ginseng, which may help to normalize myocardial conduction to slow tachyarrhythmias [2, 20]. Use caution with hypertension or in patients with marked inflammation or have Excess conditions [2, 20].

III) Urinary Incontinence

Incontinence in these animals can be due to Lung *Qi* Deficiency and Kidney *Qi* or *Yang* Deficiency and is exacerbated by the strain of diuretic drugs. Practitioners should recognize that incontinence may be a life limiting symptom as it creates an increased burden of care on clients and damages the human-animal-bond.

Therapy Options

Moxibustion: Useful in Cold animals and may be applied to: GV-4, BL-23, ST-36, SP-6, KID-1, KID-6

Acupuncture: Tonify the Bladder using acupoints: BL-26, BL-28, BL-39, 40, LI 10, ST 36, CV-3

Chinese Herbal Medicine

Suo Quan Wan warms and consolidates Kidney *Qi* [1].

Cuscuta 15 astringes Essence; nourishes the Kidney and reduces discharges, especially associated with Kidney *Yang* Deficiency [21].

Palliative Rehabilitation Techniques

Palliative rehabilitation techniques for patients with heart disease include strength/resistance training; massage (for pain and anxiety); lymphatic drainage; advice/education on home adaptations to facilitate better function; education/emotional support for the family, and social interaction for the patient [22]. Incorporating palliative rehabilitation techniques can prolong good quality of life and further support the human-animal-bond.

Therapeutic Exercise to Maintain Muscles

- Sitting-to-standing
- Laying-to-sitting/standing
- Reverse walking
- Uneven surfaces/Bosu ball/obstacle course work
- Walks (purposeful/for sniffing)
- Gentle hill walks
- Weaving on/off curbs
- Nose Work

Additional Therapies

- Sunshine therapy to support the *Shen* and the human-animal-bond
- Lymphatic and circulatory massage
- Teach owners to do massage or other simple techniques (i.e. light brushing over the body to encourage general circulation).

Hospice Tactics for Advanced Heart Disease

Patients with advanced disease need special consideration. Prioritize supplements and add treatments using a staggered approach. If possible, space medications and supplements throughout the day to avoid overwhelming the GI tract. Practitioners must do their due diligence and research potential herb-drug and herb-herb interactions and monitor closely for adverse effects (e.g., poor appetite, diarrhea). Client education is paramount, and practitioners should check in frequently with clients to ensure treatment recommendations are in concert with patient quality-of-life and client ethics.

Reminder: Gauging Distress

- Respiratory rates in sleeping patients should be <35/min [23, 24].
- Signs of distress include nasal flare, paradoxical breathing, and inability to engage with the environment/owner due to respiratory effort [4, 23, 24].

Food and Fluids: Feed small, frequent meals warmed closer to body temperature. Decrease parenteral fluids or discontinue altogether to improve quality of life.

Comfort Kits: Providing clients with a comfort kit including clear, written instructions and palliative treatments can support hospice patients. These kits empower clients to prevent emergency room visits and preserve patient well-being until the veterinarian can be consulted.

Diuretics: Consider including 1–2 doses of an injectable diuretic in the comfort kit. Patients on Lasix that decompensate can be given the prescribed oral dose hourly until clinical signs improve. If there is only a mild change in clinical signs, the prescribed dose can be given every other hour until clinical improvement. Patients can get 2 mg/kg TID, up to 6 mg/kg if really needed [23, 24].

Terminal Pain: Humans with terminal CHF report pain. Consider low dose of morphine for these patients [23].

- Dogs and cats: 0.2–0.5 mg/kg PO q 6–8 hours.
- Adverse reactions (dysphoria, respiratory depression) can be reversed with naloxone.

- These small doses can still cause nausea, diarrhea, or constipation but it is less likely to happen with oral dosing.

Respiratory Distress: Patients experiencing air hunger can be comforted through air movement from a fan at their level [24]. Short-term use of in-home oxygen may be necessary using a C or E tank with a pediatric oxygen mask or animal specific mask at 2L/min or less several times per day [24]. Lasix and magnesium sulfate can be offered via nebulizer to further palliate air hunger [24].

Sedation Options: Palliative sedation may further help with comfort care in these patients.

- Butorphanol 10 mg/mL for dogs and cats: 0.2–0.4 mg/kg IM or IV; Acepromazine 10 mg/mL for dogs and cats: 0.01–0.02 mg/kg SQ or IM [23, 24]

Body Positioning: Body position can help decrease secretion build up (i.e., head down and patient in sternal).

Conclusion

Treating CHF can be overwhelming for both practitioner and client. Having a broad understanding of progression of disease, common co-morbidities, and treatment tactics throughout all stages will enable the practitioner to better guide the client to support their pet. By providing an integrative, multi-modal approach to therapy, the practitioner can truly support the human-animal bond and impact their patients' quality of life in a positive way.

Acknowledgment

This chapter is dedicated to my teachers – my pets, Prudence and Oliver Erwin.

References

1 Xie, H. et al. (2014). *Practical Guide to Traditional Chinese Veterinary Medicine*. Chi Institute Press.
2 Marsden, S. (2020). Integrative management of cardiopulmonary disorders, lecture notes. CIVT. (delivered 13 February 2020).
3 Beebe, S. (2009 August). Treatment of congestive heart failure with conventional pharmaceuticals plus acupuncture, Chinese herbal medicine and food therapy in a Toy Poodle dog. *AJTCVM* 4 (2).
4 Wynn, S. and Fougere, B. (2007). *Veterinary Herbal Medicine*. Mosby Elsevier.

5 August, K. Palliative herbal medicine- cardiovascular system. lecture notes, Purple Moon Herbs and Studies Hospice and Palliative Care Part 1 (delivered October 2020).

6 Kim, J.-H. (2012). Cardiovascular diseases and Panax ginseng: a review on molecular mechanisms and medical applications. *J Ginseng Res* 36 (1): 16–26. doi: 10.5142/ jgr.2012.36.1.16.

7 Moey, M., Gan, X.T., Huang, C.X. et al. (2012 July 1). Ginseng reverses established cardiomyocyte hypertrophy and postmyocardial infarction-induced hypertrophy and heart failure. *Circ Heart Fail* 5 (4): 504–514. doi: 10.1161/ CIRCHEARTFAILURE.112.967489. Epub 2012 May 10. PMID: 22576957.

8 Mesquita, T.R.R. et al. (2017 May 11). Cardioprotective action of Ginkgo biloba extract against sustained β-adrenergic stimulation occurs via activation of M2/NO pathway. *Front Pharmacol* 8: 220. doi: 10.3389/fphar.2017.00220.

9 Clare, B.A. et al. (2009). The diuretic effect in human subjects of an extract of Taraxacum officinale folium over a single day. J *Altern Complement Med* 15 (8): 929–934. doi: 10.1089/acm.2008.0152.

10 Karimi, G. et al. (2011). 'Silymarin', a promising pharmacological agent for treatment of diseases. *Iran J Basic Med Sci* 14 (4): 308–317.

11 Holliday, J. and Cleaver, M. (2008). Medicinal value of the caterpillar fungi species of the genus Cordyceps (Fr.) Link (Ascomycetes). A review. *Int J Med Mushrooms* 10 (3): 219–234.

12 Liu, X. et al. (2014). Cordyceps sinensis protects against liver and heart injuries in a rat model of chronic kidney disease: a metabolomic analysis. *Acta Pharmacol Sin* 35 (5): 697–706. doi: 10.1038/aps.2013.186.

13 Sakuma, K. and Yamaguchi, A. (2012). Novel intriguing strategies attenuating to sarcopenia. *J Aging Res* 2012: 251217. doi: 10.1155/2012/251217. Epub 2012 Feb 20. PMID: 22500226; PMCID: PMC3303581.

14 Burns, K. (2013). Benefits of fish oils and fatty acids in cardiac patients with valvular disease. lecture notes, ACVIM.

15 Capuzzi, J. (2020). Disuse muscle atrophy inhibited by nutritional supplement. DVM 360 online magazine. July 2, 2020. https://www.dvm360.com/view/disuse-muscle-atrophy-inhibited-by-nutritional-supplement (viewed 16 January 2021).

16 Dohmen, L. (2018). Muscle physiology: ursolic acid herbs. Lecture notes, Sun N Fun Conference.

17 Seo, D.Y. et al. (2018). Ursolic acid in health and disease. *Korean J Physiol Pharmacol* 22 (3): 235–248. doi: 10.4196/ kjpp.2018.22.3.235.

18 Naidoo, D.B. et al. (2018 April 10). Withania somnifera modulates cancer cachexia associated inflammatory cytokines and cell death in leukaemic THP-1 cells and peripheral blood mononuclear cells (PBMC's). *BMC Complement Altern Med* 18 (1): 126. doi: 10.1186/ s12906-018-2192-y.

19 Straughn, A.R. and Kakar, S.S. (2019). Withaferin A ameliorates ovarian cancer-induced cachexia and proinflammatory signaling. *J Ovarian Res* 12: 115. doi: 10.1186/s13048-019-0586-1.

20 Bannink, E. (2020). Liu Jun Zi Tang- mechanisms of anti-emetic effect and appetite support. lecture notes MettaPets, delivered December.

21 Dharmananda, S. (2004). *A Bag of Pearls*. Institute of Traditional Medicine.

22 Edge-Hughes, L. (2021). Palliative care and physiotherapy. blog, Four Leg Rehab Inc, January 02, 2021. https://www. fourleg.com/Blog/473/Blog?b=494 (viewed 16 January 2021).

23 Bittel, E. (2016). Hospice care for congestive heart failure and dyspnea. lecture notes, AHVMA (delivered 21–24 October 2016).

24 Shanan, A. et al. (2017). *Hospice and Palliative Care for Companion Animals: Principles and Practices*. John Wiley & Sons, Inc.

20

Integrative Pain Management
Carolina Medina

Introduction

Assessment and treatment of pain in animals is essential for optimal health and well-being. Assessment of pain in animals is challenging as they are nonverbal; however, the use of validated pain scales provides an objective measurement of pain and therefore treatment success. Management of pain should focus on anticipation of pain, early intervention, and evaluation of treatment response on an individual-patient basis. A multimodal approach to managing pain, including both pharmacologic and non-pharmacologic modalities, is superior to single therapies alone.

Pain Assessment

One of the most challenging aspects of veterinary medicine is pain assessment. Since animals are nonverbal, owners and veterinary professionals must perform pain assessment. If pain is identified, a treatment plan should include assigning a pain score, appropriate pain management, and re-assessment to determine if the selected treatment is effective.

Behavior is the most accurate method for evaluating pain in animals. Attention should be paid to maintenance of normal behaviors, loss of normal behaviors, and/or development of new behaviors that could indicate an adaption to pain or a response to pain relief.

For common causes of pain in dogs and cats, as well as pain behaviors in dogs and cats, please refer to Tables 20.1–20.4.

Pain Scales

There are several species-specific pain scales to assess both acute and chronic pain in animals (Table 20.7). The use of

pain scales decreases subjectivity and observer bias, therefore resulting in more effective pain management leading to overall better patient care.

Websites to Access Pain Scale Information

Colorado State University Canine Acute Pain Scale
http://csu-cvmbs.colostate.edu/Documents/anesthesia-pain-management-pain-score-canine.pdf

University of Glasgow Canine Short Form Composite Pain Score
http://www.isvra.org/PDF/SF-GCPS%20eng%20owner.pdf

Acute post-operative pain scales for dogs include the Colorado State University Canine Acute Pain Scale, and the University of Glasgow Short Form Composite Pain Score. The Colorado State University Canine Acute Pain Scale contains psychological and behavioral indicators of pain, as well as a pain response to palpation [1]. The University of Glasgow Short Form Composite Pain Score is a validated pain scale that is considered a clinical decision-making tool for dogs in acute pain, an indicator of analgesic requirement, and it includes 30 descriptors and 6 behavioral indicators of pain [2].

UNESP-Botucatu Multidimensional Composite Pain Scale

https://static1.squarespace.com/static/56c72d078259b517148247e6/t/579dc74744024362eb01bdbc/1469957961939/UNESP+Botucatu+Multidimensional+Composite+Pain+Scale.pdf

---

(Continued)

(Continued)

Colorado State University Feline Acute Pain Scale
http://csu-cvmbs.colostate.edu/Documents/anesthe sia-pain-management-pain-score-feline.pdf

University of Glasgow Feline Facial Expression Tool
https://www.aprvt.com/uploads/5/3/0/5/5305564/ cmp_feline_eng.pdf

The UNESP-Botucatu Multidimensional Composite Pain Scale is validated in cats for acute, post-operative pain. This pain scale assesses pain expression through behavior, vocalization, and reaction to palpation of a surgical wound. In addition, psychomotor change of posture, comfort, activity, and attitude are included as well as physiological variables such as appetite and arterial blood pressure. Colorado State University developed a Feline Acute Pain Scale for acute, post-operative pain. This scale is based

Table 20.1 Common causes of pain in dogs.

- Osteoarthritis
- Fracture
- Trauma
- Surgery
- Torn cranial cruciate ligament and/or meniscus
- Intervertebral disc disease
- Cystitis, bladder/renal calculi
- Tooth root abscess
- Corneal ulcer, glaucoma
- Foreign body
- Pancreatitis
- Neoplasia
- Otitis

Table 20.2 Common causes of pain in cats.

- Degenerative joint disease
- Fracture
- Trauma
- Surgery
- Urinary obstruction, FLUTD, cystitis, bladder/renal calculi
- Aortic thromboembolism
- Tooth root abscess, resorptive lesions
- Stomatitis
- Pancreatitis
- Corneal ulcer, glaucoma
- Foreign body
- Neoplasia
- Otitis

Table 20.3 Pain behaviors in dogs.

- Excessive panting
- Changes in habits (less social, decreased appetite, changes in sleep, changes in eliminations)
- Abnormal posture (arched back, tucked abdomen, low head carriage)
- Vocalizations
- Changes in activity level (restless, hiding, difficulty standing, rising and/or walking)
- Aggression
- Self-trauma
- Self-protection (decreased weight bearing, protecting body part, not allowing to be held or pet)

Table 20.4 Pain behaviors in cats.

- Facial expressions (grimaces, flattened ears, glazed eyes, mydriasis)
- Change in habits (less social, decreased appetite, decreased grooming, changes in sleep, not using the litter box)
- Abnormal posture
- Vocalizations (meowing, growling, hissing)
- Changes in activity level (restless, decreased jumping, hiding)
- Aggression (growling, hissing, biting, pinning ears back)
- Self-trauma (excessive licking, scratching, biting)
- Self-protection

on psychological and behavioral responses, response to palpation of surgical wound, and body tension. The University of Glasgow has developed a facial expression tool to assess acute pain in cats. This facial expression scale was designed using the ear position (slope of line joining base of ear and tip of ear) and the muzzle/cheek shape. Caricatures were developed and sequenced as a facial scoring scale; one depicting the ear position and the other depicting the nose/muzzle shape. Standardized mouth and ear distances when combined showed excellent discrimination, correctly differentiating pain-free and painful cats in 98% of cases [3].

Helsinki Chronic Pain Index

https://www.fourleg.com/media/Helsinki%20 Chronic%20Pain%20Index.pdf

Canine Brief Pain Inventory
https://www.vet.upenn.edu/docs/default-source/VCIC/ canine-bpi.pdf?sfvrsn=6fd20eba_0

Liverpool Osteoarthritis in Dogs
http://siriusvet.com/storage/app/media/files/load-b-editablepdf-initlvisit-2017.pdf

There are three validated canine chronic pain scales that were created for owners to assess their dog's pain level at home; they include the Helsinki Chronic Pain Index (HCPI), the Canine Brief Pain Inventory (CBPI), and the Liverpool Osteoarthritis in Dogs (LOAD). The HCPI was validated in 2009 [4] for canine osteoarthritis, and it evaluates demeanor, behavior, pain, and locomotion. The CBPI was validated for canine osteoarthritis in 2007 [5] and osteosarcoma in 2009 [6]. It involves assessing pain severity, pain interference with function, and quality of life. The LOAD was validated to evaluate canine elbow osteoarthritis in 2009 [7], and it assesses a dog's mobility in general terms and with exercise.

Feline Musculoskeletal Pain Index

https://cvm.ncsu.edu/research/labs/clinical-sciences/comparative-pain-research/labs-comparative-pain-research-clinical-metrology-instruments-feline-musculoskeletal-pain-index

---

The Feline Musculoskeletal Pain Index (FMPI) is a chronic pain scale used to score the degree of pain associated with a chronic musculoskeletal disorder. It measures the relevant clinical features of a cat's mobility, agility, and disposition that are associated with chronic pain. The FMPI was developed for owner assessment of the severity and impact of musculoskeletal pain. It contains 17 items involving mobility, ability to perform daily activities (i.e., jumping, playing, grooming, using the litter box), and interaction with other pets and people [8].

Multimodal Pain Management

Multimodal pain management involves the use of two or more pain relieving therapies in order to maximize pain relief and minimize side effects. The goal is to affect different aspects of pain processing with the use of different pain relievers. Examples of a multimodal approach include the use of a combination of pharmaceuticals, non-pharmaceuticals, acupuncture, and rehabilitation modalities.

Pharmaceutical Analgesics (Table 20.5)

Local analgesics provide complete analgesia as they block nerve impulse conduction. They should be used with every surgical procedure as it allows for fewer anesthetics to be used.

Opioids are the most effective for managing acute pain and can play a role in managing chronic pain [9]. Full *mu* agonists elicit greater and more predictable analgesia than partial *mu* agonists or *kappa* agonists. Zorbium^{TM} is a buprenorphine transdermal (TD) solution that is FDA-approved for feline acute pain control. It delivers 4 days of pain relief from a single dose, and it is dosed at 2.7–6.7 mg/kg TD, and applied 1–2 hours prior to a surgical procedure.

Studies using both thermal threshold and surgical models demonstrated that tramadol produces a pain-modifying effect in cats via the production of the *mu*-agonist M1 metabolite [10, 11]. Caution when combined with SSRIs, TCAs, MAOIs. Tramadol in dogs has a very short half-life (1.7 hours) and negligible amounts of the opioid M1 metabolite are produced; therefore, it is not a good analgesic for dogs [12].

Many conditions that cause pain have an inflammatory component. NSAIDs are considered the hallmark for chronic pain and perioperative use due to their central and peripheral effects. Numerous studies have proven NSAIDs to be effective for pain control. Galliprant® (grapiprant) is a non-traditional, non-COX-inhibiting NSAID that works as a prostaglandin receptor antagonist. It selectively blocks the EP4 receptor, which is the primary mediator of osteoarthritic pain and inflammation. It does not inhibit production of other prostaglandins that maintain homeostasis.

Robenacoxib is a COX-2 selective NSAID which is FDA-approved for surgical pain in cats. It is effective and well-tolerated for the control of postoperative pain and inflammation in cats undergoing a spay, neuter, or declaw [13]. Meloxicam is a COX-2 selective NSAID that is FDA-approved for surgical pain and inflammation in cats undergoing a spay, neuter, or orthopedic surgery. In the UK meloxicam is approved for long-term use at a lower dose (0.01–0.03 mg/kg PO every 24 hours), as it has been found that meloxicam is effective for feline osteoarthritis and is well-tolerated in cats with stable chronic kidney disease [14].

Gabapentin produces analgesia by downregulating calcium channels and blocking the release of excitatory neurotransmitters. It alters the brain concentrations of GABA; therefore, can cause somnolence especially in high doses. In an experimental dog model of osteoarthritis, Gabapentin reduced the development of cartilage lesions and significantly reduced the expression of MMP-13, a key mediator in osteoarthritis [15].

Amantadine decreases central sensitization through blockade of NMDA receptors in the dorsal horn of the spinal cord. It also increases beta-endorphins and serotonin concentrations, and decreases the pain threshold. A study showed Amantadine is a useful adjunct therapy to NSAIDs for the treatment of canine osteoarthritic pain [16]. Caution should be taken with concurrent use of SSRIs, Tramadol, and Trazodone as it may cause serotonin syndrome.

Acetaminophen is a non-selective COX inhibitor (COX-3) that is used to treat mild to moderate pain in dogs (*never*

Table 20.5 Doses of common pharmaceutical analgesics.

Analgesic	Dose
Lidocaine 2%	Dogs: Infiltration (diluted to 0.5% concentration) 1–5 mg/kg
	Cats: Infiltration (diluted to 0.5% concentration) 2–4 mg/kg
	Dogs and Cats: Epidural 4.4 mg/kg
Bupivacaine 0.5%	Dogs:
	Infiltration 1–2 mg/kg
	Epidural 1.25 mg/kg
	Cats:
	Infiltration 1.1 mg/kg
	Epidural 1.5–2.5 mg/kg
Morphine	Dogs:
	0.5–1 mg/kg IV, IM, SQ q 2 hrs
	CRI: initial loading dose 0.3–0.5 mg/kg IV or IM, then 0.1–1 mg/kg/hr
	Cats:
	0.1–0.25 mg/kg IV, IM, SQ q 2–4 hrs
	CRI: 0.05–0.1 mg/kg/hr
Hydromorphone	Dogs:
	0.05–0.2 mg/kg IV, IM, SQ q 2–4 hrs
	CRI: initial dose 0.025–0.05 mg/kg, then 0.03 mg/kg/hr
	Cats:
	0.05–0.1 mg/kg IV, IM, SQ q 2–6 hrs
	CRI: initial dose 0.025 mg/kg, then 0.01–0.05 mg/kg/hr
Methadone	Dogs: 0.1–1 mg/kg IV, IM, SQ q 4–8 hrs
	Cats: 0.1–1 mg/kg IV, IM, SQ q 4–8 hrs
Buprenorphine	Dogs: 0.005–0.03 mg/kg IV, IM q 4–6 hrs
	Cats: 0.01–0.03 mg/kg IV, IM, OTM e 4–8 hrs
	Cats – Simbadol™ 0.24 mg/kg SQ once a day (lasts 3 days)
	Cats – Zorbium™ 2.7–6.7 mg/kg transdermal (lasts 4 days)
Galliprant™	Dogs: 2 mg/kg q 24 hr
Robenacoxib	Cats: 2 mg/kg SQ q 24 hrs, 1 mg/kg PO q 23 hrs
Gabapentin	Dogs and Cats: 10–30 mg/kg PO q 8 hrs
Amantadine	Dogs and Cats: 3–8 mg/kg PO q 12 hrs
Acetaminophen	Dogs ONLY: 10–15 mg/kg PO q 8 hrs
Methocarbamol	Dogs and Cats: 15–30 mg/kg PO q 12 hrs
Solensia™	Cats ONLY: 1 mg/kg SQ q 30 days

CRI – Constant Rate Infusion, IV – intravenous, IM –intramuscular, SQ – subcutaneous, OTM-oral transmucosal

use in cats). Two studies have shown that acetaminophen reduced the acute inflammatory reaction and pain level after orthopedic surgery in dogs [17, 18].

Methocarbamol, a centrally acting muscle relaxant, can be added to alleviate muscle spasms within the periarticular or compensatory musculature that tend to be secondary pain generators.

Solensia™ is a feline anti-nerve growth factor monoclonal antibody that is FDA-approved for the control of pain associated with osteoarthritis in cats. It is dosed at 1 mg/kg SQ q 30 days.

Synovetin™ is an injectable veterinary device containing a tin radioisotope that emits low-energy therapeutic radiation to reduce inflammation within the treated joint.

It is FDA-approved for intra-articular treatment of elbow osteoarthritis in dogs only.

Non-pharmaceutical Analgesics (Table 20.6)

Polysulfated glycosaminoglycan products are primarily chondroitin sulfate as a semisynthetic preparation from bovine trachea. Reported effects are anti-inflammatory, chondroprotective, and improved lameness [19, 20].

Omega 3 fatty acids are anti-inflammatory eicosanoids that reduce inflammatory cytokines and inhibit glycosaminoglycan loss in cartilage. Mehler found that clinical outcomes for discomfort, lameness, and joint severity at day 84 significantly improved with omega fatty acid supplement [21].

Perna canaliculus is a New Zealand green-lipped mussel that is anti-inflammatory via inhibition of 5-lipoxygenase pathway. It has been shown to significantly improve pain and mobility in dogs with osteoarthritis [22–24].

Undenatured type II collagen contains active immune modulators that reduce the secretion of enzymes that break down type II collagen thereby slowing the inflammatory response. It was found to significantly improve overall pain level and peak vertical force and vertical impulse in dogs with moderate osteoarthritis [25, 26].

A study evaluated the systemic anti-inflammatory and mobility enhancing effects of an eggshell membrane supplement in dogs with pain and mobility impairment due to osteoarthritis. Inflammatory biomarker IL-2 and pain scores were significantly lower in the eggshell membrane supplement group compared to placebo [27].

Glucosamine and chondroitin inhibit IL-1 induced COX2 and PGE2 synthesis, COX independent anti-inflammatory properties (decrease inflammatory cytokine release), inhibit metalloproteinase synthesis, increase production of proteoglycans, and cartilage repair.

Cannabidiol (CBD) decreases pain by inhibiting spinal nociceptive processing, and modulating cellular mechanisms involved in central sensitization. CBD decreases

inflammation by decreasing pro-inflammatory cytokines such as IL-1 and TNF-α, and by increasing anti-inflammatory cytokines such as IL-10. Recent clinical studies have investigated the safety of CBD for dogs and cats and found clinical improvement in clinical metrology instruments (CMIs), as well as a decrease in the veterinary assessment of pain and analgesic requirements. In one study, CBPI and Hudson activity scores showed a significant decrease in pain and increase in activity in osteoarthritic dogs with CBD administration [28]. The addition of CBD to a multimodal approach (NSAID, Gabapentin, and Amitriptyline) for the treatment of canine osteoarthritis significantly improved the CBPI and Quality of Life Index scores in another study [29].

Therapies that Provide Analgesia

Acupuncture stimulates the release of endogenous substances such as beta-endorphins, dynorphins, enkephalins, and serotonin. Studies have shown that acupuncture provides effective postoperative analgesia in dogs [30, 31]. A prospective study was conducted on 181 dogs with musculoskeletal or neurologic diseases to determine the effects of acupuncture alone or combined with analgesics for chronic pain and quality of life. Success rates for Helsinki chronic pain index, quality of life, and visual analog scales for pain and locomotion were 80% when both diseases and groups of treatment were combined. The use of acupuncture alone or in combination with analgesics reduces pain and improves quality of life in dogs with neurological and musculoskeletal diseases [32].

Transcutaneous electrical nerve stimulation (TENS) inhibits pain by releasing beta-endorphins and stimulating sensory nerves. Electrical muscle stimulation (EMS) improved lameness scores in dogs undergoing stabilization of the cranial cruciate ligament deficient stifle [33].

Low-level laser therapy decreases pain by releasing endogenous opioids, changing nerve conduction latencies, increasing cellular metabolism and circulation, promoting neovascularization, decreasing fibrosis formation, and reducing inflammation [34, 35]. Laser therapy was successful in improving lameness and pain scores, and in lowering NSAID requirement in canine elbow osteoarthritis patients [36].

Extracorporeal shockwave produces a high-energy, focused pressure wave that delivers energy to a specific focal point in the body. The pressure from this energy causes cells to release proteins that decrease inflammation and increase blood flow. It also increases serotonin in the dorsal horn, and affects the descending pain pathways. It has been shown to be an effective treatment modality for dogs with hip osteoarthritis as it significantly improved weight bearing measured by force plate analysis [37].

Table 20.6 Doses of common non-pharmaceutical analgesics.

Analgesic	Dose
Polysulfated glycosaminoglycan	4.4 mg/kg IM, SQ twice a week for 4 weeks
Omega 3 fatty acids	100–200 mg/kg/day
Perna canaliculus	22–60 mg/kg/day
Undenatured type II collagen	10 mg daily
Eggshell membrane	18–36 mg/kg/day
Glucosamine and chondroitin	60–70 mg/kg BID × 4–6 wks then QD
CBD	2 mg/kg q 12 hrs

Table 20.7 Links for pain scales associated with this chapter to be posted on book webpage.

Colorado State University Canine Acute Pain Scale

http://csu-cvmbs.colostate.edu/Documents/anesthesia-pain-management-pain-score-canine.pdf

University of Glasgow Canine Short Form Composite Pain Score

http://www.isvra.org/PDF/SF-GCPS%20eng%20owner.pdf

UNESP-Botucatu Multidimensional Composite Pain Scale

https://static1.squarespace.com/static/56c72d078259b517148247e6/t/579dc74744024362eb01bdbc/1469957961939/UNESP+Botucatu+Multidimensional+Composite+Pain+Scale.pdf

Colorado State University Feline Acute Pain Scale

http://csu-cvmbs.colostate.edu/Documents/anesthesia-pain-management-pain-score-feline.pdf

University of Glasgow Feline Facial Expression Tool

https://www.aprvt.com/uploads/5/3/0/5/5305564/cmp_feline_eng.pdf

Helsinki Chronic Pain Index

https://www.fourleg.com/media/Helsinki%20Chronic%20Pain%20Index.pdf

Canine Brief Pain Inventory

https://www.vet.upenn.edu/docs/default-source/VCIC/canine-bpi.pdf?sfvrsn=6fd20eba_0

Liverpool Osteoarthritis in Dogs

http://siriusvet.com/storage/app/media/files/load-b-editablepdf-initlvisit-2017.pdf

Feline Musculoskeletal Pain Index

https://cvm.ncsu.edu/research/labs/clinical-sciences/comparative-pain-research/labs-comparative-pain-research-clinical-metrology-instruments-feline-musculoskeletal-pain-index

Cryotherapy decreases inflammation, histamine release, and edema. It decreases pain by altering muscle spasms, reducing prostaglandin concentration, and slowing nerve conduction. It is useful post activity in the arthritic patient for 15–20 minutes. Thermotherapy increases blood flow and facilitates muscle relaxation. It can break the pain cycle associated with muscle spasms. Its use prior to exercise in arthritic patients for 5–20 minutes can be useful.

Manual therapy can also alleviate pain and includes massage, range of motion, and joint mobilization. Massage improves local blood flow in the soft tissues and decreases muscle spasms. Range of motion improves joint integrity, decreases pain, and lubricates joints. Joint mobilization is the gliding of joints in their cranial, caudal, medial and lateral directions to improve joint integrity, joint mobility, and joint lubrication [38].

Conclusion

A multimodal approach to pain management is important and includes pharmacological and non-pharmacologic analgesic strategies. Every patient is different therefore careful physical examination and review of concurrent illnesses should be taken into account when planning a pain management protocol. Incorporating more than one analgesic strategy is superior to any one alone, as this will allow targeting pain from multiple perspectives.

References

1 Epstein, M., Rodan, I., Griffenhagen, G. et al. (2015 Mar-Apr). AAHA/AAFP pain management guidelines for dogs and cats. *J Am Anim Hosp Assoc* 51 (2): 67–84. http://www.csuanimalcancercenter.org/assets/files/csu_acute_pain_scale_canine.pdf.

2 Mathews, K., Kronen, P.W., Lascelles, D. et al. (2014 Jun). Guidelines for recognition, assessment and treatment of pain: WSAVA global pain council. *J Small Anim Pract* 55 (6): E10–68. http://www.newmetrica.com/cmps.

3 Guidelines for recognition, assessment and treatment of pain. The world small animal veterinary association. www.wsava.org.

4 Hielm-Bjorkman, A. et al. (2009). Psychometric testing of the Helsinki chronic pain index by completion of a questionnaire in Finnish by owners of dogs with chronic signs of pain caused by osteoarthritis. *Am J Vet Res* 70 (6): 727–734.

5 Cimino-Brown, D. et al. (2007). Development and psychometric testing of an instrument designed to measure chronic pain in dogs with osteoarthritis. *Am J Vet Res* 68: 631–637.

6 Brown, D. et al. (2009). A novel approach to the use of animals in studies of pain: validation of the canine brief pain inventory in canine bone cancer. *Pain Med* 10 (1): 133–142.

7 Hercock, C. et al. (2009). Validation of a client-based clinical metrology instrument for the evaluation of canine elbow osteoarthritis. *J Sm An Pract* 50 (6): 266–271.

8 Enomoto, M. et al. (2022 Feb). Refinement of the Feline Musculoskeletal Pain Index (FMPI) and development of the short-form FMPI. *J Fel Med Surg* 24 (2): 142–151.

9 Epstein, M. et al. (2015). AAHA/AAFP Pain management guidelines for dogs and cats. *J Fel Med Surg* 7 (3): 251–272.

10 Pypendop, B. et al. (2009). Effects of tramadol hydrochloride on the thermal threshold in cats. *Am J Vet Res* 70 (12): 1465–1470.

11 Brondani, J. et al. (2009). Analgesic efficacy of perioperative use of vedaprofen, tramadol or their combination in cats undergoing ovariohysterectomy. *J Fel Med Surg* 11 (6): 420–429.

12 KuKanich, B. and Papich, M. (2011). Pharmacokinetics and antinociceptive effects of oral tramadol hydrochloride administration in Greyhounds. *Am J Vet Res* 72 (2): 256–262.

13 King, S. et al. (2012). Evaluation of oral robenacoxib for the treatment of postoperative pain and inflammation in cats: results of a randomized clinical trial. *Vet Sci* 2012 (1-8): Article ID 794148.

14 Gowan, R.A. et al. (2011). Retrospective case-control study of the effects of long-term dosing with meloxicam on renal function in aged cats with degenerative joint disease. *J Fel Med Surg* 13 (10): 752–761.

15 Boileau, C. et al. (2005). Oral treatment with PD-0200347, an alpha2delta ligand, reduces the development of experimental osteoarthritis by inhibiting metalloproteinases and inducible nitric oxide synthase gene expression and synthesis in cartilage chondrocytes. *Arthritis Rheum* 52 (2): 488–500.

16 Lascelles, D. et al. (2008 January–February). Amantadine in a multimodal analgesic regimen for alleviation of refractory osteoarthritis pain in dogs. *J Vet Int Med* 22 (1): 53–59.

17 Mburu, D. et al. (1988). Effects of paracetamol and acetylsalicylic acid on the post-operative course after experimental orthopaedic surgery in dogs. *J Vet Pharmacol Ther* 11 (2): 163–170.

18 Mburu, D.N. (1991). Evaluation of the anti-inflammatory effects of a low dose of acetaminophen following surgery in dogs. *Vet Pharmacol* 14 (1): 109–111.

19 Fujiki, M. et al. (2007 August). Effects of treatment with polysulfated glycosaminoglycan on serum cartilage oligomeric matrix protein and C-reactive protein concentrations, serum matrix metalloproteinase-2 and -9 activities, and lameness in dogs with osteoarthritis. *Am J Vet Res* 68 (8): 827–833.

20 de Haan, J.J. et al. (1994 May–June). Evaluation of polysulfated glycosaminoglycan for the treatment of hip dysplasia in dogs. *Vet Surg* 23 (3): 177–181.

21 Mehler, S. et al. (2016 June). A prospective, randomized, double blind, placebo-controlled evaluation of the effects of eicosapentaenoic acid and docosahexaenoic acid on the clinical signs and erythrocyte membrane polyunsaturated fatty acid concentrations in dogs with osteoarthritis. *Prostaglandins Leukot Essent Fatty Acids* 109: 1–7.

22 Pollard, B. et al. (2006 June). Clinical efficacy and tolerance of an extract of green-lipped mussel (Perna canaliculus) in dogs presumptively diagnosed with degenerative joint disease. *N Z Vet J* 54 (3): 114–118.

23 Bui, L. et al. (2003 Winter). Influence of green lipped mussels (Perna canaliculus) in alleviating signs of arthritis in dogs. *Vet Ther* 4 (4): 397–407.

24 Hielm-Bjorkman, A. et al. (2009 September). Evaluating complementary therapies for canine osteoarthritis part I: green-lipped mussel (Pernacanaliculus). *Evid Based Compl Alt Med* 6 (3): 365–373.

25 Deparle, L. et al. (2005 August). Efficacy and safety of glycosylated undenatured type-II collagen (UC-II) in therapy of arthritic dogs. *J Vet Pharmacol Ther* 28 (4): 385–390.

26 Peal, A. et al. (2007 June). Therapeutic efficacy and safety of undenatured type-II collagen (UC-II) alone or in combination with (-)-hydroxycitric acid and chromemate in arthritic dogs. *J Vet Pharmacol Ther* 30 (3): 275–278.

27 Muller, C. et al. (2019 November). Placebo-controlled pilot study of the effects of an eggshell membrane-based supplement on mobility and serum biomarkers in dogs with osteoarthritis. *Vet J* 253: 105379.

28 Gamble, L. et al. (2018 July 23). Pharmacokinetics, safety, and clinical efficacy of cannabidiol treatment in osteoarthritic dogs. *Front Vet Sci* 5: 165.

29 Brioschi, F. et al. (2020 August 26). Oral transmucosal cannabidiol oil formulation as part of a multimodal analgesic regimen: effects on pain relief and quality of life improvement in dogs affected by spontaneous osteoarthritis. *Animals (Basel)* 10 (9): E1505.

30 Cassu, R. et al. (2012). Electroanalgesia for the postoperative control of pain in dogs. *Acta Cir Bras* 21 (1): 43–48.

31 Gakiya, H. et al. (2011). Electroacupuncture versus morphine for the postoperative control of pain in dogs. *Acta Cir Bras* 25 (5): 346–351.

32 Silva, N. et al. (2017). Effect of acupuncture on pain and quality of life in canine neurological and musculoskeletal diseases. *Can Vet J* 58: 941–951.

33 Johnson, J. et al. (1997). Rehabilitation of dogs with surgically treated cranial cruciate ligament deficient stifles by use of electrical stimulation of muscles. *Am J Vet Res* 58 (12): 1473–1478.

34 Hagiwara, S., Iwasaka, H., Hasegawa, A. et al. (2007). GaAlAs (830 nm) low-level laser enhances peripheral endogenous opioid analgesia in rats. *Lasers Surg Med* 39: 797–802.

35 Schlerder da Rosa, A. et al. (2012). Effects of low-level laser therapy at wavelengths of 660 and 808 nm in experimental model of osteoarthritis. *Photochem Photobiol* 88: 161–166.

36 Looney, A.L. et al. (2018 September). A randomized blind placebo-controlled trial investigating the effects of photobiomodulation therapy (PBMT) on canine elbow osteoarthritis. *Can Vet J* 59 (9): 959–966.

37 Mueller, M. et al. (2007 June 2). Effects of radial shockwave therapy on the limb function of dogs with hip osteoarthritis. *Vet Rec* 160 (22): 762–765.

38 Coates, J. (2013). Manual therapy. In: *Canine Sports Medicine and Rehabilitation* (ed. M.C. Zink and J.B. Van Dyke), 108–114. Ames, IA: Wiley-Blackwell.

21

Integrative Approach to Neurology

Patrick Roynard

Introduction

Neurological disorders are common among companion animals, and some of the most frequently encountered are myelopathies (e.g. intervertebral disc disease [IVDD]) and seizure disorders. Clinical neurology has markedly changed in the past few decades with the spread of advanced imaging, often pre-requisite to an accurate diagnosis for disorders of the central nervous system (CNS). Conventional treatments for neurological disorders can be broadly divided into medical and surgical interventions, with decompression of the CNS being a frequent surgical goal. Various "alternative or complimentary" treatment modalities have been described in the management of small animal neurological disorders, often as an adjunct to standard medical care. Some of these modalities, such as acupuncture and physical rehabilitation for spinal cord injuries (SCIs), have already been investigated in several clinical studies and are relatively well-established practice at this time. This text does not aim at being exhaustive but rather presenting the integrative modalities most used and documented in small animal neurological disorders, along with suggestions for their implementation. The modalities are presented per neurolocalization (i.e. myelopathies, encephalopathies, neuropathies), with emphasis on the most reported indications for integrative therapies first (e.g. acupuncture and physical rehabilitation for IVDD). For more specific discussion regarding each therapeutic modality, the reader is referred to the corresponding sections and chapters of this textbook.

Myelopathies

Acupuncture for Myelopathies

Spinal Cord Injury (SCI)

Following initial spinal cord trauma, neuroscience has established an important secondary neurodegenerative process that occurs, which causes significant cord injury. Calcium entry into neurons and glial cells results in a cytokine and free radical cascade released by activated microglia and damaged mitochondrial membranes [1, 2]. Tumor necrosis factor α (TNF-α), interleukin-1β (IL-1β), matrix metalloprotease-9 (MMP-9), and nitric oxide (NO) promote the inflammatory-cascade, creating neuronal and oligodendrocyte damage. Demyelination of axons, neuronal inflammation and progressive disruption of nervous tissue follows with long-term consequences that impair SCI recovery [2, 3]. No proven pharmacological protocol providing protection from these secondary changes is currently available; however, research suggests acupuncture may inhibit this process. An experimental study of SCI in rats with sham/placebo control demonstrated acupuncture improved functional recovery after SCI compared to controls ($P < 0.01$). Acupuncture attenuated microglial activation ($P < 0.01$) and reduced expression of TNF-α ($P < 0.01$), IL-1β ($P < 0.01$), IL-6 ($P < 0.01$), MMP-9 ($P < 0.05$), NO synthase ($P < 0.001$), and cyclooxygenase-2 ($P < 0.001$). Reduced apoptotic cell death of both neurons and oligodendrocytes ($P < 0.001$) along with axonal loss and lesion size reduction on immune-histochemical staining ($P < 0.05$) demonstrated acupuncture provided neuroprotection [4].

Neuroplasticity defines the ability of nervous tissue to change structurally, resulting in functional changes. Trauma and neurologic disease alter plasticity-factors. Specific neurotrophins, such as brain-derived neurotrophic factor (BDNF) and neurotrophic factor-3 (NT-3) are endogenous plasticity promoters that may be key to recovery from SCI. These neurotrophins are downregulated in SCI [5] and SCI rodent-model studies suggest a positive correlation of BDNF and NT-3 levels with optimum functional neurologic recovery [6, 7] and reduction in neuropathic pain [8]. An SCI murine model study reported a positive correlation between electro-acupuncture's neuro-protective effects and improved locomotor function recovery with the up-regulation of BDNF and NT-3 ($P < 0.05$) [9].

Intervertebral Disc Disease (IVDD)

In the traditional Chinese veterinary medicine (TCVM) paradigm, SCIs are due to *Qi* and Blood Stagnation, and acupuncture has long been used for various myelopathies. Multiple studies document the use of acupuncture for canine IVDD, as adjunct or alternative to standard management. While several studies present methodological flaws and researcher bias (groups not matched, evaluator not blinded), a trend toward faster, more complete recovery appears to be associated with electro-acupuncture (EA), and some authors have concluded EA may have a canine thoracolumbar (TL) IVDD treatment success rate up to 83–95% [10, 11]. In one study on 50 dogs with TL-IVDD, a significantly shorter time to recover ambulation was reported with conventional treatment + EA (10.10 ± 6.49 days) versus conventional treatment alone (20.83 ± 11.99 days; $P = 0.0341$) for non-ambulatory dogs

with intact nociception (grades 3 and 4). The ability to walk without assistance for grades 3 or 4 and overall success rate were also significantly higher with EA (respectively $P = 0.047$ and 0.015) [12]. In a retrospective study (80 dogs) with paraplegia and intact nociception from TL-IVDD (grade 4), the combination of EA with prednisone was significantly ($P = 0.01$) more effective than prednisone alone to recover ambulation; allowed faster return to ambulatory status ($P = 0.011$), relieved back pain ($P = 0.001$) and decreased relapse rate ($P = 0.031$) [13]. Another study compared EA, hemilaminectomy and hemilaminectomy + EA in 40 dogs with more than 48 hours of severe neurologic deficits due to IVDD (only grades 4 and 5) confirmed by diagnostic imaging (MRI, CT, myelography). "Clinical success," defined as a patient initially classified grade 4 or 5 then classified as grade 1 or 2 within 6 months of treatment, was significantly ($P < 0.05$) higher for dogs that received EA alone (15/19, 79%) or EA and surgery (8/11, 73%) than dogs with surgery alone (4/10, 40%) [14]. Refer to Table 21.1 for grading of neurological deficits.

Besides benefiting the spinal cord itself, EA has also shown effects on vertebrae and intervertebral discs likely to be beneficial in cases of IVDD. In a randomized controlled murine study, EA inhibited Wnt-β-catenin, which may delay the degenerative process of cervical intervertebral discs [15]. Acupuncture can also improve the ability of degenerated discs to repair by reducing the amount of type I collagen in the nucleus pulposus while promoting type II collagen, necessary for proper hydration of proteoglycans leading to compression resistance [16, 17]. In an IVDD rat model, EA also increased vertebral blood flow,

Table 21.1 Grading scale for neurological deficits commonly used in canine IVDD and suggested recommendation for use of TCVM and integrative modalities.

0	Normal
1	Cervical or thoracolumbar pain, hyperesthesia with no neurological deficits:
	TCVM and other modalities (e.g. laser) as an adjunct, or alternative to standard management (activity restriction still recommended in acute/painful stage)
2	Ataxia, paresis, decreased proprioception, ambulatory:
	TCVM and other modalities (e.g. laser) ideally used as adjunct to standard management including rehabilitation (activity restriction still recommended in acute/painful stage)
3	Paresis with absent proprioception, non-ambulatory:
	TCVM and other modalities (e.g. laser), as an adjunct to standard management with recommendation for advanced imaging +/− decompressive surgery and rehabilitation
4	Paralysis, nociception present:
	TCVM as adjunct to standard management with recommendation for advanced imaging +/− decompressive surgery and intensive neuro-rehabilitation post-operatively (e.g. NMES, therapeutic exercises including land treadmill, laser)
5	Paralysis, absent nociception:
	Both TCVM, decompressive surgery and intensive neuro-rehabilitation post-operatively (e.g. NMES, therapeutic exercises including land treadmill, laser)

micro-vessel density, and number of normal spinal cord neurons. [18]

TCVM can be used for cervical IVDD and, in the author's opinion, may be one of the most rewarding conditions to treat with EA. A retrospective study (19 dogs, cervical myelopathy), used three different acupuncture protocols: dry needle acupuncture (DN) +/− EA, and Chinese herbal medicine (CHM).[1,2] All 19 dogs, which had previously failed conventional medical/surgical management (18 with IVDD, 1 with fibro-cartilaginous embolic myelopathy), reported both pain and neurological function improvement [19]. A case report also describes successful use of EA and herbals for IVDD at C3-C4 in a miniature Pinscher [20].

While the author still recommends advanced imaging and decompressive surgery when indicated for cases of presumptive IVDD, these results justify offering EA as an adjunct to the "gold standard," whether the conventional management pursued is surgical or conservative. Suggested recommendations for TCVM use based on neurological deficit grade is included in Table 21.1.

Cervical Spondylomyelopathy (CSM)

A clinical trial of 40 dogs with presumptive or diagnosed CSM comparing standard treatment (medical and surgical) vs standard treatment + EA reported an overall EA efficacy of 85% versus 20% standard treatment only (noticeably lower than classically reported) [21]. A retrospective study of 19 animals (13 dogs, 6 horses) with presumptive or diagnosed CSM reported results obtained with the following TCVM treatments: DN, EA, aqua-acupuncture (1000 µcg/ml Vitamin B-12), CHM[1] for all patients, CHM[2] in grades 2 or higher, CHM[3] in patients with cervical pain, and additional Chinese herbal medicines based on the Chinese pattern diagnosis. All animals showed improvement, except for one horse with poor tolerance of acupuncture, precluding completion of treatment [22].

As for IVDD, the author still recommends advanced imaging and surgery (if indicated) for presumptive cases of CSM, but also recommends integrating TCVM and neurological rehabilitation for ideal pain management and functional recovery.

Selection of Acupuncture Points Based on Neuroanatomical Function

For a more in-depth review of the anatomy and physiology relevant to acupuncture, the reader is referred to Section II, Chapters 4 and 6 of this textbook.

Recent studies have allowed identification of criteria associated with higher likelihood of effect when considering acupuncture points. Up to 70% of acupuncture points have been identified as motor entry points, which are locations where the motor branch of a nerve enters the muscle belly of an innervated muscle [23]. These points can be identified with neuromuscular electrical stimulation (NMES) as the point that will elicit maximal contraction of a muscle belly if stimulated. Recently, acupuncture points have also been identified as neurogenic inflammatory spots, which are areas of local tissue response caused by cutaneous neurogenic inflammation encountered in visceral disorders. They are located in the dermatome overlapping the visceral afferent innervation [24]. Features of neurogenic spots include: plasma extravasation, vasodilation in postcapillary venules of the skin, wheal-and-flare reaction and substance P from activated small diameter sensory afferents. Neurogenic spots also show hypersensitivity, high electrical conductance and small diameter nerve fiber-mediated sensation (C fibers, Aδ). Features which are classically associated with acupuncture points [25]. Overall approximately 70% of neurogenic spots were found to match acupoints. More importantly, in murine models of colitis and hypertension, acupuncture was effective when performed at acupoints that were also neurogenic spots, and ineffective at non-neurogenic spot acupoints [24].

Although it has been reported that acupuncture is more efficient when practiced according to patient TCVM Pattern diagnosis (See Section II, Chapter 5), based on these studies and personal observations, the author suggests including local points (e.g. *Jing-jia-ji* for cervical IVDD) and distal points (including specific acupoints identified as motor entry points and/or neurogenic spots) when using EA for neurological disorders (Table 21.2).

Electro-acupuncture Treatment Timing and Parameters

The author recommends acupuncture early after injury/surgery (ideally within 24–72 hours), in order to maximize benefits. Very low frequency EA (2–10 Hz) is helpful in treating neuropathic pain and is, like low frequency EA (20–40 Hz), associated with endorphins and enkephalins release. High frequency (80–120 Hz) and very high frequency (200 Hz) are associated, respectively, with dynorphin and serotonin release. Suggested protocol includes 10 minutes at low frequencies (20/40 Hz), followed by 5–10 minutes at higher (80/120 Hz) and very high frequencies (0/200 Hz), with added very low frequency (2–5 Hz) for 5–15 minutes in case of neuropathic pain, based on severity and patient's tolerance. The author suggests starting each session with "permission points" (e.g. GV-20 and bilateral *An-Shen*) to help patient compliance, and recommends EA 1–2 times/week for the first 3 weeks prior to considering progressive reduction of frequency.

Another benefit is that, acupuncture as a "passive" modality, is acceptable therapy in acute inflammation when the patient may not be a candidate for other

Table 21.2 Acupuncture points for neurological disorders and indication.

Location	Acupuncture point*	Suggested indications (emphasis on neurological disorders)
Thoracic limbs (from proximal to distal)	LI-11 (Large Intestine 11)	Thoracic limbs paresis, radial nerve disorders, elbow pain, diarrhea, clearing heat
	LI-10 (Large Intestine 10)	Thoracic limbs paresis (and paraparesis), musculocutaneous and radial nerve disorders, contralateral motor cortex disorders, elbow pain, immune regulation, diarrhea
	LI-4 (Large Intestine 4)	Thoracic limb paresis, master point for face and mouth
	PC-8 (Pericardium 8)	Thoracic limb paresis, median nerve disorders, oral disorders (e.g. stomatitis); bilateral PC-8 form the "4 roots" with bilateral KID-1
Pelvic limbs (from proximal to distal)	**SP-10 (Spleen-10)**	Paraparesis and paralysis, femoral nerve disorders, blood deficiency
	BL-40 (Bladder 40)	Paraparesis, sciatic nerve disorders, spinal and pelvic pain, pyelonephritis, urinary pain, coxofemoral joint pain, master point for lower back
	GB-34 (Gallbladder 34)	Paraparesis, sciatic nerve disorders, tendon and ligament pain, stifle pain
	ST-36 (Stomach 36)	Paraparesis, sciatic nerve disorders, contralateral motor cortex disorders, gastrointestinal or abdominal pain, nausea, vomiting, gastric ulcers
	BL-60 (Bladder 60)	Paraparesis, sciatic nerve disorders, spinal pain, tarsal pain, headache, cervical pain, hypertension
	LIV-3 (Liver 3)	Paraparesis, generalized pain, anxiety, pelvic limb lameness
	KID-1 (Kidney 1)	Paraparesis and paralysis, heel pain; bilateral KID-1 form the "4 roots" with bilateral PC-8
Truncal (paraspinal)	*Jing-jia-ji* (cervical *Hua-tuo-jia-ji*)	Cervical pain and stiffness (e.g. IVDD, cervical spondylomyelopathy)
	Hua-tuo-jia-ji	IVDD, spinal pain
	BL-23 (Bladder 23)	Spinal pain, paraparesis, urinary tract pain, pyelonephritis
	Bai-hui	IVDD, lumbosacral (LS) disease, pelvic limb pain

* acupoints that are motor entry points are bolded.

interventions (e.g., pain preventing active treadmill work or unstable vertebral fractures) or early post-operative period (Figures 21.1 and 21.2).

Rehabilitation/Physical Therapy for Myelopathies

For a more in-depth review of the anatomy and treatment modalities involved in physical rehabilitation, the reader is referred to Section VI, Chapters 13, 14, and 15 of this textbook.

Physical activity increases levels of neurotrophins and exercise has been suggested the best method to increase BDNF levels [6, 26]. Early initiation after SCI, [5, 27] type of exercise, timing and duration of session(s) have been reported to influence effects; with early treadmill training (repetitive, sustained locomotor work), increasing BDNF boosting functional recoveries in SCI [8, 28], and stroke murine models [29–31]. It is noticeable that static standing

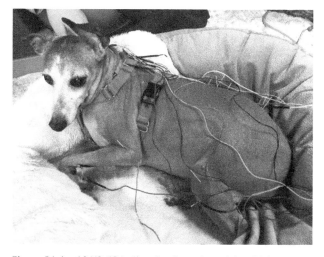

Figure 21.1 10 YO FS Italian Greyhound receiving EA for multifocal IVDD. Note the multiple leads with both truncal/local points (e.g. *Jing-jia-ji*, *Hua-tuo-jia-ji*, Bladder acupoints) and appendicular/distal points (e.g. LI-4, LI-10, ST-36, GB-34).

A

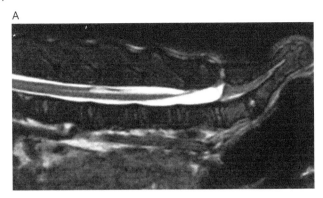

Figure 21.2 (A) T2 weighted fat-sat MR image (sagittal view) showing protrusion of the meninges and spinal cord/ nervous tissue (myelomeningocele) through bifidous spinous process at the last lumbar vertebra (spina bifida) in a six-month-old French Bulldog with congenital urinary/fecal incontinence. The spinal cord is deviated dorsally, consistent with tethered cord syndrome.

B

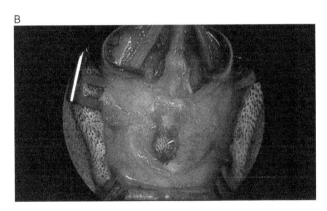

C

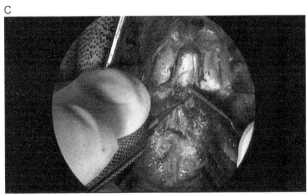

Figure 21.2 (B, C) Intra-operative images of surgical correction. After identification of the myelomeningocele (B), it is dissected down to the vertebral canal and the nervous structures (visible through the durotomy incision) are being dissected from adhesions (C) to restore normal anatomy.

and swimming did not exhibit similar benefits [32]. NT-3 is also up-regulated in the spinal cord and skeletal muscle with treadmill exercise [6, 33, 34]. Studies have shown benefits (albeit sometimes minimal) in neuroplasticity, motor and

D

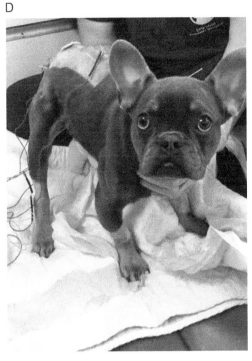

Figure 21.2 (D) Patient one-day post-operative receiving electro-acupuncture at GV-1, CV-1, ST-36, and BL-40.

sensory recovery (allodynia) when exercise is initiated early after neurologic injury [8, 32, 35], with stronger improvements noted with comprehensive, multimodal rehabilitation [36]. This suggests that exercise such as sustained gait training modulates neuro-inflammation and stimulates neurotrophins, which is potentiated when combined with other modalities, NMES, laser, and acupuncture [36–40].

Canine Models of Spinal Cord Injury

Studies in canine models of SCI support the positive association between BDNF and functional recovery [41, 42], with higher levels of BDNF being associated with improved recovery, which can be stimulated with sustained exercise in dogs [43]. However, MMP-9, a pro-inflammatory metalloproteinase, may dampen the benefits of treadmill training in promoting BDNF and NT-3 [35], highlighting the possible synergistic effect of using treatment modalities diminishing neuro-inflammation (e.g. acupuncture, laser) concomitantly to locomotor training. Hence, locomotor training (e.g. land treadmill) appears as a cornerstone for a neuro-rehabilitation program in dogs. In clinical practice, treadmill training is routinely used to initiate rhythmic locomotor movements and is relatively easy to implement (Figure 21.3). In the authors' experience, patients with a remaining degree of motor function (whether ambulatory or not) benefit most from treadmill training. Animals with severe deficits and paralysis may show limited benefits, or even detrimental in stimulating negative neuroplasticity and/or compensation.

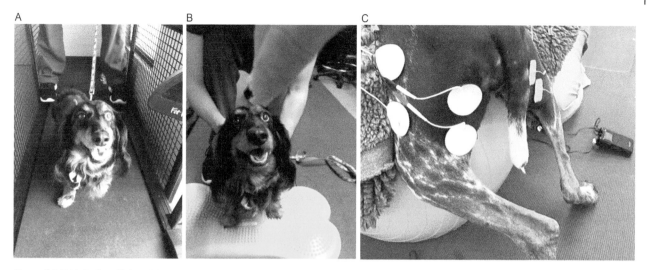

Figure 21.3 (A, B, C) 5YO MN Dachshund recovering from TL IVDD surgery and undergoing physical therapy with land treadmill (A) and balance exercises to help improve proprioception (B). (C) Dog receiving neuromuscular electrical stimulation (NMES) on quadriceps and hamstrings while engaged in an assisted standing exercise (fNMES).

Intervertebral Disc Disease (IVDD)

Several studies report the use of physical rehabilitation in dogs recovering from TL-IVDD surgery, with conflicting findings regarding results, but an overall trend toward improved recovery. Many studies are retrospective, address patients that were non-ambulatory at presentation, involve some rehabilitation even in the control group and all involve multimodal therapy in the protocols including physical exercise (e.g. land treadmill once patients can stand, NMES, balance board, laser therapy) [44–50].

A randomized, blinded, prospective clinical trial on 30 non-ambulatory paraparetic or paraplegic dogs (with pain perception) after surgery for TL-IVDD found that early initiation of intensive postoperative rehabilitation was safe and well-tolerated. No significant improvement in outcome, however, was found when comparing early intensive post-operative rehabilitation [supported standing, NMES, weight shifting/balance board exercises, underwater treadmill] to less intensive post-operative treatment (ice/hot packs, passive ROM, sling walks) [44]. The lack of significant benefits of intense neurologic rehabilitation program(s) in outcome is limited to this study, as all other published studies, albeit retrospective concluded some benefits. A retrospective study on 248 non-ambulatory dogs reported multimodal post-operative rehabilitation did not accelerate recovery, but improved functional outcome with higher chance of complete recovery and lower chance of complications [45]. Another similar retrospective study (186 dogs) reported faster and significantly higher successful outcome with multimodal rehabilitation than without, for all neurological grades (86%, 83/96 vs 52%, 47/90; P < 0.01) [46].

A larger retrospective controlled clinical study (367 paraplegic dogs) also reported significant improvement in recovery of ambulation with intensive neurorehabilitation (P < 0.001) [47]. Finally, another retrospective study of 113 dogs treated with comprehensive rehabilitation post-operatively reported that more time in formal rehabilitation (P < 0.001) and more underwater treadmill sessions (P < 0.001) increased the chances of improvement [50]. This trend is also reported in cervical IVDD, with a retrospective study (58 dogs) reporting significantly higher success with multimodal rehabilitation post-operatively (27/34 vs 15/24; P < 0.05) [51].

Degenerative Myelopathy

A retrospective study reported on the effects of varying intensities of physical rehabilitative therapy on survival and length of ambulatory status in 50 dogs with presumptive degenerative myelopathy (DM) [52]. Survival time was positively associated with the degree of physical rehabilitation therapy. Dogs that received intensive physical rehabilitation (n = 59) had longer survival time (mean 255 days) than dogs with moderate (n = 56, mean 130 days) or no (n = 57, mean 55 days) rehabilitation (P = 0.05). The authors reported that, compared to the group with intensive physiotherapy, the risk of death was 5.8 times higher (P = 0.046) for dogs with moderate physical rehabilitation and 112 times higher (P = 0.001) for dogs without physical rehabilitation [52]. Another retrospective study on 20 dogs with presumptive degenerative myelopathy (DM) receiving a combination of rehabilitation therapy and either one of two different PBMT therapy protocols showed no difference in survival time compared to historical controls for one of the groups, but there was significantly longer time to reach non-ambulatory paraparesis along with longer survival time for the group receiving intense laser therapy treatment (p < 0.05) [53]. Despite study limitations (e.g. few dogs with confirmed DM), this and physical rehabilitation are the only clinical therapies documented that suggest slower disease progression.

Botanical Medicine

A comprehensive review of all herbal indications in small animal neurology is beyond the spectrum of this chapter. For a more in-depth review of herbal medicine with actions and indications, the reader is referred to Section IV, Chapters 9–10 and Section VIII, Chapter 24 of this textbook as well as other texts published on the topic [54].

Research has shown multiple benefits of herbal formulas, such as promoting neural regeneration, seizure control, alleviating pain, reducing hemorrhage, and treating peripheral nerve injuries [55–62]. Several case reports document neurological disorders treated with herbals in dogs and cats, with a retrospective study (50 dogs, 6 cats) treated for pelvic limb paresis/paralysis reporting significantly higher success and faster recovery when using Chinese herbal medicine and EA (compared to conventional medical treatment alone) [63].

Additional Therapeutic Modalities for Myelopathies

Neuromuscular Electrical Stimulation (NMES)

NMES utilizes an electric current applied through electrodes to specific skeletal muscles or motor points, to produce contraction of the muscle [64]. It is documented in experimental and clinical research to improve the performance of both healthy and dysfunctional skeletal muscles [65–70]. NMES is used in neurologic rehabilitation after central nervous system injury to minimize disuse atrophy, reduce muscle spasticity, facilitate the feasibility of exercise training programs, stimulate motor control improvements, and improve gait [65, 71, 72].

NMES recruits motor units in a non-selective, spatially fixed, and temporally synchronous fashion, which leads to heightened muscle fatigue compared to voluntary activation [65, 73]. The non-selective recruitment of NMES creates potential to activate any fiber type at low intensities, as opposed to voluntary action. The therapeutic effect of NMES, therefore, should help attenuate the muscle's response to disuse and accelerate recovery. The ability to target larger motor units as compared to most voluntary contractions is especially useful [65]. NMES combined with active exercises provides the best functional response (e.g. engaging active muscle contraction while standing/bearing weight, potentially on different surfaces) [64, 65, 72, 74]. This highlights the importance of a multimodal approach including NMES, therapeutic exercises, and locomotor training for optimum recoveries (Figure 21.3).

Laser Therapy (PBMT)

Photobiomodulation, also called low-level laser therapy or "cold laser" therapy, may be of interest in CNS and peripheral nervous system disorders due to optimized oxidative neuronal metabolism, reduced pro-inflammatory mediators' expression and reduced glial scaring [75, 76]. Experimental studies have shown significantly improved axonal regrowth, increased axonal number and better functional recovery with laser treatment than without in murine models of SCI [77, 78]. Evidence also exists of benefits in pain management, through disruption of microtubules array and slowing axonal flow for peripheral nerve injuries, and through laser-induced spinal cord changes for chronic pain [79].

Although no adverse effects are reported in the veterinary literature, no consensus exists regarding evidence-based benefits in clinical studies. An unblinded, unrandomized prospective study of non-ambulatory dogs post TL-IVDD surgery reported shorter time to ambulation with laser (3.5 vs 14 days) [39]. However, a blinded, randomized, prospective study also evaluating laser with or without rehabilitation revealed no statistical difference in recovery [48]. Another retrospective study on rehabilitation with or without laser reported a tendency (not reaching statistical significance) for shorter time to ambulation (4.2 ± 8.55 vs 24 ± 18.49 days) [49]. Laser treatment can be started immediately after initial injury/post-surgery, and should be applied directly over the site of injury, with adjustable parameters calculated to achieve a dose and power density within therapeutic range at the targeted tissue (i.e. spinal cord) [80].

Pulsed Electro-magnetic Fields (PEMF)

Pulsed electromagnetic fields therapy may reduce postoperative pain through anti-inflammatory effects and studies on SCI models show possible neuroprotective effects. A randomized, controlled clinical trial (16 dogs) recovering from TL-IVDD surgery reported significant improvement at 6 weeks of incision-associated pain and proprioceptive placing when using PEMF 15 min every 2 hrs for 2 weeks then twice-daily for 4 weeks [81]. One study (22 dogs) with diverse cervical lesions reported 72.8% return to functionality and autonomy with multimodal rehabilitation including pulse-magnetic therapy [82].

Encephalopathies

Acupuncture for Encephalopathies

Traumatic Brain Injury (TBIs)/Cerebrovascular Events ("Strokes")/Post-operative

A rat model of cerebral ischemic stroke demonstrated, similar to SCI models, that EA improved motor impairment

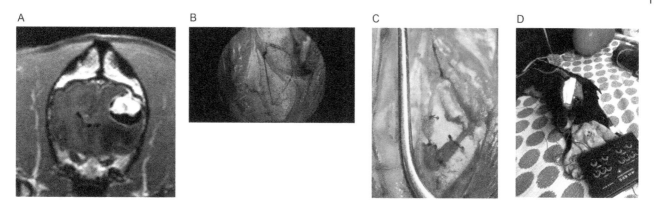

Figure 21.4 (A) MR image showing a large cystic meningioma. Surgical removal with immunotherapy ("meningioma vaccine") was elected (B) Combined approach of a modified left unilateral transfrontal craniectomy and a left rostrotentorial craniectomy. After elevation of the left temporalis muscle, the outer table of the left frontal bone and left frontal sinus was removed using an oscillating saw. The craniectomy was extended through a classical left rostrotentorial approach. (C) After tumor removal, the bone piece is replaced. (D) Since the surgical site was in the left frontal/parietal cortex (close proximity to pre-motor and motor cortex), the patient was treated post-surgically with EA on the right side at ST-36 and LI-10, among others.

following middle cerebral artery occlusion. Electro-acupuncture inhibited microglia-mediated neuro-inflammation, and significantly ($P < 0.05$) decreased levels of TNF-α, IL-1β and IL-6 in sensorimotor cortex and blood serum [83]. The author regularly uses electro-acupuncture post-operatively following brain surgery, with similar principles to the myelopathies (Figure 21.4).

Seizure Disorders

Conventional diagnosis of seizures in animals includes disorders such as idiopathic epilepsy, meningoencephalitis, hydrocephalus, toxic agents, and brain tumors. From a TCVM perspective, the pattern diagnosis is "Internal Wind" which can be related to Phlegm, *Qi*/Blood Stagnation and Deficiencies of *Jing*, *Yin* and Blood. Liver *Yin* and Blood Deficiencies may manifest as Internal Wind and are the most common TCVM Patterns in idiopathic epilepsy (IE) [84]. Approximately 25–30% of dogs with a conventional diagnosis of IE have refractory epilepsy (RE) to anti-epileptic medications (AEMs) (i.e. unsatisfactory seizure control despite ≥2 AEMs within therapeutic range). Since RE patients are not well controlled with classical treatment, they tend to be overrepresented in the population treated with alternative modalities.

One drawback of dry needle (DN) treatment for epilepsy is the requirement for frequent treatment, and most research involves EA. Although not traditionally recommended in seizure disorders (due to suspected but unverified pro-epileptic effect), recent research shows EA benefits in several models of epilepsy. There is, however, no consensus on acupoints and frequency of use. A murine study documented reduced epileptic seizures with both low (10Hz/1mA) and high frequency (100Hz/1mA) EA

($P < 0.05$) but high-frequency elicited a greater effect [85]. Low-frequency (10Hz) EA at bilateral Gallbladder 20 (GB-20) suppresses pilocarpine induced focal epilepsy by action on the μ, δ, and κ opioid receptors of the central nucleus of amygdala [86]. EA also reduces spontaneous seizures and epileptogenesis by elevating the expression of GAD(67) mRNA in the dentate gyrus granule cell layer [87], and by reducing mossy fiber sprouting and COX-2 levels in the hippocampus [88, 89].

Three publications report success using implantation of acupoints to treat seizures in dogs. Two to three mm gold wire pieces were associated with a ≥ 50% reduction in seizure frequency in 9/15 dogs (60%) with IE [90]. In a case series of 5 RE dogs, small subcutaneous gold implants placed over the calvaria on the Bladder (BL), Governing Vessel (GV) and Gallbladder (GB) meridians resulted in decreased seizure frequency in 5/5 dogs [91]. Due to artifacts on MRI with gold implants, Clemmons used 1mm × 0.5mm polylactic acid beads inserted using a modified 16-gauge needle in 10 dogs with RE. He reported significant reduction in amplitude of EEG activity, reduction of seizures by > 50% in 9/10 dogs (90%) and change in seizure characteristics from cluster seizures to singular seizures [92].

Physical Rehabilitation for Encephalopathies

Traumatic Brain Injury (TBIs)/Cerebrovascular Events ("Strokes")/Post-operative

Exercise diminishes the stroke-induced damage [93–95] and sustained locomotor training improves motor function in murine stroke model [96] and endurance in humans. A 2018 meta-analysis on stroke rehabilitation indicated that treadmill training, regardless of intensity and volume, results in a significantly greater recovery of motor function (P = 0.0001) [97]. NMES affects physiological functions of the brain, by activating specific motor centers, decreasing cortical inhibition, and increasing amplitude of motor evoked potentials in both healthy and stroke patients [98–100]. A meta-analysis and systematic review examining RCT using NMES in human stroke patients both showed significant improvements in recovery of speed of ambulation [98, 101]. Another study similarly suggests that NMES results in increased walking distances in patients with chronic stroke [74].

Botanical Medicine for Encephalopathies

Traumatic Brain Injury (TBIs)/Cerebrovascular Events ("Strokes")/Post-operative

A Chinese herbal medicine formulation, *Bu Yang Huan Wu*, has been used to improve functional recovery after strokes for hundreds of years in China [102]. This formulation has demonstrated protection via several mechanisms along with potent anti-inflammatory effects and appears well-tolerated in human patients [103]. A rodent model study indicated that it facilitated functional and neurophysiological rehabilitation via an improvement in synaptic plasticity [102]. Furthermore, a recent systematic review and meta-analysis, of 56 studies using 1,270 animals concluded that it "possessed substantial neuroprotective effects" [104].

Seizure Disorders

Some evidence for herbal management of RE includes single-herbs such as *Gastrodia elata root*, *Ginkgo biloba*, *Cannabis sativa*, formulations of *Xi Feng* and multi-herb formulations [105, 106]. The most commonly used Chinese herbal medicine for treatment of seizures is *Di Tan Tang*. It is an herbal blend which, like most Chinese herbal medicine in TCVM, contains multiple herbs, fungi, and other organic/inorganic compounds, with synergistic and balancing effects. *Di Tan Tang* includes *Citrus*, *Arisaema*, *Poria*, and *Uncaria*, which have demonstrated anti-epileptic properties in animal models [105]. Recommended dosage is 0.5 g per 5–10 kgs every 12 hrs. A prospective open-label, non-comparative clinical trial in 8 dogs with RE treated with *Di Tan Tang* at 0.1 g/kg PO q12 hrs documented an overall mean reduction in seizure frequency of 27% (P = 0.035) with 2 of the 8 dogs qualifying as responders (>50% reduction) and 2 other dogs achieving > 40% reduction [106].

Nutrition and Other Supplements

Seizure Disorders

Use of a ketogenic diet has proven effective in reducing seizure frequency in certain forms of human juvenile epilepsy. It has also been advocated in canine epileptic patients, and two studies have documented the use and benefits of medium chain triglycerides (MCTs) in epileptic dogs. A six-month prospective, randomized, double-blinded, placebo-controlled cross-over dietary trial comparing a ketogenic MCT diet with a standardized placebo diet in 21 RE dogs showed significantly lower seizure frequency with the MCT diet (2.31/month, 0–9.89/month vs 2.67/month, 0.33–22.92/month; P = 0.020). Three dogs achieved seizure freedom and seven had ≥ 50 % reduction in seizure frequency [107]. Another six-month multi-center, prospective, randomized, double-blinded, placebo-controlled crossover trial comparing an MCT oil as diet supplement with a control oil in 28 dogs also documented significantly lower seizure frequency (median 2.51/month, 0–6.67 vs 2.67/month, 0–10.45; P = 0.02) [108]. Cannabidiol (CBD) products have become popular and easily available. A randomized blinded controlled clinical trial used CBD infused oil at 2.5 mg CBD/kg PO q12 hrs for 12 weeks in dogs with IE treated with AEM(s). A significant reduction in seizure frequency (median change 33%), was reported, although the proportion of responders (>50% reduction) was similar to the placebo group [109].

Neuropathies

Acupuncture for Cranial Nerve (CN) Neuropathies

Facial Nerve (CN VII) Paresis/paralysis

A Cochrane review of the human literature reported that the quality of six randomized controlled trials (RCT) was inadequate to allow any conclusions regarding benefits of acupuncture for facial paralysis (partly due to flaws in study design and reporting). It is noticeable however that three of the six trials that compared acupuncture directly to drug therapy found a significantly (P < 0.05) higher cure rate with acupuncture treatment [110]. Another systematic review and meta-analysis of 14 RCTs over 1,541 human patients, despite mentioning a high risk of bias in methodological quality of the studies reviewed, reported a significantly (P = 0.005) increased response rate associated with acupuncture for Bell's palsy [111]. Both DN and EA can be used successfully as adjunct to standard treatment for various causes of CN VII paresis/paralysis. Several canine case reports document resolution of facial nerve paralysis after acupuncture; one case was idiopathic [112] and one occurred following dental procedure [113].

Vestibular Disorders (CN VIII)

Acupuncture and acupressure (applying pressure to acupoints) at Pericardium-6 (PC-6) has shown benefits in treating nausea and vomiting associated with vestibular disorders in humans. It significantly reduces the discomfort associated with dizziness, vertigo and motion sickness [114–120]. A human clinical trial showed immediate improvement after acupuncture for vertigo and dizziness in an emergency department [120]. Functional MRI (fMRI) studies have shown that the effect of acupuncture at PC-6 on vestibular disorders is via activation of the cerebellar vestibular neuromatrix [121] and selectively evoked neural responses in limbic-cerebellar brain areas (posterior insula, hypothalamus, and flocculonodular lobe of the cerebellum). These effects were found to be specific to PC-6 and lasting after stimulation was discontinued [121]. The stimulation of other acupoints can also exert a compensatory effect on vestibular disorders. A guinea pig model of peripheral vestibular disease demonstrated EA at ST-36 significantly (P < 0.05) reduced nystagmus frequency and head tilt, although the last criteria did not reach statistical significance [122]. Multiple canine case reports document the use of TCVM (with acupuncture and herbal medicine) for peripheral/presumptive idiopathic vestibular disease [123–125]. Both DN and EA can be used successfully as adjunct to standard treatment for dogs with vestibular disorders.

Although a modified Epley repositioning maneuver has been described to treat canine patients affected by geriatric vestibular disease, its clinical use has not been reported in enough detail to evaluate efficacy [126].

Conclusion

Integrative treatment modalities can be implemented easily as alternative or ideally complement to standard treatment in small animal neurology. Laser and acupuncture may offer alluring options to decrease neuro-inflammation and promote the best environment for neuronal recovery, while their innocuity allows safe initiation early after injury and surgery. Physical rehabilitation has become the gold standard in post-neurosurgical recovery and may offer benefits in pain management and functional recovery. Herbal medicine, nutritional therapy and other alternatives such as CBD may be of interest in management of refractory epilepsy.

Notes

1 Cervical Formula, Jing Tang Herbal Inc, Ocala, FL. USA.
2 Double P II, modified *Da Huo Luo Dan*, Jing Tang Herbal, Ocala, FL. USA.
3 Body Sore, modified *Shen Tong Fang*, Jing Tang Herbal Inc, Ocala, FL. USA.

References

1 Olby, N. (2010 September). The pathogenesis and treatment of acute spinal cord injuries in dogs. *Vet Clin North Am Small Anim Pract* 40 (5): 791–807.

2 Jeffery, N., Levine, J., Olby, N., and Stein, V. (2013 November–December). Intervertebral disk degeneration in dogs: consequences, diagnosis, treatment, and future directions. *J Vet Intern Med* 27 (6): 1318–1333.

3 Olby, N.J. and Jeffery, N.D. (2012). Chapter 29. Pathogenesis and physiology of central nervous system disease and injury. In: *Veterinary Surgery: Small Animal* (ed. K.M. Tobias and S.A. Johnston), 374–387. Saint Louis: Elsevier Saunders.

4 Choi, D., Lee, J., Moon, Y. et al. (2010 September). Acupuncture-mediated inhibition of inflammation facilitates significant functional recovery after spinal cord injury. *Neurobiol Dis* 39 (3): 272–282.

5 Spejo, A.B. and Oliveira, A.L. (2015). Synaptic rearrangement following axonal injury: old and new players. Review. *Neuropharmacology* 96: 113–123.

6 Houle, J.D. and Cote, M.P. (2013). Axon regeneration and exercise-dependent plasticity after spinal cord injury. *Ann NY Acad Sci* 1279: 154–163.

7 Ying, Z., Roy, R.R., Zhong, H. et al. (2008). BDNF exercise interactions in the recovery of symmetrical stepping after a cervical hemisection in rats. *Neuroscience* 155: 1070–1078.

8 Hutchinson, K.J., Gómez-Pinilla, F., Crowe, M.J. et al. (2004). Three exercise paradigms differentially improve sensory recovery after spinal cord contusion in rats. *Brain* 127: 1403–1414.

9 Tu, W.Z., Jiang, S.H., Zhang, L. et al. (2017 July 31). Electro-acupuncture at Governor Vessel improves neurological function in rats with spinal cord injury. *Chin J Integr Med*. doi: 10.1007/s11655-017-2968-9. Epub ahead of print. PMID: 28762132.

10 Janssens, L. and De Prins, E. (1989). Treatment of thoracolumbar disk disease in dogs by means of acupuncture: a comparison of two techniques. *J Amer Ani Hosp Assoc* 25: 169–174.

11 McCaskill, L. (2018 August). A retrospective study of the use of traditional Chinese veterinary medicine in the treatment of reoccurring canine intervertebral disc disease. *American Journal of Traditional Chinese Veterinary Medicine* 13 (2): 39–48. 10p.

12 Hayashi, A., Matera, J., and Fonseca Pinto, A. (2007). Evaluation of electroacupuncture treatment for thoracolumbar intervertebral disc disease in dogs. *J Amer Vet Med Assoc* 231: 913–918.

13 Han, H. et al. (2010). Clinical effect of additional electroacupuncture on thoracolumbar intervertebral disc

herniation in 80 paraplegic dogs. *Am J Chin Med* 38 (6): 1015–15.

14 Joaquim, J. et al. (2010). Comparison of decompression surgery. Electroacupuncture, and decompressive surgery followed by electroacupuncture for the treatment of dogs with intervertebral disc disease with long-standing neurologic deficits. *J Amer Vet Med Assoc* 236: 1225–1229.

15 Liao, J. et al. (2014). Effects of electro-acupuncture on Wnt-B-catenin signal pathway in annulus fibrous cells in intervertebral disc in rats with cervical spondylosis. [In Chinese]. *Zhongguo Zhen Jiu* 34 (12): 1203–1207.

16 Innes, J.F. and Melrose, J. (2015). Chapter 1: embryology, innervation, morphology, structure, and function of the canine intervertebral disc. In: *Advances in Intervertebral Disc Disease in Dogs and Cats* (ed. J.M. Fingeroth and W.B. Thomas), 3–7. Ames: Wiley Blackwell.

17 Wang, X. et al. (2009). Effect of acupuncture at cervical Huatuo Jiaji on type I and II collagen and pulpiform nucleus ultrastructure in rat cervical intervertebral discs. *Shanghai Zhenjiu Zazhi* 28 (11): 674–677.

18 Jiang, D. et al. (2015). Electro-acupuncture improves microcirculation and neuronal morphology in the spinal cord of a rat model of intervertebral disc protrusion. *Neural Regen Res* 10 (2): 237–243.

19 Liu, C., Chang, F., and Lin, C. (2016 September 30). Retrospective study of the clinical effects of acupuncture on cervical neurological diseases in dogs. *J Vet Sci* 17 (3): 337–345.

20 Hayashi, A., Matera, J., da Silva, T. et al. (2007). Electro-acupuncture and Chinese herbs for treatment of cervical intervertebral disc disease in a dog. *J Vet Sci* 8 (1): 95–98.

21 Sumano, H. et al. (2000). Treatment of Wobbler syndrome in dogs with electroacupuncture. [Article in German]. *Dtsch tieraztl Wschr* 107: 231–235.

22 Xie, H. and Rimar, F. (2010). Effect of a combination of acupuncture and herbal medicine on wobbler syndrome in dogs and horses. In: *Traditional Chinese Veterinary Medicine-Empirical Techniques to Scientific Validation* (ed. X. Yang and H. Xie), 101–112. Reddick: Jing-tang Publishing.

23 Lee, M., Longenecker, R., Lo, S., and Chiang, P. (2019 February 1). Distinct neuroanatomical structures of acupoints kidney 1 to kidney 8: a cadaveric study. *Med Acupunct* 31 (1): 19–28. doi: 10.1089/acu.2018.1325. Epub Feb 7, 2019. PMID: 30805076; PMCID: PMC6386779.

24 Kim, D.H., Ryu, Y., Hahm, D.H. et al. (2017). Acupuncture points can be identified as cutaneous neurogenic inflammatory spots. *Sci Rep* 7: 15214. doi: 10.1038/s41598-017-14359-z.

25 Li, A., Zhang, J., and Xie, W. (2004). Human acupuncture points mapped in rats are associated with excitable muscle/skin-nerve complexes with enriched nerve endings. *Reviews Brain Res* 1012: 154–159.

26 Weishaupt, N., Blesch, A., and Fouad, K. (2012). BDNF: the career of a multifaceted neurotrophin in spinal cord injury. *Exp Neurol* 238 (2): 254–264. ISSN 0014-4886. doi: 10.1016/j.expneurol.2012.09.001. Should be Kim et al 2017.

27 Weishaupt, N., Li, A., Di Pardo, S., and Sipione, K. (2013). Fouad, synergistic effects of BDNF and rehabilitative training on recovery after cervical spinal cord injury. *Behav Brain Res* 239: 31–42. ISSN 0166-4328. doi: 10.1016/j.bbr.2012.10.047.

28 Joseph, M.S., Tillakaratne, N.J.K., and de Leon, R.D. (2012). Treadmill training stimulates brain-derived neurotrophic factor mRNA expression in motor neurons of the lumbar spinal cord in spinally transected rats. *Neuroscience* 224: 135–144. ISSN 0306-4522. doi: 10.1016/j.neuroscience.2012.08.024.

29 Yong, M.S., Kim, S.G., and Cheon, S.H. (2017). Effects of skilled reach training with affected forelimb and treadmill exercise on the expression of neurotrophic factor following ischemia-induced brain injury in rats. *J Phys Ther Sci* 29: 647–650.

30 Himi, N., Takahashi, H., Okabe, N. et al. (2016). Exercise in the early stage after stroke enhances hippocampal brain-derived neurotrophic factor expression and memory function recovery. *J Stroke Cerebrovasc Dis* 25: 2987–2994.

31 Ahn, J.H., Choi, J.H., Park, J.H. et al. (2016). Long-term exercise improves memory decits via restoration of myelin and microvessel damage, and enhancement of neurogenesis in the aged gerbil hippocampus after ischemic stroke. *Neuro Rehabil NeuralRepair* 30: 894–905.

32 Fu, J., Wang, H., Deng, L., and Li, J. (2016). Exercise training promotes functional recovery after spinal cord injury. *Neural Plast* 4039580. doi: 10.1155/2016/4039580. Epub 2016Dec6.

33 Gómez-Pinilla, F., Ying, Z., Roy, R.R. et al. (2002). Voluntary exercise induces a BDNF-mediated mechanism that promotes neuroplasticity. *J Neurophysiol* 88: 2187–2195.

34 Gómez-Pinilla, F., Ying, Z., Opazo, P. et al. (2001). Differential regulation by exercise of BDNF and NT-3 in rat spinal cord and skeletal muscle. *Eur J Neurosci* 13: 1078–1084.

35 Hansen, C.N., Fisher, L.C., Deibert, R.J. et al. (2013). Elevated MMP-9 in the lumbar cord early after thoracic spinal cord injury impedes motor relearning in mice. *J Neurosci* 7: 13101–13111.

36 Yang, X., Liu, B., and Ouyang, B. (2014). Effect of acupuncture combined with rehabilitative training on neural functional recovery of stroke patients during recovery phase: a randomized controlled trial. *World J Acupunct Mox* 24: 17–23.

37 de Freitas, G.R., Santo, C.C.D.E., de Machado-Pereira, N.A.M.M. et al. (2018). Early cyclical neuromuscular

electrical stimulation improves strength and trophism by Akt pathway signaling in partially paralyzed biceps muscle after spinal cord injury in rats. *Phys Ther* 98: 172–181.

38 Canton, S., Momeni, K., Ramanujam, A. et al. (2016). Neuromotor response of the leg muscles following a supine, stand retraining with/without neuromuscular electrical stimulation training intervention for individuals with SCI: a case series. In: *Proceedings of the 2016 38th Annual International Conference of the IEEE Engineering in Medicine and Biology Society (EMBC)*. Piscataway, NJ: IEEE, 3143–3146.

39 Draper, W.E., Schubert, T.A., Clemmons, R.M., and Miles, S.A. (2012). Low-level laser therapy reduces time to ambulation in dogs after hemilaminectomy: a preliminary study. *J Small Anim Pract* 53: 465–469.

40 Zheng, J., Wu, Q., Wang, L., and Guo, T. (2018). A clinical study on acupuncture in combination with routine rehabilitation therapy for early pain recovery of post-stroke shoulder-hand syndrome. *Exp Ther Med* 15: 2049–2053.

41 Han, S., Wang, B., Jin, W. et al. (2015). The linear-ordered collagen scaffold-BDNF complex significantly promotes functional recovery after completely transected spinal cord injury in canine. *Biomaterials* 41: 89–96.

42 Lee, S.H., Kim, Y., Rhew, D. et al. (2016). Impact of local injection of brain-derived neurotrophic factor-expressing mesenchymal stromal cells (MSCs) combined with intravenous MSC delivery in a canine model of chronic spinal cord injury. *Cytotherapy S* 1465–3249: 30540-30540.

43 Brass, E.P., Peters, M.A., Hinchcliff, K.W. et al. (2009). Temporal pattern of skeletal muscle gene expression following endurance exercise in Alaskan sled dogs. *J Appl Physiol* 107: 605–612.

44 Zidan, N., Sims, C., Fenn, J. et al. (2018). A randomized, blinded, prospective clinical trial of postoperative rehabilitation in dogs after surgical decompression of acute thoracolumbar intervertebral disc herniation. *J Vet Intern Med* 32: 1133–1144. doi: 10.1111/jvim.15086.

45 Hodgson, M.M., Bevan, J.M., Evans, R.B., and Johnson, T.I. (2017). Influence of in-house rehabilitation on the postoperative outcome of dogs with intervertebral disk herniation. *Vet Surg* 46: 566–573. doi: 10.1111/vsu.12635.

46 Jeong, I.S., Piao, Z., Rahman, M.M. et al. (2019). Canine thoracolumbar intervertebral disk herniation and rehabilitation therapy after surgical decompression: a retrospective study. *J Adv Vet Anim Res* 6 (3): 394–402. Published 2019 Aug 18. doi: 10.5455/javar.2019.f359.

47 Martins, Â., Gouveia, D., Cardoso, A. et al. (2021 October 22). A Controlled clinical study of intensive neurorehabilitation in post-surgical dogs with severe acute intervertebral disc extrusion. *Animals (Basel)* 11

(11): 3034. doi: 10.3390/ani11113034. PMID: 34827767; PMCID: PMC8614363.

48 Bennaim, M., Porato, M., Jarleton, A. et al. (2017). Preliminary evaluation of the effects of photobiomodulation therapy and physical rehabilitation on early postoperative recovery of dogs undergoing hemilaminectomy for treatment of thoracolumbar intervertebral disk disease. *Am J Vet Res* 78: 195–206. doi: 10.2460/ajvr.78.2.195.

49 Bruno, E., Canal, S., Antonucci, M. et al. (2020). Perilesional photobiomodulation therapy and physical rehabilitation in post-operative recovery of dogs surgically treated for thoracolumbar disk extrusion. *BMC Vet Res* 16: 120. doi: 10.1186/s12917-020-02333-3.

50 Hady, L.L. and Schwarz, P.D. (2015). Recovery times for dogs undergoing thoracolumbar hemilaminectomy with fenestration and physical rehabilitation: a review of 113cases. *J Vet Med Ani Heal* 7: 278–289.

51 Jeong, I., Rahman, M., Choi, G. et al. (2019). A retrospective study of canine cervical disk herniation and the beneficial effects of rehabilitation therapy after ventral slot decompression. *Veterinarni Medicina* 64: 251–259.

52 Kathmann, I., Cizinauskas, S., Doherr, M.G. et al. (2006). Daily controlled physiotherapy increases survival time in dogs with suspected degenerative myelopathy. *J Vet Intern Med* 20: 927–932.

53 Miller, L.A., Torraca, D.G., and De Taboada, L. (2020 April). Retrospective observational study and analysis of two different photobiomodulation therapy protocols combined with rehabilitation therapy as therapeutic interventions for canine degenerative myelopathy. *Photobiomodul Photomed Laser Surg* 38 (4): 195–205. doi: 10.1089/photob.2019.4723. PMID: 32301669; PMCID: PMC7187977.

54 Wynn, S.G. and Fougère, B.J. (2007). Veterinary herbal medicine: a systems-based approach. *Vet Herb Med* 291–409. doi: 10.1016/B978-0-323-02998-8.50024-X. Epub 2009 May 15. PMCID: PMC7151902.

55 Chen, A., Wang, H., Zhang, J. et al. (2008). BYHWD rescues axotomized neurons and promotes functional recovery after spinal cord injury in rats. *J Ethnopharmacol* 117 (3): 451–456.

56 Wang, L. and Jiang, D. (2009). Neuroprotective effect of Buyang Huanwu decoction on spinal ischemia/reperfusion injury in rats. *J Ethmopharmacol* 124 (2): 219–223.

57 Seo, T., Baek, K., and Kwon, K. (2009). Shengmai-san-mediated enhancement of regenerative responses of spinal cord axons after injury in rats. *J Pharmacol Sci* 110 (4): 483–492.

58 Huang, Y.M., Zhao, Y.Q., and Tian, W. (2007 Aug). Experimental study on the effect of Suifukang in promoting repair and regeneration of nerve fibers in spinal cord. *Chin J Integr Tradit Western Med* 27 (8): 724–727.

59 Zhu, H., Wan, J., Wang, Y. et al. (2014). Medicinal compounds with antiepileptic/anticonvulsant activities. *Epilepsia* 55 (1): 3–16.

60 Zhang, Y., Wang, C., Wang, L. et al. (2014 January 20). A novel analgesic isolated from a Traditional Chinese Medicine. *Curr Biol* 24 (2): 117–123.

61 Wei, S., Zhang, P., Yang, D. et al. (2008). Traditional Chinese medicine and formulas for improving peripheral nerve regeneration. *Zhongguo Zhong Yao Za Zhi* 33 (17): 2069–2072.

62 Shu, B., Li, X., Xu, L. et al. (2010). Effects of Yiqi Huayu decoction on brain-derived neurotrophic factor expression in rats with lumbar nerve root injury. *Zhong Xi Yi Jie He Xue Bao* 8 (3): 280–286.

63 Cahyono, T. (2020). Comparison of conventional medical treatment to electro-acupuncture combined with Chinese herbal medicine for the treatment of hind limb paresis and paralysis in dogs and cats: a retrospective study. *Am J Trad Chin Vet Med* 15 (1): 43–56.

64 Knutson, J.S., Fu, M.J., Sheffler, L.R., and Chae, J. (2015). Neuromuscular electrical stimulation for motor restoration in hemiplegia. *Phys Med Rehabil Clin N Am* 26 (4): 729–745. ISSN 1047-9651, ISBN 9780323413480. doi: 10.1016/j.pmr.2015.06.002.

65 Bickel, C.S., Gregory, C.M., and Dean, J.C. (2011). Motor unit recruitment during neuromuscular electrical stimulation: a critical appraisal. *Eur J Appl Physiol* 111: 2399–2407.

66 Johnston, T.E., Smith, B.T., Mulcahey, M.J. et al. (2009). A randomized controlled trial on the effects of cycling with and without electrical stimulation on cardiorespiratory and vascular health in children with spinal cord injury. *Arch Phys Med Rehabil* 90: 1379–1388.

67 Mahoney, E.T., Bickel, C.S., Elder, C. et al. (2005). Changes in skeletal muscle size and glucose tolerance with electrically stimulated resistance training in subjects with chronic spinal cord injury. *Arch Phys Med Rehabil* 86: 1502–1504.

68 Stevens, J.E., Mizner, R.L., and Snyder-Mackler, L. (2004). Neuromuscular electrical stimulation for quadriceps muscle strengthening after bilateral total knee arthroplasty: a case series. *J Orthop Sports Phys Ther* 34: 21–29.

69 Lewek, M., Stevens, J., and Snyder-Mackler, L. (2001). The use of electrical stimulation to increase quadriceps femoris muscle force in an elderly patient following a total knee arthroplasty. *Phys Ther* 81: 1565–1571.

70 Ruther, C.L., Golden, C.L., Harris, R.T., and Dudley, G.A. (1995). Hypertrophy, resistance training, and the nature of skeletal muscle activation. *J Strength Cond Res* 9: 155–159.

71 Stein, R.B., Everaert, D.G., Thompson, A.K. et al. (2010). Long-term therapeutic and orthotic effects of a foot drop stimulator on walking performance in progressive and non progressive neurological disorders. *Neurorehabil Neural Repair* 24 (2): 152–167. doi: 10.1177/1545968309347681.

72 Harvey, L.A. (2016). Physiotherapy rehabilitation for people with spinal cord injuries. *J Physiother* 62: 4–11.

73 Gregory, C.M. and Bickel, C.S. (2005). Recruitment patterns in human skeletal muscle during electrical stimulation. *Phys Ther* 85: 358–364.

74 Pereira, S., Mehta, S., McIntyre, A. et al. (2012). Functional electrical stimulation for improving gait in persons with chronic stroke. *TopStroke Rehabil* 19: 491–498.

75 Hamblin, M.R. (2017). Mechanisms and applications of the anti-inflammatory effects of photobiomodulation. *AIMS Biophys* 4: 337–361. doi: 10.3934/biophy.2017.3.337.

76 Hashmi, J.T., Huang, Y.Y., Osmani, B.Z. et al. (2010). Role of low-level laser therapy in neurorehabilitation. *PMR* 2: S292–S305. doi: 10.1016/j.pmrj.2010.10.013.

77 Wu, X., Dmitriev, A.E., Cardoso, M.J. et al. (2009). 810 nm Wavelength light: an effective therapy for transected or contused rat spinal cord. *Lasers Surg Med* 41: 36–41. doi: 10.1002/lsm.20729.

78 Byrnes, K.R., Waynant, R.W., Ilev, I.K. et al. (2005 March). Light promotes regeneration and functional recovery and alters the immune response after spinal cord injury. *Lasers Surg Med* 36 (3): 171–185. doi: 10.1002/lsm.20143. PMID: 15704098.

79 Chow, R., Armati, P., Laakso, E.L. et al. (2011 June). Inhibitory effects of laser irradiation on peripheral mammalian nerves and relevance to analgesic effects: a systematic review. *Photomed Laser Surg* 29 (6): 365–381. doi: 10.1089/pho.2010.2928. Epub 2011 Apr 1. PMID: 21456946.

80 Godine, R.L. (2017). Neurological conditions. In: *Laser Therapy in Veterinary Medicine* (ed. R.J. Riegel and J.C. Godbold). doi: 10.1002/9781119220190.ch17.

81 Zidan, N., Fenn, J., Griffith, E. et al. (2018). The effect of electromagnetic fields on post-operative pain and locomotor recovery in dogs with acute, severe thoracolumbar intervertebral disc extrusion: a randomized placebo-controlled, prospective clinical trial. *J Neurotrauma* 35: 1–11. doi: 10.1089/neu.2017.5485.

82 Inês Rodrigues Gonçalves, F., Neves Rocha Martins, A.P., and Ferreira Alves, M.M. (2016). Functional neurorehabilitation in dogs with cervical neurologic lesion. *Vet Sci Tech* 7: 1–6.

83 Liu, W., Wang, X., Yang, S. et al. (2016 April 15). Electroacupuncture improves motor impairment via inhibition of microglia-mediated neuroinflammation in the sensorimotor cortex after ischemic stroke. *Life Sci* 151: 313–322.

84 Chrisman, C. (2011). Seizure disorders. In: *Traditional Chinese Medicine for Neurological Diseases* (ed. H. Xie, C. Chrisman, and L. Travisanello), 71–112. Reddick, FL: Jing Tang Publishing.

85 Kang, X., Shen, X., and Xia, Y. (2013). Electroacupuncture-induced attenuation of experimental epilepsy: a comparative evaluation of acupoints and stimulation parameters. *Evid Based Complement Alternat Med* 2013: 149612.

86 Yi, P., Lu, C., Jou, S., and Chang, F. (2015 July 7). Low-frequency electroacupuncture suppresses focal epilepsy and improves epilepsy-induced sleep disruptions. *J Biomed Sci* 22: 49.

87 Guo, J., Liu, J., Fu, W. et al. (2008 January 10). The effect of electroacupuncture on spontaneous recurrent seizure and expression of GAD(67) mRNA in dentate gyrus in a rat model of epilepsy. *Brain Res* 1188: 165–172.

88 Liu, C.H., Lin, Y.W., Hsu, H.C. et al. (2014). Electroacupuncture at ST36-ST37 and at ear ameliorates hippocampal mossy fiber sprouting in kainic acid-induced epileptic seizure rats. *Biomed Res Int* 2014: 756019. https://doi.org/10.1155/2014/756019.

89 Liao, E.T., Tang, N.Y., Lin, Y.W., and Liang Hsieh, C. (2017 March 28). Long-term electrical stimulation at ear and electro-acupuncture at ST36-ST37 attenuated COX-2 in the CA1 of hippocampus in kainic acid-induced epileptic seizure rats. *Sci Rep* 7 (1): 472.

90 Goiz-Marquez, G., Caballero, S., Solis, H. et al. (2009 February). Electroencephalographic evaluation of gold wire implants inserted in acupuncture points in dogs with epileptic seizures. *Res Vet Sci* 86 (1): 152–161.

91 Klide, A., Farnbach, G., and Gallagher, S. (1987). Acupuncture therapy for the treatment of intractable, idiopathic epilepsy in five dogs. *Acupunct Electrother Res* 12: 71–74.

92 Clemmons, R. (2015). PLA Bead Treatment of refractory epilepsy in dogs. 2015 ACVIM Forum Research Reports Program. *J Vet Intern Med* 29: 1257–1283.

93 Endres, M., Gertz, K., Lindauer, U. et al. (2003). Mechanisms of stroke protection by physical activity. *Ann Neurol* 54: 582–590.

94 Wang, R.Y., Yang, Y.R., and Yu, S.M. (2001). Protective effects of treadmill training on infarction in rats. *Brain Res* 922: 140–143.

95 Waagfjord, J., Levangie, P.K., and Certo, C.M. (1990). Effects of treadmill training on gait in a hemiparetic patient. *Phys Ther* 70: 549–558.

96 Zhang, Q., Wu, Y., Sha, H. et al. (2012). Early exercise affects mitochondrial transcription factors expression after cerebral ischemia in rats. *Int J Mol Sci* 13: 1670–1679.

97 Abbasian, S. and Mm, M.R. (2018). Is the intensity or duration of treadmill training important for stroke patients? *A Meta-analysis J StrokeCerebrovasc Dis* 27: 32–43.

98 Hong, Z., Sui, M., Zhuang, Z. et al. (2018). Effectiveness of neuromuscular electrical stimulation on lower limbs of patients with hemiplegia after chronic stroke: a systematic review. *Arch Phys Med Rehabil* 99 (5): 1011–1022.e1. https://doi.org/10.1016/j.apmr.2017.12.019.

99 Smith, G.V., Alon, G., Roys, S.R., and Gullapalli, R.P. (2003). Functional MRI determination of a dose-response relationship to lower extremity neuromuscular electrical stimulation in healthy subjects. *Exp Brain Res* 150: 33–39.

100 Han, B.S., Jang, S.H., Chang, Y. et al. (2003). Functional magnetic resonance image finding of cortical activation by neuromuscular electrical stimulation on wrist extensor muscles. *Am J Phys Med Rehabil* 82: 17–20.

101 Robbins, S.M., Houghton, P.E., Woodbury, M.G., and Brown, J.L. (2006). The therapeutic effect of functional and transcutaneous electric stimulation on improving gait speed in stroke patients: a meta-analysis. *Arch Phys Med Rehabil* 87: 853–859.

102 Pan, R., Cai, J., Zhan, L. et al. (2017 March 28). Buyang Huanwu decoction facilitates neurorehabilitation through an improvement of synaptic plasticity in cerebral ischemic rats. *BMC Complement Altern Med* 17 (1): 173.

103 Li, J., Liu, A., Li, H. et al. (2014). Buyang huanwu decoction for healthcare: evidence-based theoretical interpretations of treating different diseases with the same method and target of vascularity. *Evid Based Complement Alternat Med* 2014: 506783.

104 Wei, R., Teng, H., Yin, B. et al. (2013). A systematic review and meta-analysis of buyang huanwu decoction in animal model of focal cerebral ischemia. *Evid Based Complement Alternat Med* 2013: 138484.

105 Schachter, S.C., Acevedo, C., Acevedo, K.A. et al. (2008). Complementary and alternative medical therapies. In: *Epilepsy: A Comprehensive Textbook*, 2e (ed. J. Engel and T.A. Pedley), 1407–1414. Philadelphia: Wolters Kluwer Health/Lippincott Williams & Wilkins.

106 Dewey, C.W., Gridley, A., and Fletcher, A. (2020 August). Evaluation of the Chinese Herbal Formula Di Tan Tang as an oral add-on therapy for dogs with presumptive refractory idiopathic epilepsy: an open label investigation in 8 dogs. *Am Journal of Traditional Chinese Veterinary Medicine* 15 (2): 1–6.

107 Law, T.H., Davies, E.S., Pan, Y. et al. (2015). A randomised trial of a medium-chain TAG diet as treatment for dogs with idiopathic epilepsy. *Br J Nutr* 114 (9): 1438–1447. https://doi.org/10.1017/S000711451500313X.

108 Berk, B.A., Law, T.H., Packer, R.M.A. et al. (2020 May). A multicenter randomized controlled trial of medium-chain triglyceride dietary supplementation on epilepsy in dogs. *J Vet Intern Med* 34 (3): 1248–1259. doi: 10.1111/

jvim.15756. Epub 2020 Apr 15. PMID: 32293065; PMCID: PMC7255680.

109 McGrath, S., Bartner, L.R., Rao, S. et al. (2019). Randomized blinded controlled clinical trial to assess the effect of oral cannabidiol administration in addition to conventional antiepileptic treatment on seizure frequency in dogs with intractable idiopathic epilepsy. *J Am Vet Med Assoc* 254 (11): 1301. doi: 10.2460/javma.254.11.1301.

110 Chen, N., Zhou, M., He, L. et al. (2010 August 4). Acupuncture for Bell's palsy. *Cochrane Database Syst Rev* 2010 (8): CD002914. https://doi.org/10.1002/14651858.CD002914.pub5.

111 Li, P., Qiu, T., and Qin, C. (2015 May 14). Efficacy of acupuncture for Bell's Palsy: a systematic review and meta-analysis of randomized controlled trials. *PLoS One* 10 (5): e0121880.

112 Jeong, S., Kim, H., Lee, C.H. et al. (2001). Use of acupuncture for the treatment of idiopathic facial nerve paralysis in a dog. *Veterinary Record* 148 (20): 632–633.

113 Abdel-Rahman, H., Jun, H., Song, K. et al. (2008). Alternative treatment for facial nerve paralysis in a dog. *J Vet Clin* 25 (6): 526–528.

114 Hu, S., Stern, R., and Koch, K.L. (1992). Electrical acustimulation relieves vection-induced motion-sickness. *Gastroenterology* 102: 1854–1858.

115 Hu, S., Stritzel, R., Chandler, A., and Stern, R. (1995). P6 acupressure reduces symptoms of vection-induced motion sickness. *Aviat Space Environ Med* 66: 631–634.

116 Streitberger, K., Ezzo, J., and Schneider, A. (2006 October 30). Acupuncture for nausea and vomiting: an update of clinical and experimental studies. *Auton Neurosci* 129 (1–2): 107–117.

117 Alessandrini, M., Napolitano, B., Micarelli, A. et al. (2012 December). P6 acupressure effectiveness on acute vertiginous patients: a double blind randomized study. *J Altern Complement Med* 18 (12): 1121–1126.

118 He, J., Jiang, L., Peng, T. et al. (2016). Acupuncture points stimulation for Meniere's disease/syndrome: a promising therapeutic approach. *Evid Based Complement Alternat Med* 2016: 6404197.

119 White, A. (2016). Acupuncture for ear, nose and throat conditions. In: *Medical Acupuncture: A Western Scientific Approach* (ed. J. Filshie, A. White, and M. Cummings), 505–506. Philadelphia: Elsevier.

120 Chiu, C., Lee, T., Hsu, P. et al. (2015 June 9). Efficacy and safety of acupuncture for dizziness and vertigo in emergency department: a pilot cohort study. *BMC Complement Altern Med* 15: 173.

121 Yoo, S., Teh, E., Blinder, R., and Jolesz, F. (2004). Modulation of cerebellar activities by acupuncture stimulation: evidence from fMRI study. *Neuroimage* 22: 932–940.

122 Hu, S., Zhang, Z., and Xu, J. (1985). The effect of electroacupuncture on the vestibular compensation in the guinea pig. [Article in Chinese]. *Zhen Ci Yan Jiu* 10 (1): 21–23.

123 Fowler, M. (2011). TCVM treatment of severe canine geriatric vestibular disease. *Proceedings of the 13th Annual International TCVM Conference, Traditional Chinese Veterinary Medicine for Neurological Disease*s, 217–220.

124 King, D. (2011). Treatment of Head tilt/vestibular disease with acupuncture and Chinese Herbal Medicine in a Chinese Pug. *Proceedings of the 13th Annual International TCVM Conference, Traditional Chinese Veterinary Medicine for Neurological Diseases*, 211–215.

125 Yamate, M. (2013). Acute peripheral vestibular syndrome in a dog (what's your diagnosis?). *Am J Trad Chin Vet Med* 8 (1): 73–76.

126 Kraeling, M. (2014 March). Proposed treatment for geriatric vestibular disease in dogs. *Top Companion Anim Med* 29 (1): 6–9. doi: 10.1053/j.tcam.2014.04.004. Epub 2014 Apr 16. PMID: 25103883.

22

Integrative Oncology
Kendra Pope

Introduction

Cancer is currently the most common natural cause of death in dogs and cats in the United States [1]. One in three cats and one in three dogs will develop cancer in their lifetime, with rates increasing to one in two dogs over the age of ten [2, 3]. Cancer is not a reportable disease in animals and availability and performance of longitudinal epidemiologic studies is lacking, therefore updated information regarding current accuracy of these statistics is unknown. At the time of publication of this chapter, the risk of developing cancer in a male human lifetime is 1 in 2; female human lifetime is 1 in 3 [4]. Since 1999, cancer has surpassed heart disease as the primary cause of death in the Unites States for people under the age of 85 [5] and as of 2019, cancer has become the leading cause of death worldwide, regardless of age, accounting for nearly one in six deaths in 2020 [6]. As our companion animals have been moved indoors alongside us, exposed to similar environmental toxins and lifestyle changes including inactivity, obesity, highly processed, high carbohydrate diets, it would be expected that incidence rates in our companion animals would mimic those in humans.

Integrative oncology is the practice of medicine that reaffirms the importance of the relationship between the practitioner and patient, focuses on the whole patient, is informed by evidence, and makes use of all appropriate therapeutic approaches, healthcare professionals, and disciplines to achieve optimal health and healing [7]. Several National Cancer Institute (NCI)-designated comprehensive cancer centers have formally established integrative medicine centers within their hospitals, offering integrative approaches such as acupuncture, massage, music therapy, meditation, physical therapy, nutrition, and more to oncology patients [8]. Human oncology patients report using integrative modalities to take a proactive approach to their health and medical care, improve survival and manage treatment side effects [8, 9]. Pet parents of animals with cancer reportedly seek nontraditional modalities commonly alongside conventional oncology care. Reports show up to 76% of veterinary cancer patients receive at least some type of treatment commonly referred to as complementary and alternative [10]. An additional finding to note is that the majority of pet parents chose not to discuss these treatments with their primary oncologist, citing fear of being told to discontinue treatment [10]. Ongoing education of both veterinary students and veterinarians to the possible benefits as well as risks of integrative medicine in the oncology patient is paramount to supporting our clients, improving outcomes, and improving quality of life in our patients during treatment.

Integrative Therapy

Nutrition

Role of Diet in Cancer

The impact of diet on the development of cancer as well as the role of nutrition in the treatment of cancer is well researched although hotly debated in human oncology. Research continues to investigate varying approaches to oncologic nutrition, with recommendations remaining individualized and tailored for every patient. Whole food, minimally processed diets, rich in phytonutrients and low in carbohydrates are a generally agreed upon approach in human oncology, with further recommendations regarding whole grains, elimination of animal products, amount of fats or carbohydrates remaining controversial. Limited data exists within veterinary oncology investigating the role nutrition plays in the development or treatment of cancer.

The role of diet in the prevention of cancer was investigated in a population of Scottish terriers, a breed predisposed to the development of transitional cell carcinoma [11]. This survey study evaluated each dog's diet a year prior to diagnosis and compared data to non-neoplastic counterparts. A statistically significant decrease in risk of developing transitional cell carcinoma occurred in dogs fed green-leafy and yellow-orange vegetables as well as for dogs fed vegetables at least three times per week [11]. Few studies have examined the effects of dietary substrate (protein, fat, carbohydrate) and plant based dietary intake and cancer [12]. Two epidemiological studies revealed contradictory information to human findings, showing dogs with increased protein intake having increased survival times following diagnosis and intake of fat and carbohydrate not relevant to progression of the disease [13, 14]. Although more recent epidemiological data shows that more than 50% of owners of pets with cancer incorporate a nontraditional feeding program after diagnosis [15], additional studies have not been performed to evaluate the role of dietary modifications in the treatment of cancer, with current data guiding clinical decisions greater than twenty years old.

Protein, Carbohydrate and Fat Ratios

Currently, feeding recommendations for the veterinary cancer patient is driven by known metabolic derangements of tumorous tissues as well as identified abnormalities in amino acid, fatty acid, substrate and vitamin/mineral imbalances. The well-researched derangement of cancer cells to increase metabolic pathways that utilize glucose coupled with a limited fatty acid metabolism is known as the Warburg effect, after Otto Warburg's seminal work suggesting glycolysis as the primary pathway for energy production in neoplastic cells [12]. This altered glucose metabolism concurrent with insulin resistance and hyperlactatemia support the recommendation for minimizing carbohydrate levels in veterinary cancer patients [16]. Alterations in fatty acid ratios as well as lipid metabolism in veterinary cancer patients, support the addition of dietary unsaturated fatty acids to minimize loss of lean body mass as well as possibly reduce tumor growth rate [12]. Current nutritional recommendations suggest providing foods with an omega-6:omega-3 ratio as close to 1:1 as possible alongside concurrent omega-3 supplementation. Alterations in protein metabolism, as well as inhibitory effects of certain amino acids like arginine against neoplastic cell proliferation [17] support recommendations to increase protein levels in excess of adult maintenance requirements, assuming renal and hepatic function is adequate to tolerate increased amounts. As cancer progresses, alterations in normal patient metabolism may occur causing simultaneous loss of both protein and fat stores with concurrent cytokine stimulation and insulin resistance, known as cancer cachexia. Cachexic patients need high energy in the form of fat, and additional carbohydrates may need to be reintroduced at this stage [18].

Highly Processed Foods

The high temperatures used in commercial pet food processing facilitate chemical reactions in proteins and carbonyl groups of reducing sugars which result in the formation of advanced glycation end products (AGEs). The release of these byproducts into systemic circulation has been associated with multiple degenerative diseases such as cardiovascular disease, osteoarthritis, autoimmune, and cancer. In a study quantifying the amount of these end products found in commercial pet foods, canned pet foods contained the most, followed by pelleted and extruded foods. Average daily intake (mg/kg body weight$^{0.75}$) of byproducts was 122 times higher for dogs and 38 times higher for cats than average intake for adult humans [19]. These inflammatory byproducts are currently under investigation for their effects on animal health and are the reasons to advocate for minimally processed and fresh food diets in patients with conditions such as cancer.

For additional information regarding the byproducts of commercial pet food processing, specifically those related to Malliard Reaction products and AGEs, please refer to Chapter 12 in Section V (Integrative Nutrition) of this textbook [20–22].

Dietary Modification for Cancer Patients

As each veterinary patient has their unique metabolic requirements and nutritional needs, feeding recommendations for every oncologic patient should be tailored and individualized. Using a foundational recommendation of high protein, low carbohydrate, supplemented with omega-3 fatty acids and as minimally processed as the owner can provide should serve as a basis that can be modified for the specific needs of each patient.

Dietary Supplements

Vitamin D3

Vitamin D3 (cholecalciferol) has been examined for its benefits as a preventive agent and as a treatment for many types of cancer. In animal models, dietary vitamin D3 demonstrates chemo-preventative effects against breast cancer equivalent to those elicited by calcitriol without causing hypercalcemia [23]. The anticancer effect of vitamin D3 is thought to be due to induction of cell differentiation and antiproliferation. A positive feedback signaling loop between the serine-protein kinase ATM (ataxia telangiectasia mutated) and the VDR (vitamin D receptor) was identified as critical for cancer chemoprevention by vitamin D3.

In a 2016 veterinary study, low serum vitamin D3 levels were shown to be associated with an increased risk of developing cancer in canine patients [24]. The optimal serum vitamin D3 level was determined to be 100–120 ng/mL based on iPTH and c-CRP variations plateauing at this level. In the author's practice, serum vitamin D3 levels are routinely monitored and supplementation with oral vitamin D3 initiated with a target serum range of 100–120 ng/mL, although higher serum concentrations have been maintained in individual patients with no accompanying hypercalcemia to date. In a recent study, oral vitamin D3 supplementation at five times the recommended allowance (2–3 ug/kg) was not effective for rapidly raising serum 25(OH)D concentrations in healthy, adult dogs, although supplementation was well tolerated and caused no toxicity [25]. A current clinical trial is underway investigating oral vitamin D3 supplementation as part of a multi-herb treatment regimen for dogs with hemangiosarcoma [26].

Omega-3 Fatty Acids

Preliminary findings suggest fish oil supplementation increases chemotherapy efficacy, improves survival, and helps to maintain weight and muscle mass in patients with various cancers [27, 28]. An EPA-enriched oral supplement improved tolerability of chemotherapy in patients with advanced colorectal cancer and when combined with chemotherapy, fish oil supplementation may delay tumor progression in patients with colorectal cancer [29]. Omega-3 fatty acids are thought to have anticoagulant effects at doses greater than three grams in humans, however, results from clinical studies are mixed [30, 31]. In a study of 32 dogs with lymphoma fed kibble-based diets supplemented with omega-3 fatty acids and arginine, an increase in disease free interval and survival time was noted to be longer than those in the control group [32]. The amount of EPA in the fish oil diet (on a DM basis) was 29 g/kg of diet (13.2 g/lb of diet), and that of DHA was 24 g/kg of diet (10.9 g/ lb of diet) [32].

The Antioxidant Debate

Use of antioxidants during conventional cancer treatment is among the most controversial areas in integrative oncology. Agents including anthracyclines, platinum compounds, alkylating agents and radiation therapy exert their anticancer effects through the generation of free radicals or reactive oxygen species. The theoretical concern exists that antioxidants may render these treatments less effective. A secondary hypothesis also exists that antioxidants may improve efficacy of chemo/radiation therapy by increasing tumor response and decreasing toxicity to normal cells. This is supported by evidence that chemo/radiation therapy can reduce levels of normal tissue antioxidants. Systematic reviews on antioxidant use with chemo/radiation therapy in humans have shown similar mixed conclusions. Heterogenous patient populations, variations in administration/dosages/genetic coding, as well as patient antioxidant status are hurdles to a consensus in the available literature regarding safety [33–35].

In a review article evaluating 33 published papers and 2,446 human patients, various antioxidants were evaluated to determine their effect on chemotherapeutic toxicity. The majority (73%) of studies reported evidence of decreased toxicities, nine (27%) reported no difference in toxicities between the two groups, and five (15%) reported the antioxidant group completed more full doses of chemotherapy or had less-dose reduction than control groups. With the exception of one, all of the antioxidant supplemented groups, reported tumor responses that were the same or better than the control. One study (3%), however, reported increased toxicity (myelosuppression) in the antioxidant (vitamin A) group versus control; although controls had a significantly increased risk of disease progression and death compared to the vitamin A group [35]. Additional systematic reviews and meta-analyses have reported similar results [33, 36].

Routine examples of current use of pharmaceutical and nutraceutical antioxidants alongside chemotherapy should also be noted. Mesna, a chemotherapy adjuvant, is used alongside cyclophosphamide and ifosfamide to prevent sterile hemorrhagic cystitis and hematuria through its free radical scavenging activity. Dexrazoxane, used for its cardioprotective effects against doxorubicin or as an antidote when extravascular injection has occurred, minimizes cardiac damage and tissue necrosis via free radical scavenging and antioxidant activity. Denamarin®, a nutraceutical shown to delay hepatotoxicity with lomustine administration, minimizes hepatotoxicity through prevention of glutathione depletion [37]. These agents are used routinely as antioxidants, showing similar results to those reported in larger studies of lessened toxicities from conventional treatments without concern for negative implications to conventional therapies. It should also be noted that not all chemotherapy agents work via the creation of free radicals. Common classes of antineoplastic agents and degree of dependence on formation of free radicals for anticancer activity is detailed in Table 22.1.

The use of the single high dose antioxidant beta-carotene may be an exception, including supplementation alongside radiation therapy. In a report on 540 head and neck cancer patients undergoing radiation therapy, patients were randomly assigned into two arms, one receiving supplementation with α-tocopherol (400 IU/d) and β-carotene (30 mg/d) while the second arm was receiving placebo. Patients were administered these supplements throughout radiation and for three years thereafter. Patients in the treatment group reported significantly less side effects, however, rate of local recurrence was significantly higher in the supplement arm (hazard ratio, 1.37; 95% CI, 0.93 to 2.02) [38]. In a meta-analysis of twelve trials evaluating effects of antioxidant supplementation on primary cancer incidence and mortality, beta carotene supplementation was also found

Table 22.1 Production of free radicals as mechanism of action of anticancer activity.

Dependence on free radicals	Class	Example
High	Anthracylines	Doxorubicin, Daunorubicin
	Alkylating agents	Cyclophosphamide, Ifosfamide, Procarbazine, Dacarbazine, Melphalan
	Platinum containing compounds	Carboplatin, Cisplatin
	Topoisomerase 1 inhibitors	Irinotecan
	Topoisomerase 2 inhibitors	Etoposide
	Proteosome inhibitors	Bortezomib
Low	Purine/Pyrimidine analogues	6-Mercaptopurine, 6-Thioguanine, Rabacfosadine (Tanovea®)
	Antimetabolites	Methotrexate, L-asparaginase
	Monocloncal antibodies	Rituximab
	Vinca alkaloids	Vincristine, Vinblastine
	Taxanes	Paclitaxel
	Corticosteroids	Prednisone, Dexamethasone
Insufficient data	Antiangiogenic agents	Bevacizamab+
	Tyrosine-kinase inhibitors	Imatinib+, dasitinib+, nilotinib+ toceranib (Palladia®)

+ Preclinical data suggests that mechanism of action may in part be related to oxidative stress.
Modified from Abrams and Weil, 2014.

to increase cancer incidence and cancer mortality among smokers [39]. Additional trials evaluating the use of antioxidants concurrently with radiation therapy have not found similar concerning results with other antioxidants. Agents such as selenium, vitamin E and vitamin C have demonstrated anticarcinogenic effects, regression of radiation induced fibrosis, and protection against radiation induced proctitis [39–41].

Botanicals

Herbal Formulas

Among the 520 new drugs approved in the United States between 1983 and 1994, 157 were derived from natural products; accounting for more than 60% of antibacterial and anticancer drugs developed (Table 22.2) [34].

The use of combinations of medicinal herbs according to traditional practices (e.g. Traditional Chinese Medicine (TCM), Ayurvedic Medicine, Western Herbal Medicine) are commonly used in the treatment of patients with cancer, both human and animal. Herbal medicines are chosen for various reasons with multiple goals in mind, alongside conventional therapy, or when declined or when no longer an option. Each herb and botanical agent have tens to thousands of active constituents, which increase exponentially when combined with other herbs into commonly used formulas, allowing the targets and goals of therapy to be multifactorial.

Addressing cancer-related clinical signs, adverse treatment side effects, modulating pain/inflammation/immune function, mitigating or reversing multidrug resistance, and improving quality of life are a few of the many possible goals when using herbal formulas for cancer patients.

Medicinal herbs commonly used in the treatment of cancer are comprised of various chemical constituents. Some of the many categories include: alkaloids (e.g. berberine, matrine, colchicine), flavonoids (e.g. baicalein, wogonin, luteolin, apigenin, tectorigenin), terpenoids (e.g. oridonin, ursolic acid, oleanolic acid, artemisinin, saikogenin), anthraquinones, polyphenols, organic acids (e.g. ursolic acid, oleanolic acid), polysaccharides, and saponins (e.g. saikosaponin, pulsatilla saponins). Studies indicate that the active compounds from these herbs regulate a wide range of signaling pathways, kinase activity and gene expression, which are involved in cell proliferation, cell cycle arrest, apoptosis, invasion, and metastasis as well as modulation of tumor microenvironments [42, 43].

As cancer is a complex systemic disease, effective herbal approaches must not be directed to the Western/conventional diagnosis, but rather to the patient and their specific presentation, clinical signs, and needs. A tailored, personalized approach addressing underlying/chronic medical issues, as well as pattern imbalances and root causes taught in traditional schools of herbal medicine will create the most effective herbal plan.

Table 22.2 Chemotherapy agents derived from natural products.

Natural derivative	Mechanism of action	Chemotherapeutic agents(s)
Pacific Yew tree (*Taxus brevifolia*)	Microtubule disruption; taxanes	Paclitaxel, docetaxel
Red or pink periwinkle (*Catharanthus roseus*)	Microtubule disruption; vinca alkaloids	Vincristine, vinblastine, vinorelbine
Xi Shu Tree "Happy Tree" (*Campotheca acuminata*)	Topoisomerase inhibition; alkaloid	Camptothecin
Mayapple (*Podophyllum peltatum*)	Topoisomerase II inhibitor; podophyllotoxin	Etoposide, teniposide
Streptococcus paucities var. *caesius*	Topoisomerase II inhibitor	Doxorubicin, Daunorubicin
Streptomyces yeast species	Inhibition of RNA and protein synthesis; mTOR inhibitor	Actinomycin C, Mitomycin, Rapamycin

Adapted from Abrams and Weil, 2014.

Turmeric

Turmeric (*Curcuma longa*) is a rhizomatous plant in the ginger family that is native to South Asia but is cultivated in tropical areas around the world. The rhizome is used as a spice in regional cuisines, and as a coloring agent in food and cosmetics. It has long been used in traditional medicine for improving circulation and digestion. Turmeric extracts are widely marketed as dietary supplements to improve arthritis, memory, and cancer prevention, among others.

Turmeric, as well as its most well-studied polyphenol extract, curcumin, have powerful antioxidant, anti-inflammatory, and antitumor activity, documented to inhibit more than seventy oncogenes. Curcumin has been shown to inhibit transformation, proliferation, invasion, angiogenesis, and metastasis of tumors. It also downregulates many abnormal cell signaling proteins used by cancer cells to become more virulent and spread. More than 100 proteins, enzymes and receptors, including NF-Kβ, VEGF, TNF-α, COX-2, IL-1, 6, and 8, STAT 3 and 5, and 5-LOX have been found to be switched off by curcumin [44]. It inhibits gastric and bowel cancers [44–47] and is used as part of most cancer protocols. Curcumin, used as a single constituent extract, carries a risk of interference with cytochrome P450 enzymes and therefore chemotherapy drugs such as alkylating agents, doxorubicin and toceranib phosphate (Palladia®), as well as those that can enhance bleeding tendencies or gastrointestinal toxicity should be cautioned in combination. Further investigation is required to determine the optimal dosing strategies to achieve desired effects. Suggested dosing varies on formulation and intended use and are listed below in Box 22.1. Currently, there are no clinical trials or published research investigating the use of turmeric or curcumin in veterinary cancer patients.

Box 22.1 Turmeric Dosing

<u>Dried Herb</u>: 50–60 mg/kg divided daily (optimally TID) or to maximal palatability tolerance

<u>Decoction</u>: 5–30 gm per cup of water, administered at a rate of ¼ – ½ cup for 10 kg, divided daily (optimally TID)

<u>Tincture</u> (usually in 45–60% alcohol) 1:2 – 1:3: 1.0–3.0 ml per 10 kg, divided daily (optimally TID) and diluted or combined with other herbs. Higher doses may be appropriate if the herb is used singly and is not combined in a formula

<u>Curcumin</u>: 50–250 mg TID (canine), 50–100 mg QD (feline), 1200–2400 mg daily (equine)

Reference: Adapted from [48]. Wynn SG, Fougère BJ, 2007.

Milk Thistle

Milk thistle (*Silybum marianum*) is a plant originally native to Southern Europe and Asia, but now found throughout the world. Silymarin, which is derived from the milk thistle plant, is primarily used to manage liver disease, but additional studies suggest antioxidant and anticancer effects. Found in veterinary products such as Denamarin and Denosyl (Nutramax Laboratorites), this synthetic formulation has been shown to delay onset of chemotherapy-induced hepatotoxicity in patients receiving lomustine chemotherapy [37].

Silibinin, a flavonoid isolated from milk thistle, demonstrated antioxidant and anti-inflammatory effects by inhibiting release of hydrogen peroxide and production of tumor necrosis factor alpha [49]. Other studies indicate the flavonoids in milk thistle exert anticancer effects by arresting G1 and S phases of the cell cycle [50]. Generally well tolerated and considered safe in combination with most medications, there are limited concerns for combination with chemo-radiation therapy.

Cannabis

The *Cannabis sativa* plant has been used in herbal remedies for centuries. Over 480 biologically active components have been identified in cannabis, with the two best-studied being *delta-9-tetrahydrocannabinol* (often referred to as THC), and *cannabidiol* (CBD). Various other cannabinoids are being studied for their medicinal and therapeutic effects.

At the time of publication, the US Drug Enforcement Administration (DEA) lists cannabis and its cannabinoids as Schedule I controlled substances, meaning they cannot legally be prescribed, possessed, or sold under federal law. The use of cannabis to treat some medical conditions is legal under state laws in many jurisdictions for licensed physicians, however, veterinarians are not included in these regulations. Dronabinol, a synthetic form of THC, is approved by the FDA for cancer treatment-related conditions such as nausea. Recently, the FDA has approved Epidiolex, which contains a purified form of CBD for the treatment of seizures associated with Lennox-Gastaut syndrome, Dravet syndrome or tuberous sclerosis in humans one year of age and older [51]. There are currently no FDA approved cannabis products for veterinary patients.

Studies from the 1970s discovered that dogs have the highest number of THC receptors in the brain, even more so than humans. For this reason, human dosing strategies should not be extrapolated to canine patients and considered safe. Although considered to have a high margin of safety, with no human deaths ever recorded, deaths in dogs have been seen after ingestion of food products containing concentrated medical-grade THC butter. The minimum lethal oral dose for dogs for THC is more than 3 g/kg [52]. Hemp-based CBD extracts have been found to be effective in treating refractory epilepsy and osteoarthritis in dogs [53–55]. Varying dosing strategies have been reported ranging from 2 mg/kg BID to 20–50 mg per day [53–56]. In vivo trials have proven efficacy of CBD in inducing apoptosis in various canine neoplastic cell lines. [57] CBD is a potent competitive inhibitor of cytochrome p450, even more so than Bergapten found in grapefruit juice, and therefore should be cautioned when used alongside medications that are metabolized by these same pathways such as chemotherapy and antiepileptic agents. [58, 59] A study evaluating the safety and efficacy of CBD oil use during chemotherapy in dogs with lymphoma is currently underway [60]. For additional information regarding use of cannabis in the veterinary patient as well as rapidly changing regulations in this growing field, visit https://veterinarycannabissociety.org.

Medicinal Mushrooms

Various medicinal mushroom species have been researched and utilized for their cancer prevention and treatment properties for centuries. More than 100 species of medicinal mushrooms are used in Asia routinely, including *Ganoderma lucidum* (Reishi), *Trametes versicolor* or *Coriolus versicolor* (Turkey Tail), *Lentinus edodes* (Shiitake), and *Grifola frondosa* (Maitake). Studies have examined the effects of mushrooms on immune response pathways and on direct antitumor mechanisms. Innate immune effects are believed to be mediated primarily by the presence of high-molecular-weight polysaccharides, known as beta-glucans, although other constituents may be involved [61]. Beta-glucans have been found to stimulate monocytes, natural killer cells, and dendritic cells, leading to their reported benefits in immune system response, improved quality of life, increased survival, increased apoptosis and reduction in side effects of conventional treatment [62, 63].

A previous clinical trial investigating the benefits of polysaccharopeptide (PSP), a single extract of the turkey tail mushroom, showed survival benefits for dogs diagnosed with hemangiosarcoma (HSA) following splenectomy [64]. However, the prospective follow-up study which evaluated the use of PSP alone versus doxorubicin/placebo or doxorubicin/PSP, post-splenectomy, did not improve survival in dogs with splenic HSA [65]. Underpowering of the original trial or use of single extract versus full spectrum mushroom product were some possible explanations hypothesized for these results. Although clear data around dosing is not available, the author suggests the following dosing strategy for patients; 25–50 mg/kg daily as starting dosing with escalations as high as 100–200 mg/kg daily for aggressive support.

Generally well tolerated, the most common side effects of these products are gastrointestinal in nature. Mushroom cell walls contain chitin and are not digestible without being first processed or heated. Traditional techniques of hot water extractions are generally recommended to maintain the highest level of beta-glucans. The fruiting bodies of the mushrooms are considered to contain the highest quantity of beta-glucans when compared to the mycelium.

Herb-Drug Interactions

Available data indicates that human cancer patients use herb and dietary supplements more often than the general population, citing reasons such as improving health, reducing the risk of recurrence, and reducing side effects of cancer treatments [66]. Similar trends would be expected in veterinary oncology, but it is important to note that these herbs and dietary supplements contain biologically active compounds that may potentially interact with conventional cancer treatments, including chemotherapy and radiation. The basic mechanisms of herb-drug interactions (HDIs) are similar to other drug-drug interactions and can be divided into pharmacokinetic and pharmacodynamic categories. Direct toxicity to organs from herbal agents as well as toxicity from adulterated or contaminated products may also contribute to HDIs. It is also important to note that not all HDIs are negative, as neutral and positive HDIs also exist.

Pharmacokinetic interactions, which describe how herbs can influence the absorption, distribution, metabolism, and excretion of other drugs, often involve actions of microsomal enzymes of the cytochrome P450 (CYP) family and membrane transporters such as P-glycoprotein (P-gp). Compounds derived from botanicals are known to interfere with CYP enzymes and transporters, with CYP 3A4 most frequently implicated in HDIs, as it is responsible for oxidations of greater than thirty-five percent of currently prescribed anticancer drugs [67]. The second major mechanism of HDIs is in relation to a botanical agent's affinity for membrane transporters P-glycoprotein, multidrug resistance-associated protein-1, and breast cancer resistance protein; the three major classes of drug transporters expressed in the liver and kidneys [67]. Chemical constituents found in botanicals are substrates for the same transporters and therefore confer possible interactions. The most notable herb-drug interaction is with *Hypericum perforatum* (St. John's Wort), which interferes with both CYP isoenzymes as well as P-gp, and therefore is a well-known herb to avoid with many medications, including chemotherapy agents.

Pharmacodynamic studies comprise the interactions between drugs and herbs resulting in changes in their physiologic effects. In cancer care, medications that are prone to pharmacodynamic interactions include chemotherapeutic agents, anticoagulants, hormones, and immunosuppressive agents. Not all interactions, however, will be detrimental as many can be additive or synergistic and may enhance efficacy or reduce toxicity [66].

To fully appreciate the clinical relevance of HDIs, both the drug and the herb must be studied together in vivo. Very few herbs and drugs have been studied in this way, and much of the current knowledge rests on data from in vitro, lab animal, and in silico models. In a large review article evaluating a total of sixty-six clinical pharmacokinetic interaction studies, clinical herb-drug interactions were examined for six popular herbal drugs (echinacea, garlic, gingko, ginseng, goldenseal, milk thistle). Collectively, the available evidence indicated that, at commonly recommended doses, none of these herbs act as potent or moderate inhibitor or inducer of CYP enzymes or P-gp [68]. Another large review article evaluated available evidence for herb-drug interactions with Chinese herbal medicine in cancer therapy and identified 168 articles. Little direct evidence for negative interactions could be found, whereas some indirect evidence for benefit was identified. The authors concluded that in this dilemma, it is not reasonable to discard the potential usefulness of the traditional wisdom of herbal medicine, which has the backing of thousands of years of clinical experience but rather, a platform, or vocabulary, be created so that Western physicians and herbal medicine practitioners can discuss and manage the concomitant use of herbal medicine and chemotherapy agents [69]. In another large study evaluating traditional Chinese medicine (TCM) in cancer care, a large database was created by separating each TCM formula into its constituent herbs and then checked against an existing single-herb/western drug interactions database. A total of 1,361,535 TCM prescriptions were analyzed, with only 251 total interactions (0.18%) reported, however, clinically relevant interactions that required prescription change occurred a total of four (<0.001%) times [70]. Additional in vivo studies are needed to aid in identifying clinically relevant HDIs, however, a number of clinically relevant pharmacokinetic interactions have been identified of which the reader should be aware and are outlined in Table 22.3.

Due to differences in regulations surrounding herbs and dietary supplements, it is recommended to exercise caution regarding adulteration and contamination of available products (e.g. heavy metal levels in Chinese herbs, lack of advertised ingredients in place of unlabeled contaminants). Working alongside a trained herbalist with an understanding of botanical sourcing and quality control is paramount in the treatment of oncology patients and will eliminate concerns for contaminants of agents and pharmaceuticals unknowingly being administered to patients with often suboptimal health status.

Advanced Therapies in Integrative Oncology

A few advanced therapies which may help improve patient outcomes are included in this area for consideration in an integrative oncology program. Although extensive discussion and limitations on topics (i.e. hyperbaric oxygen therapy, medical ozone therapy) are necessary due to chapter length, resources for advanced training are listed in Table 22.4.

Intravenous Vitamin C (IVC)

Vitamin C, or ascorbic acid, has had a prominent role in oncology and the integrative treatment of cancer for many decades, although consistent dosing strategies, clinical response, and standardized treatment recommendations are not available in human or veterinary literature. Pharmacologic ascorbate, when used as a cancer intervention, can function as a bi-oxidant, displaying varying mechanisms of action based on dose administered [71]. At low and physiological concentrations, ascorbate is a potent free radical scavenger, protecting cells against oxidative damage

Table 22.3 Specific botanicals to caution during chemotherapy.

Botanical	Concurrent chemotherapy/condition (suspected effect)
Ephedra	Avoid with all cardiovascular chemotherapy (synergistic increase in blood pressure)
Gingko	Caution with camptothecins, cyclophosphamide, TK inhibitors, epipodophylotoxins, taxanes, and vinca alkaloids (CYP3A4 and CYP2C19 inhibition); discourage with alkylating agents, antitumor antibiotics, and platinum agents (free-radical scavenging)
Ginseng	Discourage in patients with estrogen-receptor positive breast cancer and endometrial cancer (stimulation of tumor growth)
Green tea	Discourage with erlotinib and pazopanib (CYP1A2 induction)
Japanese arrowroot	Avoid with methotrexate (ABCC and OAT transporter inhibition)
St. John's wort	Avoid with all concurrent chemotherapy (CYP2B6, CYP2C9, CYP2C19, CYP2E1, CYP3A4, and ABCB1 induction)
Valerian	Caution with tamoxifen (CYP2C9 inhibition), cyclophosphamide, and teniposode (CYP2C19 inhibition)
Kava kava	Avoid in all patients with preexisting liver disease, with evidence of hepatic injury (herb-induced hepatotoxicity), and/or in combination with hepatotoxic chemotherapy; caution with camptothecins, cyclophosphamide, TK inhibitors, epipodophylotoxins, taxanes, and Vinca alkaloids (CYP3A4 induction)

Adapted from Abrams and Weil, 2014.

Table 22.4 Resources for advanced training in integrative oncology.

Modality	Organization	Website
Intravenous vitamin C therapy	International IV Nutritional Therapy Global Physician Education	https://www.ivnutritionaltherapy.com
	Riordan Clinic	https://riordanclinic.org
Mistletoe therapy	Physician's Association for Anthroposophic Medicine	https://anthroposophicmedicine.org
Hyperbaric oxygen therapy	Veterinary Hyperbaric Association*	https://www.vhavet.org
Medical ozone therapy	Dr. Frank Shallenberger's Ozone Therapy Training & Certification Course*	http://www.oxygenhealingtherapies.com
	O3 Vets*	http://www.O3vets.com

* Specific courses/certifications available for veterinarians.

[72]; as well as a biological response modifier, increasing extracellular collagen production and strengthening extracellular matrix [73]. Conversely, in extracellular concentrations greater than 1 mM, pharmacological ascorbate leads to pro-oxidant effects that are preferentially toxic toward tumor cells due to the lack of catalase, an enzyme required to cease production of hydrogen peroxide or lipid hydroperoxides [74–77]. This preferential cytotoxicity has been well documented in varying tumor cell lines in vitro [78] including those in canine osteosarcoma cell lines [71].

These peroxides are shown to induce an incredibly wide variety of anticancer mechanisms. [74–77, 79] Quality of life improvement for human cancer patients treated with pharmacologic ascorbate is associated with reduced pain, fatigue, insomnia, nausea, and vomiting as well as improved appetite and tolerance to chemotherapy and/ or radiation therapy [76, 80, 81]. Well-designed clinical trials proving efficacy of direct tumor responsiveness to pharmacologic ascorbate, however, are not widely available in human oncology and do not exist in the veterinary literature.

Conflicting opinions exist surrounding the use of pharmacologic ascorbate during chemotherapy and radiation therapy due to theoretical concerns that ascorbate may inactivate free radicals created by conventional cancer treatment. These concerns have largely not been supported through clinical research, and numerous reports actually suggest that pharmacological ascorbate may increase the efficacy of several chemotherapeutic drugs and radiation in vitro [82–85]. Possible exceptions exist and are noted to follow. One glioma mouse model treated with a single fraction (4.5 Gy) of whole brain radiation, receiving intraperitoneal injections of low dose ascorbate (1 mg/kg) within 2 hours following radiation and for 37 days to follow revealed tumor progression was faster in tumor-bearing mice treated with radiation and daily ascorbate than in those treated with radiation alone [86]. Evidence exists for direct inactivation of a chemotherapy drug, bortezomib, in vitro; however, clinical trials have not been performed to determine if such reactions occur in vivo [87]. In addition, it has been observed that cells exposed to dehydroascorbic acid might be protected against arsenic trioxide or tumor necrosis factor-related apoptosis-inducing ligand (TRAIL) in vitro, requiring further investigations to determine if this also occurs in vivo. [88, 89] Additional points of consideration include that various chemotherapeutic agents act via different mechanisms of action, not all of which are via oxidative mechanisms [90]. If the chemotherapeutic agent does not act via oxidative mechanisms, concurrent low dose pharmacological ascorbate administration may not be an issue and may actually be synergistic [80]. The relatively short half-life of ascorbate in circulation due to rapid renal clearance is notable, estimated at less than 2 hours in humans and approximately 3.5 hours in dogs [71]. This allows further avoidance of interactions by targeted timing of conventional treatment and ascorbate infusions. At the time of chapter publication, a pilot study is currently enrolling patients to evaluate the benefits of pharmacological ascorbate concurrently with carboplatin chemotherapy in dogs with appendicular osteosarcoma following amputation [91].

Adverse effects from pharmacological ascorbate are rare, but reports of mild gastrointestinal upset, theoretical calcium oxalate crystalluria, and hemolytic anemia in patients with G6PDH deficiency (not readily identified in veterinary populations), do exist [92]. Recently, 7 dogs and 1 cat were reported to receive 125–1,000 mg/lb of pharmacological ascorbate IV for 3 consecutive days for the adjuvant treatment of multiple cancers, with one self-limiting episode of diarrhea observed [93]. These results were echoed in a more recent study of 550 mg/kg or 2,200 mg/kg pharmacological ascorbate IV infusion over 6 hours revealing one episode of vomiting during the higher dose infusion, and another showing nausea/ptyalism [71].

Due to limitations in length of this chapter, readers are referred to a comprehensive review of the history, mechanisms of action, safety, available literature, dosing and considerations for use of pharmacologic ascorbate in the veterinary oncology patient [85]. Resources for advanced training in intravenous vitamin C therapy are available in Table 22.4.

Mistletoe Therapy

Mistletoe (*viscum album*) is a semi-parasitic plant that grows on various host trees. Extracts of this plant are used for a variety of conditions including cancer, HIV, hepatitis, and degenerative joint disease. Oral preparations as well as tinctures are available as dietary supplements and homeopathic remedies, however, parenterally administered formulations are the ones referred to in this section. Mistletoe extracts are one of the most widely used and studied complementary and alternative cancer therapies in the world, with common use documented over the last 100 years. In much of Europe, mistletoe extracts are the most prescribed drugs for patients with cancer alongside conventional medications and pharmaceuticals [94] with palliative care use approved in several European countries.

Mistletoe extracts are believed to contain various compounds with numerous immunomodulatory and cytotoxicity activities, as well show evidence of proapoptotic effects, roles in antiangiogenesis, and DNA stabilization. The mistletoe lectins, as well as viscotoxins, are believed to be the substances most responsible for these activities, with additional constituents such as polysaccharides, membrane lipids, flavonoids, and triterpenes considered responsible for the antioxidant, anti-inflammatory, and antinociceptive responses [95–98]. The most common adverse effects from mistletoe treatment include injection site reactions, chills, and fever. Local reactions at the injection site commonly include induration, swelling, itching, hyperthermia, or pain, which generally resolve after the beginning of treatment [99]. According to the manufacturers, mistletoe extracts should be avoided in cases of known allergies to mistletoe preparations, in chronic granulomatous diseases, florid autoimmune diseases, and in immunosuppressive therapy. In the case of acute inflammatory or highly febrile diseases, application should be paused until the signs of inflammation have subsided.

Special caution should be taken when simultaneously treating with other immunomodulating drugs (e.g. interferons, interleukins), due to the risk of overstimulation. Because mistletoe extracts inhibit CYP3A4 in vitro, a theoretical interaction with drugs metabolized by this enzyme exists; however, numerous published studies support the safety of mistletoe in combination with conventional cancer treatments [100–106].

Numerous published articles support efficacy of mistletoe extracts in human cancer patients, reporting improved survival outcomes, tumor control, and improved quality of life [102, 107–111]. Even though mistletoe's potential beneficial effect on cancer survival has been described in numerous studies, benefits are still considered preliminary and further research is needed to evaluate mistletoe's impact on survival [112, 113]. At the time of chapter publication, a phase 1 open label dose escalating trial evaluating the benefits of mistletoe in human patients with advanced solid tumors is currently enrolling in the United States at the Johns Hopkins School of Medicine [114].

Table 22.5 Summary of clinical studies available for the use of mistletoe therapy in animals.

Population	Study design	Intervention	Outcome	Source
53 horses with 444 sarcoid tumors	Prospective, randomized (2:1), double blind, placebo-controlled trial	1 ml (escalating dosage to 20 mg/mL) SQ M/W/F *Viscum album ssp. Austriacus* (Iscador® P) for 15 weeks; Control received 1 ml 0.9% saline same frequency and duration	Complete regression 27 (37.5%) treatment, 9 (20.9%) control; Partial regression 21 (29.2%) treatment, 8 (18.6%) control; Stabilization 11 (15.3%) treatment, 7 (16.3%) control, Deteriorization 13 (18.1%) treatment, 19 (44.2%) control after 12 months	Clottu O et al. Treatment of Clinically Diagnosed Equine Sarcoid with a Mistletoe Extract (Viscum album austriacus). J Vet Intern Med 2010; 24:1483–1489.
44 cats with fibrosarcoma	Prospective, nonrandomized, noncontrolled, multicenter, observational (case series)	Surgery + 0.5mg PO BID *Viscum album Quercus* (Iscador® Qu), duration of treatment not clear	Disease free median survival 447 days; Recurrence = 8 (29%), No Recurrence = 36 (65%); Surgical margins were not significant to outcome; treatment well tolerated	Biegel U et al. Mistletoe extracts (Viscum album) as an adjuvant therapy concept in feline fibrosarcoma. *Klinische Anwendung und Prüfung.* unknown year/volume. 475–485.
17 dogs with transmissible venereal tumor (8 treatment, 9 historical controls)	Prospective, nonrandomized, historical controls	SQ injections three times weekly at varying dosing of *Viscum album pyrus malus* (Weleda®) for four months; Month 1: 10 mg/mL; Month 2:1 mg/mL alternating with 20 mg/mL; Month 3: 0.1 mg/mL; Month 4: 0.01 mg/mL; Concurrent Vincristine 0.5–0.7 mg/m2 IV every 7 days until complete remission or 6 months	Duration of chemotherapy reduced by pretreatment with Viscum album in treatment (26.3 days) over control (53.4 days); Incidence of leukopenia was greater in control (67%) over treatment (12.4%); Incidence of relapse within 6 months of treatment was higher in control (22%) over treatment (0%)	Lefebvre G et al. Treatment of transmissible venereal tumor (TVT) in dogs with viscum album (Mistletoe) associated to chemotherapy *Clinica Veterinaria.* 2007;70,78–86.

Literature demonstrating safety and efficacy of mistletoe therapy in veterinary patients exist, describing utility for equine sarcoids [115], canine transmissible venereal tumors [116], and feline fibrosarcomas [117]. Veterinary studies describing the use of mistletoe extracts in companion animals with cancer are summarized in Table 22.5. Resources for advanced training in mistletoe therapy are available in Table 22.4.

Conclusion

The systemic and individualized nature of each cancer diagnosis contributes to the complexity in understanding and treating this disease. The plethora of integrative treatment modalities and tools that are available with evidence of benefit further support an interdisciplinary approach to successfully support a cancer diagnosis. Due to limitations in length of this chapter, additional integrative oncology topics such as targeted and functional medicine diagnostics, repurposed drugs for use in oncology and oxygen therapies such as hyperbaric and medical ozone were not described here but are worth investigation into their efficacy and clinical application. Understanding the importance of integrative medicine in oncological care is paramount, as client demands promote their use and growing evidence provides scientific support for efficacy. Limitations in clinical research have always existed surrounding natural medicine due to complexity of botanical agents, lack of funding for nonproprietary and non-patentable agents, as well as individualized and tailored approaches not based on Western diagnoses. These challenges create unique hurdles for conventional research methods that will require outside of the box thinking to develop well designed clinical trials that will influence clinical practice for the veterinary integrative oncology patient.

References

1 Gardner, H.L., Fenger, J.M., and London, C.A. (2016). Dogs as a model for cancer. *Annu Rev Anim Biosci* 4: 199–222. doi: 10.1146/annurev-animal-022114-110911. Epub 2015 Nov 9. PMID: 26566160; PMCID: PMC6314649.

2 Bronson, R.T. (1982). Variation in age at death of dogs of different sexes and breeds. *Am J Vet Res* 43: 2057–2059.

3 Pang, L.Y. and Argyle, D.J. (2016 July). Veterinary oncology: biology, big data and precision medicine. *Vet J* 213: 38–45. doi: 10.1016/j.tvjl.2016.03.009. Epub March 11, 2016. PMID: 27240913.

4 Howlader, N., Noone, A.M., Krapcho, M. et al. (eds.) (2019 April). SEER cancer statistics review, 1975–2016. National Cancer Institute. Bethesda, MD. https://seer.cancer.gov/csr/1975_2016. based on November 2018 SEER data submission, posted to the SEER web site (accessed 22 September 2022).

5 Twombly, R. (2005 March 2). Cancer surpasses heart disease as leading cause of death for all but the very elderly. *J Natl Cancer Inst* 97 (5): 330–331. doi: 10.1093/jnci/97.5.330.

6 Ferlay, J., Ervik, M., Lam, F. et al. (2020). Global cancer observatory: cancer today. International Agency for Research on Cancer, Lyon. https://gco.iarc.fr/today (accessed February 2021).

7 Deng, G.E., Frenkel, M., Cohen, L. et al. (2009). Evidence-based clinical practice guidelines for integrative oncology: complementary therapies and botanicals. *J Soc Integr Oncol* 7 (3): 85–120.

8 Vail, D.M., Thamm, D.H., and Liptak, J.M. (2007). Chapter 17: Integrative oncology. In: *Withrow & MacEwen's Small Animal Clinical Oncology*, 6e (ed. D.M. Vail, H. Thamm, and J. Liptak), 330–339. St. Louis, Mo: Saunders Elsevier.

9 Raditic, D.M. and Bartges, J.W. (2014). Evidence-based integrative medicine in clinical veterinary oncology. *Vet Clin Small Anim* 44: 831–853. doi: 10.1016/j.cvsm.2014.06.002.

10 Lana, S.E., Kogan, L.R., Crump, K.A. et al. (2006 September–October). The use of complementary and alternative therapies in dogs and cats with cancer. *J Am Anim Hosp Assoc* 42 (5): 361–365. doi: 10.5326/0420361. PMID: 16960039.

11 Raghavan, M., Knapp, D.W., Bonney, P.L. et al. (2005 July 1). Evaluation of the effect of dietary vegetable consumption on reducing risk of transitional cell carcinoma of the urinary bladder in Scottish Terriers. *J Am Vet Med Assoc* 227 (1): 94–100. doi: 10.2460/javma.2005.227.94. PMID: 16013542.

12 Vail, D.M., Thamm, D.H., and Liptak, J.M. (2007). Chapter 16: Supportive care for the cancer patient. In: *Withrow & MacEwen's Small Animal Clinical Oncology*, 6e (ed. D.M. Vail, H. Thamm, and J. Liptak), 286–329. St. Louis, Mo: Saunders Elsevier.

13 Sonnenschein, E.G., Glickman, L.T., Goldschmidt, M.H., and McKee, L.J. (1991 April 1). Body conformation, diet, and risk of breast cancer in pet dogs: a case-control study. *Am J Epidemiol* 133 (7): 694–703. doi: 10.1093/oxfordjournals.aje.a115944. PMID: 2018024.

14 Shofer, F.S., Sonnenschein, E.G., Goldschmidt, M.H. et al. (1989 January). Histopathologic and dietary prognostic factors for canine mammary carcinoma. *Breast Cancer Res Treat* 13 (1): 49–60. doi: 10.1007/BF01806550. PMID: 2706327.

15 Rajagopaul, S., Parr, J.M., Woods, J.P. et al. (2016 September). Owners' attitudes and practices regarding nutrition of dogs diagnosed with cancer presenting at a referral oncology service in Ontario, Canada. *J Small Anim Pract* 57 (9): 484–490. doi: 10.1111/jsap.12526. Epub June 30, 2016. PMID: 27357412.

16 Hand, M.S., Thatcher, C.D., Remillard, R.L. et al. (2010). Chapter 30: Cancer. In: *Small Animal Clinical Nutrition*, 5e (ed. M.S. Hand, C.D. Thatcher, and R.L. Remillard et al.), 587–607. Topeka Kan: Mark Morris Institute.

17 Ho, V.W., Leung, K., Hsu, A. et al. (2011 July 1). A low carbohydrate, high protein diet slows tumor growth and prevents cancer initiation. *Cancer Res* 71 (13): 4484–4493. doi: 10.1158/0008-5472.CAN-10-3973. Epub 2011 Jun 14. PMID: 21673053.

18 Armstrong, S. (2013 January). Nutrition and cancer how diet and supplementation play a role in prevention and treatment. *Integrative Veterinary Care Journal*. https://ivcjournal.com/the-role-of-diet-supplementation-in-cancer-care (accessed 15 June 2022).

19 van Rooijen, C., Bosch, G., van der Poel, A.F. et al. (2014 September 3). Quantitation of Maillard reaction products in commercially available pet foods. *J Agric Food Chem* 62 (35): 8883–8891. doi: 10.1021/jf502064h. Epub August 20, 2014. PMID: 25088431.

20 ACLM. (2021). The benefits of plant based nutrition. American College of Lifestyle Medicine. Lifestylemedicine.org.

21 Prasad, C., Davis, K., Imrhan, V. et al. (2017). Advanced glycation end products and risks for chronic diseases: intervening through lifestyle modification. *Am J Lifestyle Med* 13 (4): 384–404. doi: 10.1177/1559827617708991.

22 Gentzel, J. (2013). Does contemporary canine diet cause cancer: a review. *Vet World* 6 (9): 632–639. doi: 10.14202/vetworld.2013.632-639. https://www.researchgate.net/publication/287738382_Does_contemporary_canine_diet_cause_cancer_A_review.

23 Krishnan, A.V., Swami, S., and Feldman D. (2013 July). Equivalent anticancer activities of dietary vitamin D and calcitriol in an animal model of breast cancer: importance

of mammary CYP27B1 for treatment and prevention. *J Steroid Biochem Mol Biol* 136: 289–295. doi:10.1016/j.jsbmb.2012.08.005. Epub 2012 Aug 23.

24 Selting, K.A., Sharp, C.R., Ringold, R. et al. (2016). Serum 25-hydroxyvitamin D concentrations in dogs – correlation with health and cancer risk. *Vet Comp Oncol* 14 (3): 295-305.

25 Young, L.R. and Backus, R.C. (2016 July 29). Oral vitamin D supplementation at five times the recommended allowance marginally affects serum 25-hydroxyvitamin D concentrations in dogs. *J Nutr Sci* 5: e31. doi: 10.1017/jns.2016.23. PMID: 27547394; PMCID: PMC4976120.

26 Bannink, E. and Marsden S. Investigation of a traditional Chinese medicine herbal therapy protocol for treatment of dogs with Stage II splenic hemangiosarcoma after splenectomy. *Metta Pets*. https://www.mettapets.info/hsa-study-protocol-benefits-and-req (accessed June 2022).

27 Murphy, R.A., Mourtzakis, M., Chu, Q.S. et al. (2011). Supplementation with fish oil increases first-line chemotherapy efficacy in patients with advanced nonsmall cell lung cancer. *Cancer* 117 (16): 3774–3780.

28 Murphy, R.A., Mourtzakis, M., Chu, Q.S. et al. (2011 April 15). Nutritional intervention with fish oil provides a benefit over standard of care for weight and skeletal muscle mass in patients with nonsmall cell lung cancer receiving chemotherapy. *Cancer* 117 (8): 1775–1782.

29 Camargo Cde, Q., Mocellin, M.C., Pastore Silva Jde, A. et al. (2016). **Fish oil** supplementation during chemotherapy increases posterior time to tumor progression in colorectal cancer. *Nutr Cancer* 68 (1): 70–76.

30 Heller, A.R., Fischer, S., Rossel, T. et al. (2002). Impact of n-3 fatty acid supplemented parenteral nutrition on haemostasis patterns after major abdominal surgery. *Br J Nutr* 87 (Suppl 1): S95–101.

31 Pryce, R., Bernaitis, N., Davey, A.K. et al. (2016 September 20). The use of fish oil with warfarin does not significantly affect either the international normalised ratio or incidence of adverse events in patients with atrial fibrillation and deep vein thrombosis: a retrospective study. *Nutrients* 8 (9) pii: E578.

32 Ogilvie, G.K., Fettman, M.J., Mallinckrodt, C.H. et al. (2000 April 15). Effect of fish oil, arginine, and doxorubicin chemotherapy on remission and survival time for dogs with lymphoma: a double-blind, randomized placebo-controlled study. *Cancer* 88 (8): 1916–1928. PMID: 10760770.

33 Block, K. (2004). Antioxidants and cancer: furthering the Debate. *Integr Cancer Ther* 3 (4): 342–348.

34 Abrams, D. and Weil, A. (2014). *Integrative Oncology*, 2e. Oxford University Press.

35 Block, K.I., Koch, A.C., Mead, M.N. et al. (2008 September 15). Impact of antioxidant supplementation on chemotherapeutic toxicity: a systematic review of the evidence from randomized controlled trials. *Int J Cancer* 123 (6): 1227–1239. doi: 10.1002/ijc.23754. PMID: 18623084.

36 Stargrove, M.B., Treasure, J., and McKee, D.L. (2008). *Herb Nutrient and Drug Interactions: Clinical Implications and Therapeutic Strategies*. St. Louis Missouri: Mosby Elsevier.

37 Skorupski, K.A., Hammond, G.M., Irish, A.M. et al. (2011 July–August). Prospective randomized clinical trial assessing the efficacy of Denamarin for prevention of CCNU-induced hepatopathy in tumor-bearing dogs. *J Vet Intern Med* 25 (4): 838–845. doi: 10.1111/j.1939-1676.2011.0743.x. Epub 2011 Jun 20. PMID: 21689156.

38 Bairati, I., Meyer, F., Gélinas, M. et al. (2005 August 20). Randomized trial of antioxidant vitamins to prevent acute adverse effects of radiation therapy in head and neck cancer patients. *J Clin Oncol* 23 (24): 5805–5813. doi: 10.1200/JCO.2005.05.514. Epub July 18, 2005. PMID: 16027437.

39 Bardia, A., Tleyjeh, I.M., Cerhan, J.R. et al. (2008 January). Efficacy of antioxidant supplementation in reducing primary cancer incidence and mortality: systematic review and meta-analysis. *Mayo Clin Proc* 83 (1): 23–34. doi: 10.4065/83.1.23. PMID: 18173999.

40 Kennedy, M., Bruninga, K., Mutlu, E.A. et al. (2001 April). Successful and sustained treatment of chronic radiation proctitis with antioxidant vitamins E and C. *Am J Gastroenterol* 96 (4): 1080–1084. doi: 10.1111/j.1572-0241.2001.03742.x. PMID: 11316150.

41 Delanian, S., Porcher, R., Balla-Mekias, S., and Lefaix, J.L. (2003 July 1). Randomized, placebo-controlled trial of combined pentoxifylline and tocopherol for regression of superficial radiation-induced fibrosis. *J Clin Oncol* 21 (13): 2545–2550. doi: 10.1200/JCO.2003.06.064. PMID: 12829674.

42 Zhang, Y., Liang, Y., and He, C. (2017). Anticancer activities and mechanisms of heat-clearing and detoxicating traditional Chinese herbal medicine. *Chin Med* 12: 20. Published July 12, 2017. doi: 10.1186/s13020-017-0140-2.

43 Nie, J., Zhao, C., Deng, L.I. et al. (2016). Efficacy of traditional Chinese medicine in treating cancer. *Biomed Rep* 4 (1): 3–14. doi: 10.3892/br.2015.537.

44 Aggarwal, B.B. and Harikumar, K.B. (2009). Potential therapeutic effects of curcumin, the anti-inflammatory agent, against neurodegenerative, cardiovascular, pulmonary, metabolic, autoimmune and neoplastic diseases. *Int J Biochem Cell Biol* 41 (1): 40–59.

45 Kunnumakkara, A.B., Guha, S. et al. (2009). In vitro and in vivo studies indicate curcumin potential for

preventing and/or treating colorectal cancer. *Curr Colorectal Cancer Rep* 5: 5–14.

46 Anand, P., Sundaram, C. et al. (2008). Curcumin and cancer: an "Old-Age" disease with an "Age Old" solution. *Cancer Lett* 267: 133–164.

47 Sharma, R.A., McLelland, H.R. et al. (2001). Pharmacodynamic and pharmacokinetic study of oral curcuma extract in patients with colorectal cancer. *Clin Cancer Research* 7 (7): 1894–1900.

48 Wynn, S.G. and Fougère, B.J. (2007). Chapter 24: Materia Medica. In: *Veterinary Herbal Medicine* (ed. S.G. Wynn and B. Fougere), 654. St. Louis, MO: Mosby Elsevier.

49 Li Volti, G., Salomone, S., Sorrenti, V. et al. (2011 July 14). Effect of silibinin on endothelial dysfunction and ADMA levels in obese diabetic mice. *Cardiovasc Diabetol* 10: 62.

50 Tyagi, A. et al. (2002). Antiproliferative and apoptotic effects of silibinin in rat prostate cancer cells. *Prostate* 53: 211–217.

51 https://www.fda.gov/news-events/public-health-focus/fda-regulation-cannabis-and-cannabis-derived-products-including-cannabidiol-cbd (accessed September 2022).

52 Fitzgerald, K.T., Bronstein, A.C., and Newquist, K.L. (2013 February). Marijuana poisoning. *Top Companion Anim Med* 28 (1): 8–12. doi: 10.1053/j.tcam.2013.03.004. PMID: 23796481.

53 Garcia, G.A., Kube, S., Carrera-Justiz, S. et al. (2022 July 29). Safety and efficacy of cannabidiol-cannabidiolic acid rich hemp extract in the treatment of refractory epileptic seizures in dogs. *Front Vet Sci* 9: 939966. doi: 10.3389/fvets.2022.939966. PMID: 35967998; PMCID: PMC9372618.

54 Verrico, C.D., Wesson, S., Konduri, V. et al. (2020 September 1). A randomized, double-blind, placebo-controlled study of daily cannabidiol for the treatment of canine osteoarthritis pain. *Pain* 161 (9): 2191–2202. doi: 10.1097/j.pain.0000000000001896.

55 Gamble, L.J., Boesch, J.M., Frye, C.W. et al. (2018 July 23). Pharmacokinetics, safety, and clinical efficacy of cannabidiol treatment in osteoarthritic dogs. *Front Vet Sci* 5: 165. doi: 10.3389/fvets.2018.00165. PMID: 30083539; PMCID: PMC6065210.

56 Verrico, C.D., Wesson, S., Knoduri, V. et al. (2020 September 1). A randomized, double-blind, placebo-controlled study of daily cannabidiol for the treatment of canine osteoarthritis pain. *Pain* 161 (9): 2191–2202. doi: 10.1097/j.pain.0000000000001896. PMID: 32345916; PMCID: PMC7584779.

57 Henry, J.G., Shoemaker, G., Prieto, J.M. et al. (2021 June). The effect of cannabidiol on canine neoplastic cell proliferation and mitogen-activated protein kinase activation during autophagy and apoptosis. *Vet Comp*

Oncol 19 (2): 253–265. doi: 10.1111/vco.12669. Epub January 14, 2021. PMID: 33247539.

58 Jiang, R., Yamaori, S., Okamoto, Y. et al. (2013). Cannabidiol is a potent inhibitor of the catalytic activity of cytochrome P450 2C19. *Drug Metab Pharmacokinet* 28 (4): 332–338. doi: 10.2133/dmpk.dmpk-12-rg-129. Epub January 15, 2013. PMID: 23318708.

59 Devitt-Lee, A. CBD-drug interactions: Role of cytochrome P450. https://www.projectcbd.org/medicine/cbd-drug-interactions/p450 (accessed September 2022).

60 Lejeune, A. A pilot study to determine the safety and efficacy of CBD oil use during chemotherapy in dogs with lymphoma, call for study subjects. https://research.vetmed.ufl.edu/clinical-trials/small-animal/a-pilot-study-to-determine-the-safety-and-efficacy-of-cbd-oil-use-during-chemotherapy-in-dogs-with-lymphoma (accessed 15 May 2022).

61 Mao, T., van De Water, J., Keen, C.L. et al. (1999). Two mushrooms, Grifola frondosa and *Ganoderma lucidum*, can stimulate cytokine gene expression and proliferation in human T lymphocytes. *Int J Immunother* 15 (1): 13–22.

62 Aleem, E. (2013 June). β-Glucans and their applications in cancer therapy: focus on human studies. *Anticancer Agents Med Chem* 13 (5): 709–719. doi: 10.2174/1871520611313050005. PMID: 23140353.

63 Jeitler, M., Michalsen, A., Frings, D. et al. (2020). Significance of medicinal mushrooms in integrative oncology: a narrative review. *Front Pharmacol* 11. doi: 10.3389/fphar.2020.580656.

64 Brown, D.C. and Reetz, J. (2012). Single agent polysaccharopeptide delays metastases and improves survival in naturally occurring hemangiosarcoma. *Evid-Based CAM* 2012: 8. Article ID 384301. https://doi.org/10.1155/2012/384301.

65 Gedney, A., Salah, P., Mahoney, J.A. et al. (2022 April 20). Evaluation of the anti-tumour activity of Coriolus versicolor polysaccharopeptide (I'm-Yunity) alone or in combination with doxorubicin for canine splenic hemangiosarcoma. *Vet Comp Oncol*. doi: 10.1111/vco.12823. Epub ahead of print. PMID: 35442554.

66 Yeung, K.S., Gubili, J., and Mao, J.J. (2018). Herb-drug interactions in cancer care. *Oncology (Williston Park)* 32 (10): 516–520.

67 Goey, A.K., Mooiman, K.D., Beijnen, J.H. et al. (2013 November). Relevance of in vitro and clinical data for predicting CYP3A4-mediated herb-drug interactions in cancer patients. *Cancer Treat Rev* 39 (7): 773–783. doi: 10.1016/j.ctrv.2012.12.008. Epub February 8, 2013. PMID: 23394826.

68 Hermann, R. and von Richter, O. (2012 September). Clinical evidence of herbal drugs as perpetrators of

pharmacokinetic drug interactions. *Planta Med* 78 (13): 1458–1477. doi: 10.1055/s-0032-1315117. Epub August 1, 2012. PMID: 22855269.

69 Cheng, C.W., Fan, W., Ko, S.G. et al. (2010 September–October). Evidence-based management of herb-drug interaction in cancer chemotherapy. *Explore (NY)* 6 (5): 324–329. doi: 10.1016/j.explore.2010.06.004. PMID: 20832765.

70 Chen, K.C., Lu, R., Iqbal, U. et al. (2015 December). Interactions between traditional Chinese medicine and western drugs in Taiwan: a population-based study. *Comput Methods Programs Biomed* 122 (3): 462–470. doi: 10.1016/j.cmpb.2015.09.006. Epub September 10, 2015. PMID: 26470816.

71 Musser, M.L., Mahaffey, A.L., Fath, M.A. et al. (2019 Nov 07). In vitro cytotoxicity and pharmacokinetic evaluation of pharmacological ascorbate in dog. *Front Vet Sci*. https://doi.org/10.3389/fvets.2019.00385.

72 Poljšak, B. and Ionescu, J. (2009). Pro-oxidant vs. antioxidant effects of vitamin C. In: *Handbook of Vitamin C Research: Daily Requirements, Dietary Sources and Adverse Effects* (ed. H. Kucharski and J. Zajac), 153–183. Nova Science Publishers.

73 Cameron, E., Pauling, L., and Leibovitz, B. (1979). Ascorbic acid and cancer: a review. *Cancer Res* 39 (3): 663–681.

74 Chen, Q., Espey, M.G., Krishna, M.C. et al. (2005). Pharmacologic ascorbic acid concentrations selectively kill cancer cells: action as a pro-drug to deliver hydrogen peroxide to tissues. *Proc Natl Acad Sci U S A* 102 (38): 13604–13609. doi: 10.1073/pnas.0506390102.

75 Chen, Q., Espey, M.G., Sun, A.Y. et al. (2007). Ascorbate in pharmacologic concentrations selectively generates ascorbate radical and hydrogen peroxide in extracellular fluid in vivo. *Proc Natl Acad Sci U S A* 104 (21): 8749–8754. doi: 10.1073/pnas.0702854104.

76 Ma, Y., Chapman, J., Levine, M. et al. (2014). High-dose parenteral ascorbate enhanced chemosensitivity of ovarian cancer and reduced toxicity of chemotherapy. *Sci Transl Med* 6 (222): 222ra18. doi: 10.1126/scitrans-lmed.3007154.

77 Mikirova, N.A., Casciari, J.J., and Riordan, N.H. (2010). Ascorbate inhibition of angiogenesis in aortic rings ex vivo and subcutaneous Matrigel plugs in vivo. *J Angiogenes Res* 2 (1): 2. doi: 10.1186/2040-2384-2-2.

78 Ohno, S., Ohno, Y., Suzuki, N. et al. (2009). High-dose vita- min C (ascorbic acid) therapy in the treatment of patients with advanced cancer. *Anticancer Res* 29 (3): 809–815.

79 Verrax, J. and Calderon, P.B. (2008). The controversial place of vitamin C in cancer treatment. *Biochem Pharmacol* 76 (12): 1644–1652. doi: 10.1016/j.bcp.2008.09.024.

80 Carr, A.C. and Cook, J. (2018). Intravenous vitamin C for cancer therapy: identifying the current gaps in our knowledge. *Front Physiol* 9: 1182. doi: 10.3389/fphys.2018.01182.

81 Du, J., Cieslak, J.A., III, Welsh, J.L. et al. (2015). Pharmacological ascorbate radiosensitizes pancreatic cancer. *Cancer Res* 75 (16): 3314–3326. doi: 10.1158/0008-5472.CAN-14-1707.

82 Prasad, K.N., Sinha, P.K., Ramanujam, M., and Sakamoto, A. (1979). Sodium ascorbate potentiates the growth inhibitory effect of certain agents on neuroblastoma cells in culture. *Proc Natl Acad Sci U S A* 76 (2): 829–832. doi: 10.1073/pnas.76.2.829.

83 Kurbacher, C.M., Wagner, U., Kolster, B. et al. (1996). Ascorbic acid (vitamin C) improves the antineoplastic activity of doxorubicin, cisplatin, and paclitaxel in human breast carcinoma cells in vitro. *Cancer Lett* 103 (2): 183–189. doi: 10.1016/0304-3835(96)04212-7.

84 Herst, P.M., Broadley, K.W.R., Harper, J.L., and McConnell, M.J. (2012). Pharmacological concentrations of ascorbate radiosensitize glioblastoma multiforme primary cells by increasing oxidative DNA damage and inhibiting G2/M arrest. *Free Radic Biol Med* 52 (8): 1486–1493. doi: 10.1016/j.freerad-biomed.2012.01.021.

85 Pope, K.V. (2021 Fall). Clinical utility of pharmacological ascorbate in veterinary oncology. *J AHVMA* 64: 18–29.

86 Grasso, C., Fabre, M.S., Collis, S.V. et al. (2014 December 15). Pharmacological doses of daily ascorbate protect tumors from radiation damage after a single dose of radiation in an intracranial mouse glioma model. *Front Oncol* 4: 356. doi: 10.3389/fonc.2014.00356. PMID: 25566497; PMCID: PMC4266032.

87 Zou, W., Yue, P., Lin, N. et al. (2006). Vitamin C inactivates the proteasome inhibitor PS-341 in human cancer cells. *Clin Cancer Res* 12 (1): 273–280. doi: 10.1158/1078-0432.CCR-05-0503.

88 Perez-Cruz, I., Cárcamo, J.M., and Golde, D.W. (2007). Caspase-8 dependent TRAIL-induced apoptosis in cancer cell lines is inhibited by vitamin C and catalase. *Apoptosis* 12 (1): 225–234. doi: 10.1007/s10495-006-0475-0.

89 Karasavvas, N., Cárcamo, J., Stratis, G., and Golde, D. (2005). Vitamin C protects HL60 and U266 cells from arsenic toxicity. *Blood* 105 (10): 4004–4012. doi: 10.1182/blood-2003-03-0772.

90 Simone, C.B., II, Simone, N.L., Simone, V., and Simone, C.B. (2007). Antioxidants and other nutrients do not interfere with chemotherapy or radiation therapy and can increase kill and increase survival, part 1. *Altern Ther Health Med* 13 (1): 22–28.

91 Musser, M. Pilot study of high-dose ascorbate combined with carboplatin for canine osteosarcoma (OSA). Lloyd Veterinary Medical Center, College of Veterinary of

Medicine, Iowa State University website. https://tinyurl.com/OSA-vitC-carboplatin (accessed 27 March 2021).

92 Pope, K. (2021 Fall). Clinical utility of pharmacological ascorbate in veterinary oncology. *AHVMA J* 64: 18–29.

93 Pope, K.V. (2017). Safety and dosing of intravenous ascorbic acid (vitamin C) in tumor-bearing dogs. In: *Proceedings of the Veterinary Cancer Society Conference*, 111. Portland, OR.

94 NCI National Cancer Institute (2023 Jan 13). Mistletoe extracts (PDQ®)–patient version. https://www.cancer.gov/about-cancer/treatment/cam/hp/mistletoe-pdq (accessed 2022).

95 Thies, A., Nugel, D., Pfüller, U., and Schumacher, U. (2005). Influence of mistletoe lectins and cytokines induced by them on cell proliferation of human melanoma cells in vitro. *Toxicology* 207: 105–116. doi: 10.1016/j.tox.2004.09.009.

96 Eggenschwiler, J., von Balthazar, L., Stritt, B. et al. (2007). Mistletoe lectin is not the only cytotoxic component in fermented preparations of *Viscum album* from white fir (*Abies pectinata*). *BMC Complement Altern Med* 7: 1–7. doi: 10.1186/1472-6882-7-14.

97 Schaller, G., Urech, K., and Giannattasio, M. (1996). Cytotoxicity of different viscotoxins and extracts from the European subspecies of *Vis- cum album* L. *Phyther Res* 10: 473–477. doi: 10.1002/(SICI)1099-1573(199609)10:6<473:AID-PTR879>3.0.CO;2-Q.

98 Szurpnicka, A., Kowalczuk, A., and Szterk, A. (2020). Biological activity of mistletoe: in vitro and in vivo studies and mechanisms of action. *Arch Pharm Res* 43 (6): 593–629. doi: 10.1007/s12272-020-01247-w.

99 Safety of mistletoe therapy. https://www.mistletoe-therapy.org/scientific-information/safety#c259 (accessed 1 May 2022).

100 Kienle, G.S. and Kiene, H. (2010). Review article: influence of Viscum album L (European mistletoe) extracts on quality of life in cancer patients: a systematic review of controlled clinical studies. *Integr Cancer Ther* 9: 142–157. doi: 10.1177/1534735410369673.

101 Piao, B.K., Wang, Y.X., Xie, G.R. et al. (2004). Impact of complementary mistletoe extract treatment on quality of life in breast, ovarian and non-small cell lung cancer patients. A prospective randomized controlled clinical trial. *Anticancer Research* 24: 303–310.

102 Bock, P.R., Friedel, W.E., Hanisch, J. et al. (2004). Efficacy and safety of long-term complementary treatment with standardized European mistletoe extract (Viscum album L.) in addition to the conventional adjuvant oncologic therapy in patients with primary non-metastasized mammary carcinoma. Results of a multi-center, comparative, epidemiological cohort study

in Germany and Switzerland. *Arzneimittelforschung* 54: 456–466. doi: 10.1055/s-0031-1296999.

103 Friedel, W.E., Matthes, H., Bock, P.R., and Zanker, K.S. (2009). Systematic evaluation of the clinical effects of supportive mistletoe treatment within chemo- and/or radiotherapy protocols and long-term mistletoe application in nonmetastatic colorectal carcinoma: multicenter, controlled, observational cohort study. *J Soc Integr Oncol* 7: 137–145.

104 Tröger, W., Jezdic, S., Zdrale, Z. et al. (2009). Quality of life and neutropenia in patients with early stage breast cancer: a randomized pilot study comparing additional treatment with mistletoe extract to chemotherapy alone. *Breast Cancer* 16: 35–45.

105 Matthes, H., Friedel, W.E., Bock, P.R., and Zanker, K.S. (2010). Molecular mistletoe therapy: friend or foe in established anti-tumor protocols? A multicenter, controlled, retrospective pharmaco-epidemiological study in pancreas cancer. *Curr Mol Med* 10: 430–439. doi: 10.2174/156652410791317057.

106 Tröger, W., Zdrale, Z., Tisma, N., and Matijasevic, M. (2014 September). Additional therapy with a mistletoe product during adjuvant chemotherapy of breast cancer patients improves quality of life: an open randomized clinical pilot trial. *Evid Based Complementary Altern Med* 2014: 01. doi: 10.1155/2014/430518.

107 Ostermann, T., Raak, C., and Bussing, A. (2009). Survival of cancer patients treated with mistletoe extract (Iscador): a systematic literature review. *BMC Cancer* 9: 451.

108 Horneber, M.A., Bueschel, G., Huber, R. et al. (2008). Mistletoe therapy in oncology. *Cochrane Database Syst Rev* 2008 (2): CD003297.

109 Kienle, G.S. and Kiene, H. (2007). Complementary cancer therapy: a systematic review of prospective clinical trials on anthroposophic mistletoe extracts. *Eur J Med Res* 12: 103–119.

110 Ostermann, T. and Bussing, A. (2012). Retrolective studies on the survival of cancer patients treated with mistletoe extracts: a meta-analysis. *Explore (NY)* 8: 277–281.

111 Schad, F., Atxner, J., Buchwald, D. et al. (2014). Intratumoral mistletoe (*Viscum album* L) therapy in patients with unresectable pancreas carcinoma: a retrospective analysis. *Integr Cancer Ther* 13: 332–340.

112 Kienle, G.S., Berrino, F., Bussing, A. et al. (2003). Mistletoe in cancer—a systematic review on controlled clinical trials. *Eur J Med Res* 8: 109–119.

113 Bar-Sela, G., Wollner, M., Hammer, L. et al. (2013). Mistletoe as complementary treatment in patients with advanced non-small-cell lung cancer treated with carboplatin-based combinations: a randomised phase II study. *Eur J Cancer* 49: 1058–1064.

114 Paller, Channing. Sidney Kimmel Comprehensive Cancer Center at Johns Hopkins. Trial of Mistletoe Extract in Patients With Advanced Solid Tumors. https://clinicaltrials.gov/ct2/show/NCT03051477 (accessed May 2022).

115 Clottu, O. et al. (2010). Treatment of clinically diagnosed equine sarcoid with a mistletoe extract (Viscum album austriacus). *J Vet Intern Med* 24: 1483–1489.

116 Lefebvre, G. et al. (2007). Treatment of transmissible venereal tumor (TVT) in dogs with viscum album (Mistletoe) associated to chemotherapy. *Clinica Veterinaria* 70: 78–86.

117 Biegel, U., Klocke, P., Ruess-Melzer et al. Mistletoe extracts (Viscum album) as an adjuvant therapy concept in feline fibrosarcoma. *Klinische Anwendung und Prüfung, Die Mistel in der Tumortherapie, Bd* 3: 475–485. unknown year/volume.

23

Integrative Management of Abnormal Small Animal Behavior
Cynthia McDowell

Introduction

Inappropriate behaviors in pets have serious physical, emotional, and monetary consequences. Studies estimate 40% of pet dogs and cats in the United States exhibit problem behaviors constituting the number one and two reasons for relinquishment to shelters, respectively [1–3]. Commonly reported behaviors in both include aggression, destructiveness, inappropriate elimination, and compulsive disorders; with dogs additionally reporting anxiety and unruliness [2].

Veterinarians are key to behavior wellness programs. Every veterinary visit should screen common issues such as abnormalities associated with elimination, sleep, eating, and vocalization along with human/animal interactions (e.g. mouthiness, growling, biting, property destruction) [1, 2, 4, 5]. Behavior specific questions alert caregivers to early symptoms which can be more easily treated and prevent adverse outcomes that threaten the human animal bond [1, 4]. The primary care veterinarian bears ethical responsibility to provide diagnostic and treatment options, offer the inclusion of a veterinary behavior specialist and maintain oversight of these patients. Goals to stabilize the patient, prevent disease progression, and resolve the abnormality are paramount [1]. The integrative veterinarian is in a unique position to triangulate behavioral and conventional treatment with complimentary therapies, such as traditional Chinese veterinary medicine (TCVM) to expand treatment options and improve patient outcomes [6–15].

Integrative Medicine Diagnostic Approach

Conventional

History
The behavior history determines the five "**W**'s" of the problem behavior: **W**hat? **W**here? **W**hen? **W**ho (is present)? and **W**hy? [4] A standardized, thorough behavior questionnaire insures collection of all significant information (examples on webpage). Inclusion of daily routines, family dynamics, environment, behavior frequencies and triggers help characterize the problem along with details on behavior modification/training attempted and its success [1, 4, 5]. The completed questionnaire reviewed before the behavior visit enables in-person consultation to be more productive and relevant to the behavior concerns (Web 23.1, sample questionnaires. Overall, Karen L, 2013 / with permission of Elsevier) [1, 4].

Observation
Direct observation of the patient's personality and behavior occurs during the consultation or while viewing video recordings of the pet in the home environment, if safe to do so [1, 4]. Indirect observation occurs through descriptions of the pet from family members. Conclusions about the pet's personality, motivation and mental state requires knowledge of species communicative body and facial postures [1, 4, 5]. Staff and owners must be familiar with species specific postures and expressions. (www.ZoomRoomOnline.com).

Integrative Veterinary Medicine, First Edition. Edited by Mushtaq A. Memon and Huisheng Xie.
© 2023 John Wiley & Sons, Inc. Published 2023 by John Wiley & Sons, Inc.
Companion Website: www.wiley.com/go/memon/veterinary

All stimuli and context (social and environmental) that trigger the behavior are determined [1, 4]. Owners may struggle to identify specific triggers if behaviors have advanced from episodic occurrences to more serious generalized patterns. In these situations, stimuli, or context causing increased intensity of the generalized behavior are determined [1].

Diagnosis

The complete behavior diagnosis is a descriptive phrase containing three components: the observed behavior, the behavior trigger(s) and the psychologic cause. For example, to determine the behavior diagnosis for "fear-based aggression toward children"; aggression is the observed behavior, children are the trigger stimulus and fear is the root cause. The observed behavior and trigger stimuli are gleaned from history and observation. The psychologic etiology is determined by satisfying criteria of a given psychologic behavior etiology (Table 23.1, Web 23.2). The three-part behavior diagnosis may not always be possible. The first component "observed behavior" is always known; however, the trigger stimuli and/or psychologic cause might remain unknown.

Medical Co-morbidities

Medical abnormalities can be primary, contributory, or occult causes of behavior problems requiring vigilance in treating known or suspected conventional diseases. Behavior issues are the only symptoms of some diseases such as cognitive dysfunction or pain [4]. Standard medical history, examination, and conventional database including at minimum a complete blood cell count, serum biochemistry profile, thyroid test, urinalysis, and survey radiographs are crucial to every behavior evaluation [1, 4].

Traditional Chinese Veterinary Medicine (TCVM)

Shen

Behavior abnormalities are considered a disturbance of the *Shen* (Spirit or Mind) [16]. *Shen* processes all incoming sensory and intuitive information and supervises the physical and mental reactions to that information [17]. *Shen* oversees and interprets the seven emotions (joy, anger, sadness, grief, fright, apprehension, worry) and regulates the five spirits (*Hun, Po, Yi, Zhi, Shen*) [18]. Signs of *Shen* Disturbance include abnormal behavior (e.g. restless, nervous, anxiety, insomnia, forgetful, hyperactivity, frightful, inability to focus) [16].

TCVM Patterns of Shen *Disturbance*

The *Shen*, though associated with the mind, is housed in the heart and requires nourishment from the heart *Yin* and blood to remain healthy [16]. The heart belongs to Fire and with imbalance is prone to excesses of heat, phlegm or fire, and deficiencies of blood, *Yin* and *Qi* [16]. Excess patterns result from heart heat/fire (hot foods, environmental factors, liver *Qi* stagnation) or non-substantial phlegm obstructing the heart orifice (secondary to heat, cold, damp, or spleen *Qi* deficiency) [16, 17]. Deficient patterns include heart blood, heart *Qi*, and/or heart *Yin*. Kidney *Jing* deficiency should be considered in behavior problems of young or senior patients as kidney *Jing* supports body fluids essential to manifest and anchor *Shen*. Mixed patterns result when excesses of fire, phlegm or liver *Qi* stagnation combine with depletion of blood, *Yin* or *Qi* (Table 23.2) [19].

Table 23.1 Common behavior terminology, phenotype, and definition [1]. Overall, Karen L, 2013 / with permission of Elsevier.

Behavior etiology	Behavior phenotype	Definition
Various	Aggression	Action(s) that reduces the freedom or fitness of another such as a growl, lunge, snap, nip, bite, tense body posture, or facial expression. (Expanded web table containing 12 aggression trigger/etiology categories)
Anxiety	Various	State of heightened monitoring with increased vigilance/scanning and sympathetic arousal in the absence of stimuli
Fear	Various	Response to stimuli characterized by withdrawal, passive and active avoidance, and sympathetic arousal
Phobia	Various	Profound, non-graded, extreme, often per-acute exaggerated fear response to a consistent stimuli manifest as intense, active avoidance/escape
Various	Compulsive and repetitive behaviors	Inappropriate repetitive, stereotypic motor, locomotor, grooming, ingestive, or hallucinogenic behaviors

For more information readers are directed to the expanded version (Web 23.2. Overall, Karen L, 2013 / with permission of Elsevier) containing additional behavior etiologies and phenotypes: Overactivity, Hyperactivity, Hyper-reactivity, Inappropriate Elimination, Nuisance Behavior, Geriatric Behavior, Abnormal Cognition

Table 23.2 *Shen* Disturbance TCVM Patterns, clinical signs, acupuncture, and Chinese herbal medicine treatments [7].

TCVM pattern	Clinical signs	Acupuncture points and Chinese herbal medicine
Phlegm/fire flaring upward	Tongue: red or deep red Coating: yellow or thick yellow and dry coating Pulse: surging, rapid	GV-14, *Tai-yang*, *Er-jian*, *Wei-jian*, ST-44, HT-9, PC-9, *An-shen*, *Da-feng-men*, HT-7, PC-6, ST-40, SI-3, LIV-3, LIV-2 *Zhen Xin San*[a]
Fire with *Yin* deficiency	Tongue: red or deep red, with cracked lines Coating: none to scant or peeled off and dry Pulse: thready, fast, and weak	HT-7, BL-15, *An-shen*, *Da-feng-men*, KID-3, BL-23, SP-6 *Er Yin Jian*[a]
Heart *Qi* deficiency	Tongue: pale and wet Coating: white Pulse: weak or irregular	*An-shen*, *Da-feng-men*, HT-7, PC-6, CV-17, BL-14, BL-15, BL-43, BL-44 Heart *Qi* Tonic[a]
Heart *Yin*/blood deficiency	Dry skin or dandruff Tongue: red or pale, with crack lines Coating: none to scant or peeled off and dry Pulse: thready, weak	*An-shen*, *Da-feng-men*, HT-7, PC-6, BL-14, BL-15, BL-44, BL-43, BL-17, SP-10, KID-3, SP-6 *Shen* Calmer[a]

[a] Dr Xie's Jing Tang Herbal Inc, Ocala, FL USA.

Integrative Treatment

Goals/Triage/Prognosis/Compliance

Successful treatment of a behavior problem depends upon clear communication that creates owner compliance. The owner must understand the behavior and that oral treatments are tools to facilitate success with the behavior modification exercises that create healthy brain synapses and healthy behaviors. The clinician must understand an owner's goals of treatment, objectively triage the patient, and give a reasonable prognosis [4, 20].

If the behavior presents a danger to other animals or people, the trigger is unidentified/uncontrollable or the owner is considering relinquishment of the animal; then immediate measures must provide safe management of the pet, perhaps even short-term hospitalization [20]. Sadly, if the owner is unable or unwilling to manage the pet creating safety or quality of life concerns, euthanasia may be the most humane option.

In all cases, whether mild or extreme, recommendations for behavior problems must be well-documented, reviewed verbally, provided in written form, and include judicious patient follow-up [20]. Long-term and intermediate goals established at the onset of treatment include benchmarks of improvement as well as an endpoint. A notebook of progress sheets for quick entry journaling of daily treatments and behavior scores will aid owner compliance and give the clinician a tool to follow at-home progress (Web 23.3 – daily progress sheet).

Medical Treatment of Co-morbidities

Treatment of co-morbid disease, whether TCVM or conventional, is crucial in resolving behavior problems. Even seemingly unrelated medical issues cause a stress response contributory to behavior imbalances [4]. Conventional treatment modalities may offer rapid intervention of acute problems whereas TCVM modalities may lessen conventional medications of chronic disease.

Behavior Modification

Behavior modification treatment begins with three foundational components: 1) discontinue all punishment, coercive and confrontational techniques, 2) establish a daily routine of food, water, exercise, attention, and sleep, and 3) daily practice of deference and relaxation exercises (Table 23.3 and Web 23.4 (Overall, Karen L, 2013 / with permission of Elsevier)). If possible, trigger stimuli are prevented to stop nerve signaling (associated with the behavior) which becomes stronger with each repetition. If the trigger stimuli cannot be prevented, then every attempt should be made to lessen the intensity through environmental management. In cases of aggression, trigger prevention is absolutely non-negotiable [1]. Only after success with the above should behavior modification exercises specific to the behavior (found in behavior textbooks) be attempted if still needed. Behaviorists informally state that 90% of behavior problems resolve with these foundational principles and practices.

Table 23.3 Foundational behavior protocols: Deference in this table and Relaxation in expanded web table [1]. Overall, Karen L, 2013 / with permission of Elsevier.

DEFERENCE

Benefits

- Improve relationship and trust
- Generalized calm and relaxed behavior
- Foundational for learning appropriate behaviors
- Pet has a tool to seek and take guidance
- Owner has a tool to prevent or divert undesired behaviors

Results

- Pet learns when calm, quiet, attentive, and deferring to human that attention and reward follow

Tips

- Make this enjoyable!
- NO punishment
- IGNORE undesirable behaviors, stop, walk away
- Practice daily
- End session while pet is relaxed
- Allow pet to learn at individual pace
- Small improvements are BIG triumphs!

Deference Protocol

Goal

- Pet sits calmly and looks at human for anything desired or needed

How

- Establish eye contact along with a sit
- Immediate treat reward is the "salary" to reinforce
- Use small pieces of highly palatable SOFT treat (not kibble)

Do's and Don'ts

- **Don't** stare; staring is threatening
- **Do** look at the pet
- **Do** smile
- **Do** give verbal praise with treat reward

Tips

- Pets with aggressive tendencies threatened by eye contact may require beginning without eye contact while keeping the pet in your view
- Encourage anxious pets that avoid eye contact by raising the treat hand to your forehead, then reward eye contact with a treat from the opposite, lower hand

---

Pharmaceutical Treatment

Psychogenic medications may enhance an animal's ability to learn, decrease stress, and decrease behaviors of destruction [1]. Owners hesitant to use these medications due to cost, side effects, or fear of personality changes may accept short-term or intermittent usage and should be encouraged to do so if the welfare of the animal depends upon it. Behavior medications decrease reactivity or fear through modulation of the neurotransmitters serotonin (5-HT), dopamine, noradrenaline, and/or gamma-aminobutyric acid and their

related metabolites [1]. Prescription medications commonly used are antidepressants, anti-anxiety agents, and anxiolytics that fall into three main classes: benzodiazepines, tricyclic antidepressants, and selective serotonin reuptake inhibitors [1]. Episodic occurrences of fear or anxiety benefit from intermittent usage of short-acting, fast-onset anxiolytics. Generalized or frequent behaviors interfering with daily routines benefit from the addition of daily antidepressant type medications. The six most commonly used psychogenic medications by the author, their usage and dosages are listed in Table 23.4 [5]. Before dispensing, the clinician should be

Table 23.4   Common behavior pharmaceuticals, oral doses*, indications, side effects Adapted from [5]. Horwitz, Debra F, 2018.

Drug	Onset	Canine dose	Feline dose	Indications	Comments/side effects
Alpha-2 agonist					
Clonidine	60–120 mins	0.01–0.05 mg/kg q12–24 h or PRN		Canine anxiety/fear disorders with high sympathetic arousal and/or impulsivity	Hypotension, sedation, paradoxical increased excitement; canine only
Anticonvulsant					
Gabapentin		5–30 mg/kg q 8–12h, 30–60 mg single dose 1–1.5 h before stressful event	2.5–10 mg/kg q 8–24h, 50–100 mg/cat 1–2 h before stressful event	Sedation for veterinary visits, neuropathic pain	Sedation, contraindicated in renal dysfunction
Benzodiazepine					
Alprazolam	c. 60 mins	0.02–0.1 mg/kg, q 6–8 hr or PRN	0.02–0.1 mg/kg q 8–24 h or PRN 0.125mg/cat q 8 hr	Anxiety, fear, phobia, feline urine marking	Sedation, lethargy, increased appetite, paradoxical agitation/excitement, disinhibition of aggression
Selective serotonin reuptake inhibitor					
Paroxetine	1–4 wks	0.5–2.0 mg/kg q 24 hr	0.25–1.0 mg/kg q 24 h	Feline urine marking, anxiety, over-grooming, anxious aggression	Constipation, urinary retention, lethargy, gastrointestinal effects, irritability
Tricyclic antidepressant					
Amitriptyline	1–4 wks	1.0–2.0 mg/kg q 12 h	0.5–1.0 mg/kg q 12–24 h	Feline urine marking, reactivity, anxiety, anxious, aggression, self-trauma/over-grooming	Tachycardia, constipation, mydriasis, urinary retention, sedation, avoid in epileptics, overdosage at 15 mg/kg
5-HT2A antagonist					
Trazodone	c. 45–90 mins	3.0–5.0 mg/kg q 8–12 h (maximum dose 300 mg/day) or PRN	25–100 mg/cat PRN or q 12–24 h; peak effect 90–120 min	Anxiety disorders, separation anxiety, thunderstorm or fireworks sensitivity, veterinary visits, handling/transport/hospitalization stress	Risk of serotonin syndrome with other serotonergic drugs, paradoxical excitement, sedation, gastrointestinal effects

PRN= as needed; *Given doses are typical ranges; all doses should be tailored to the specific patient/condition with appropriate additional sources utilized for additional dosing information. Adverse reactions are possible at any dose; always monitor for adverse responses. Additional drugs included in expanded Web Table 23.5.

familiar with indications, side effects, contraindications and require owner informed consent. [1, 4, 5] The reader is directed to an expanded list of psychogenic medications for additional consideration (Web 23.5 (Adapted from [5]. Horwitz, Debra F, 2018)).

TCVM Pattern Treatment

TCVM treatment of behavior disorders focuses on calming *Shen*, clearing any heat, fire, damp, or phlegm, moving *Qi* stagnation and tonifying any deficiencies of blood, *Yin* or *Qi*. TCVM treatment modalities include acupuncture, Chinese herbal medicine, *Tui-na*, and food therapy as accepted by the owner and pet (Tables 23.2, 23.5, 23.6, Web

23.6 (Xie, H et al., 2014; [22]. Xie et al., 2008) – 23.11 ([21]. Fowler et al., 2014 / Chi University)). Studies of laboratory, human and companion animals demonstrating efficacy of TCVM in behavior disorders, suggest that these modalities lessen the need for both daily and intermittent psychogenic medication [6–15].

Food Therapy for Shen Disturbance

Food therapy plays an important role in treating the causes of Shen disturbance in dogs and cats. According to principles of TCVM, heat conditions are treated with foods that have cooling properties and deficient conditions with foods that have appropriate tonifying properties (Table 23.6) [22].

Table 23.5 *Tui-na* techniques, benefits, protocol [19]. Xie, H et al., 2014; [22]. Xie et al., 2008.

Tui-Na technique	Benefit	Protocol
Moo-fa	Opens orifices, calms spirit and awakens brain; extent and duration of treatment varies and should be long enough to create a relaxed state but short enough to avoid distraction by surrounding stimuli	Encircling orbit including BL-1, GB-14, GB-1, and ST-1 Midline of head from *Long-hua* to *Da-feng-men* Encircling ear base from TH-21, SI-19, TH-17 to *An-shen*
Mo-fa	Harmonizes middle *Jiao*, regulates *Qi*, moves Stagnation	From head/neck to shoulder/pectoral area along Stomach Channel/Conception Vessel From head to rear along gall bladder channel
After mastery of relaxation with *Moo-fa/ Mo-fa* Additional *Tui-na* may be added: *Nie-fa*	Invigorates blood and *Qi*; benefits deficiency; invigorates heart, pericardium, spleen, liver and kidney channels	Midline from shoulder to lumbar area from BL-14 to BL-23
An-fa	Invigorates blood and *Qi*; unblocks obstructions; moves liver *Qi*, clears heat and phlegm	ST-36 to stimulate *Qi*; ST-40 clear phlegm *Er-jian* to clear heat TH-5/PC-6 to open heart orifice
Tui-fa	Improves blood circulation; moves liver *Qi*	Over costal regions to move liver *Qi*

Table 23.6 List of foods to consider that satisfy multiple criteria for treating *Shen* disturbance using food therapy [19]. Xie, H et al., 2014 / Chi University.

	Cooling	Move *Qi*	Tonify heart blood	Tonify heart *Yin*	Calm *Shen*	Tonify spleen *Qi*	Dry, damp, and clear phlegm
Beef	*	*	*	*		*	
Duck	*	*		*	*		
Heart			*				
Liver			*				
Lean pork	*	*		*			
Rabbit	*	*		*	*		
Turkey	*	*		*			
Whitefish	*	*		*			
Tofu	*	*		*			*
Chicken eggs	*	*	*				
Barley	*		*				*
Oats			*		*	*	
Brown rice	*				*	*	
Mung beans	*	*		*	*		
Celery	*				*		*
Cooked dark green leafy vegetables	*	*	*				
Shitake mushrooms	*	*			*	*	*

Table 23.6 (Continued)

	Cooling	Move *Qi*	Tonify heart blood	Tonify heart *Yin*	Calm *Shen*	Tonify spleen *Qi*	Dry, damp, and clear phlegm
Spinach	*			*	*		
Yams	*	*		*		*	
Apples	*	*			*		*
Dates	*	*	*			*	
Figs	*	*	*			*	
Lemon	*			*	*		*
Pears	*	*					*
Rhubarb	*			*	*		
Watermelon	*	*		*			
Fennel root	*	*			*		
Sweet basil	*	*			*		

Careful selection of various foods can treat the excess patterns of heart phlegm/fire and liver *Qi* stagnation and the deficiency patterns of heart *Qi*, blood, and *Yin* (Web 23.7 ([21]. Fowler et al., 2014 / Chi University)–23.11). The reader is directed to sample canine and feline recipes that address TCVM patterns of *Shen* disturbance (Web 23.12). When using whole food diets for dogs and cats, the clinician must keep in mind to provide balanced macro and micronutrients according to National Research Council recommendations.

Integrative Clinical Case Examples

Clinical Cases

Case 1: A 12-yr old neutered male Golden Retriever presented for abnormal behavior associated with thunderstorm fear which included panting, pacing, and drooling. The dog had a history of kidney and degenerative joint disease treated with commercial dry kibble prescription diet and intermittent oral non-steroidal anti-inflammatory drug. Owners reported that he insisted on being the center of attention, was frequently vocal, startled easily, preferred cool places, and had decreased stamina with compromised mobility in his rear limbs (the reader is directed to the website – Web 23.13, for integrative treatment strategies for this case).

Case 2: A six-year old female spayed Beagle-mix presented for problematic behaviors of aggression and noise sensitivities. Her barking and lunging at other dogs, vehicles, and unfamiliar people had become uncontrollable as well as her panting, drooling, and shaking in response to loud noises such as thunder, gun-fire, and vehicles. She was active with good stamina, sometimes

preferred cool places, ate dry commercial dog food, and drank water frequently. She sought attention from others but quickly retreated and snapped if approached. The dog had recently received long-acting heartworm preventive injection, oral intestinal dewormer, and the family was in the process of moving (the reader is directed to the website Web 23.13 for integrative treatment strategies for this case).

Conclusion

A problem behavior may be a contextually problematic normal behavior, a psychologic pathology, or due to a primary medical condition. Whatever the cause, the behavior must be addressed to prevent escalation of the abnormality and possible pet relinquishment. Strategic integration of TCVM, conventional and behavioral medicine can yield improved patient outcomes.

References

1 Overall, K.L. (2013). *Clinical Behavioral Medicine for Small Animals*. St. Louis, MO: Mosby Year Book Inc.

2 Stelow, E. (2018). Diagnosing behavior problems. *Vet Clin North Am Small Anim Pract* (Elsevier) 48: 339.

3 Salman, Mo D., et al. (2000). "Behavioral reasons for relinquishment of dogs and cats to 12 shelters." *Journal of Applied Animal Welfare Science* 3.2(2000): 93–106.

4 Landsberg, G., Hunthausen, W., and Ackerman, L. (2013). *Behavior Problems of the Dog & Cat*. London: Sauders Elsevier.

5 Horwitz, D.F. (2018). *Canine and Feline Behavior*. Hoboken, NJ: John Wiley &Sons, Inc.

6 Mayo, E. (2013 February). Behavioral disorders and acupuncture. *Am J Tradit Chin Vet Med* 8 (1): 49–55.

7 Ma, A. and Xie, H. (2020 August). Can successful behavior modification be accomplished through traditional Chinese veterinary medicine treatment? *Am J Tradit Chin Vet Med* 15 (2): 61–66.

8 Harris, L.A. (2007). Treatment of a mare with behavioral problems with Chinese herbal medicine. *Am J Tradit Chin Vet Med* 2 (1): 63–67.

9 Fong, P. and Xie, H. (2019 February). Comparison of the sedation effects of dry needle acupuncture of An-shen versus intramuscular butorphanol in 24 companion dogs. *Am J Tradit Chin Vet Med* 14 (1): 5–10.

10 Ying, W., Bhattacharjee, A., and Wu, S.S. (2019 February). Effect of laser acupuncture on mitigating anxiety in acute stressed horses: a randomized, controlled study. *Am J Tradit Chin Vet Med* 14 (1): 33–40.

11 Mier, H. (2021 February). Effectiveness of aqua-acupuncture for reducing stress of canine patients in veterinary clinics. *Am J Tradit Chin Vet Med* 16 (1): 41–50.

12 McDowell, C. and Shiau, D.-S. (2022 February). Effectiveness of integrated medical treatment for thunderstorm aversion: a case series of 23 dogs. *Am J Tradit Chin Vet Med* 17 (1): 13–25.

13 Xie, H. and Sivula, N. (2016 February). Review of veterinary acupuncture in clinical trials. *Am J Tradit Chin Vet Med* 11 (1): 49–60.

14 Koh, R. (2018 February). Traditional Chinese veterinary medicine for cognitive dysfunction syndrome. *Am J Tradit Chin Vet Med* 13 (1): 65–78.

15 Fowler, M. (2013 February). Use of modified Chai Hu Shu Gan Wan for treatment of liver *Qi* stagnation and liver yang rising in two lionesses. *Am J Tradit Chin Vet Med* 8 (1): 63–67.

16 Xie, H. and Preast, V. (2013). *Traditional Chinese Veterinary Medicine Fundamental Principles*, 2e. Reddick, FL: Chi Institute Press.

17 Xie, H., Wedemeyer, L., Chrisman, C.L., and Trevisanello, L. (2014). *Practical Guide to Traditional Chinese Veterinary Medicine Small Animal Medicine*. Reddick, FL: Chi Institute Press.

18 Skiwski, S.J. (2011 August). The fire element and *Shen* disturbances in dogs and cats. *Am J Tradit Chin Vet Med* 6 (2): 67–74.

19 Xie, H., Wedemeyer, L., and Chrisman, C.L. (2014). *Practical Guide to Traditional Chinese Veterinary Medicine Emergencies and Five Element Syndromes*. Reddick, FL: Chi Institute Press.

20 Martin, K.M., Martin, D., and Shaw, J.K. (2014). Small animal behavior triage: a guide for practitioners. *Vet Clin North Am Small Anim Pract* (Elsevier) 44 (3): 379–399.

21 Xie, H., Ferguson, B., and Deng, X. (2008). *Application of Tui-na in Veterinary Medicine*, 2e. Reddick, FL: Chi Institute, 91–94.

22 Fowler, M. and Xie, H. (2020). *Integrative and Traditional Chinese Veterinary Medicine Food Therapy*. Reddick, FL: Chi University Press.

24

Clinical Application of Chinese Herbal Medicine

Judith E. Saik

Introduction

The clinical application of Chinese herbal medicine in veterinary practice should have a similar clinical approach for their use as the many other therapeutic modalities that a veterinarian uses daily. Knowledge of an herb's therapeutic properties, as well as contraindications are as important in the practice of herbal medicine as when dispensing pharmaceuticals. A complete history, good physical exam, and appropriate conventional diagnostics are cornerstones on which to add any medical modality to an integrative practice, including Chinese herbal medicine. In addition to the foundational diagnostics, the traditional Chinese veterinary medicine (TCVM) practitioner adds a TCVM examination to their clinical evaluation. This exam, based on Chinese medicine theory, determines an individual's pattern of disease based on unique features some of which can be pulse form, tongue appearance, coolness/heat of extremities and personality constitution. With the addition of a TCVM Pattern diagnosis (e.g., Kidney *Qi* Deficiency, Liver *Qi* Stagnation, Bladder Damp Heat), the Chinese veterinary herbalist can then form a diagnostic conclusion of the pathological changes to a body caused by a disease and then optimally select an herb or herbal formula that best treats the clinical disease that their patient presents with.

Five Common Mistakes to Avoid When Prescribing Chinese Herbal Medicine

For optimal prescribing of Chinese herbal medications, there are five common mistakes to avoid [1]. The first is treating the symptoms rather than the TCVM Pattern. As conventionally trained veterinarians, it is natural to treat the clinical signs presented, and this will probably help alleviate presenting problems for a short time. It will, however, not provide long-term disease resolution as the root imbalance has not been addressed. The second common mistake is using too many herbs at one time. Limit the herbal prescriptions to three or less formulas to treat the primary pattern. Third is to treat the TCVM Pattern that is identified during the clinical TCVM exam. Avoid trying to prescribe a host of herbs to treat the many symptoms that are being observed by the caretaker. With proper herbal selection, the multitude of symptoms described by an owner mostly disappear when the primary pattern is addressed. Fourth is expecting the herbal medicine to work as quickly as conventional pharmaceuticals, many of which can have significant serum blood levels in less than an hour. Chinese herbal medicine is gentler and can take longer for a physio-chemical response. The fifth mistake is to restrain from developing "tunnel vision." It is tempting to focus on the presenting clinical signs and forget everything else that may affect an animal such as environment, emotions, constitution, and diet.

General Guidance for Herbal Therapy

Goals

There are four general goals for herbal therapy [2]. The first is to cure a disease. Examples might include soft tissue injury, UTI (urinary tract infection), IBD (inflammatory bowel disease). If the disease can't be cured, the second category would be to stabilize a condition (e.g., *Bi* syndrome, chronic renal disease, congestive heart failure – Grades 1–2). Third is to use herbal medicine as an adjunct therapy (e.g., diabetes, seizures, Cushing's disease). Fourth is to promote quality of life in severe terminal disease (e.g., cancer, end-stage renal, and heart disease).

Integrative Veterinary Medicine, First Edition. Edited by Mushtaq A. Memon and Huisheng Xie.
© 2023 John Wiley & Sons, Inc. Published 2023 by John Wiley & Sons, Inc.
Companion Website: www.wiley.com/go/memon/veterinary

Herbal Medicine Dosing

Herbal medicine therapeutic dosing covers a broad range and is dependent on a number of variables such as safety index, TCVM Pattern, age, vitality, and disease severity, just to name a few. The recommended doses below do not need to be strictly followed; these are general guidelines [2].

Companion Animal*: **Low dose** for long term/maintenance (0.5 g/20# BW, BID) – four weeks for results; **Medium dose** for most cases (0.5 g/10# BW, BID) – two weeks for results; **High Dose** for short term, usually Excess conditions (1 g/10#BW, BID) – 1–7 days

Equine*: **Maintenance**/prevention dose (7.5 g, BID) – long-term use/1 year (i.e., Body Sore[a] for performance horse aches); **Mild conditions** (15 g, BID) – 1–3 months (i.e., Shen Calmer[a] for stall anxiety); **Severe conditions** (30–60 g, BID) 1–4 weeks (i.e., Hot Hoof II[a] for laminitis); **Life threatening** (200 g BID) 1–5 days (i.e., *Yu Jin San* for acute colitis)

* = **Non-concentrated** formulas

Selection of Chinese Herbal Medicine Based on Clinical Conditions

 ### Cardiovascular-Hematopoietic Conditions

(Web Cases 1 and 2)

Congestive Heart Failure (CHF): Chinese herbal medicines may be combined with conventional medication for the most effective treatment. There are six TCVM Patterns of CHF: Heart *Qi* Deficiency, Deficiency of Heart *Qi/Yin*, Heart + Kidney *Yang* Deficiency, Heart *Yang* Deficiency, *Qi*-Blood Stagnation, Collapse of *Yang Qi*. The first three patterns are the most common (95%), with the other three more rare (Box 24.1).

Box 24.1

Heart *Qi* Deficiency – *Yang Xin Tang*/Heart *Qi* Tonic[a]

Heart *Qi/Yin* Deficiency – *Sheng Mai Yin, Zhi Gan Cao Tang*

Heart + Kidney *Yang* Deficiency – *Zhen Wu Tang*

Qi-Blood Stagnation – *Fu Fang Dan Shen Pian*/ Compound *Dan Shen*[a]

Heart *Yang* Deficiency – *Bao Yuan Tang*

Collapse of *Yang Qi* – *Shen Fu Tang* Plus

Anemia: Herbal selection for common TCVM Patterns of anemia (Box 24.2).

Box 24.2

Qi Deficiency – *Gui Pi Tang/Dang Gui Bu Xue*

Blood Deficiency – *Si Wu Tang* or *Gui Pi Tang*

Blood Deficiency (with Stagnation) – *Dang Gui*

Qi-Blood Deficiency – *Ba Zhen Tang*/Eight Treasures[a]

Bleeding/Hemorrhage: Acute trauma with bleeding can be treated with the Chinese patented formula, *Yunnan Bai Yao* capsules. Dosing for companion animals is 1 capsule per 10–20 pounds 4 times daily (1–2 days) in severe cases; for horses give 1 bottle of powder (4 g or 1 box of 16 capsules), 3 times daily in severe cases. A single small red pill is in center of the foil package and can be used for shock (given alone or with capsules) [1].

Edema/Ascites: Ascites is most commonly seen in small animals with heart/iver disease or neoplasia. Edema is observed after trauma or with poor circulation. The herbal medicines may not act as quickly as pharmaceuticals but are safer and helpful for weaning an animal (or reducing dose) of drugs (Box 24.3) [1].

Box 24.3

Water-fluid Retention – *Wu Ling San/Wu Pi Yin/Wu Pi Yin* Plus[a]

Spleen *Qi* Deficiency +/– *Qi* Stagnation – *Shi Pi Yin*

Spleen/Kidney *Yang* Deficiency – *Zhen Wu Tang*

Dermatological Conditions

(Web Cases 3 and 4)

Pruritis/Eruptions/Erosions/Dermatitis: This group of skin conditions is common, difficult to effectively control and frequently recurs. In TCVM, pruritis is associated with the master pathogen "Wind" which attacks the body surface causing itching. Wind tends to combine with Heat (*Yang* pathogen) to become Wind-Heat or Wind-Toxin or with Damp to become Damp-Heat. Wind-Heat and Damp-Heat are the major pathogens of skin diseases. Chinese herbal medicine formulas for this group of conditions have several basic actions: clear Heat (inflammation) and detoxify, clear Wind to relieve itching, minimize scab crusted eruptions, nourish Blood, and calm anxiety by increasing the smooth flow of *Qi* and Blood (Box 24.4) [3].

Box 24.4

External Wind (skin allergy) – *Qu Feng Zhi Yang*/External Wind[a]

Wind-Heat – *Shi Yi De Xiao Fang*/Wind Toxin[a]

Damp Heat – *Qing Shi Re Tang*/Damp Heat Skin[a]

Liver Damp Heat (dermatitis) – *Long Dan Xie Gan*

Blood Deficiency (with pruritis) – *Si Wu Xiao Feng*

Blood/*Yin* Deficiency (chronic itching) – *Qu Xie Fang*/Dandruff Formula[a]

Blood/*Yin* Deficiency and Damp (chronic itching) – *Wu Shen San*

Yin Deficiency (pruritis worse at night) – *Yang Yin Zhi Yang*

Wheals, Hives, and Urticaria: This can include sudden wheals on the head/neck/body, itching and swelling of eyelids/lips. The Chinese herbal medicines used to clear Heat, address Wind-toxin and detoxify are *Xiao Huang San* or Lung Wind *Huang*[a].

Endocrine Disorders

(Web Cases 5–7)

Cushing's Disease: Herbal medicine can often be used without conventional medications in mild cases or as an adjunct to pharmaceuticals in more severe cases to lower drug doses. There are three common TCVM Patterns for dogs (Box 24.5).

Box 24.5

Dog, Horse

Yin Deficiency – *Mai Men Dong*/Ophiopogon[a]

Qi-Yin Deficiency – *Xia Xiao Fang*/Rehmannia 11[a]

Yang Deficiency – *Jin Gui Shen Qi*/Rehmannia 14[a]

Horse

Qi Deficiency + Damp – *Er Chen Tang*/Phlegm Fat Formula[a]

Cushing's/Equine Metabolic Syndrome: There are four TCVM Patterns to consider for horses when adding Chinese herbal medicine to therapeutic management of cases. Early in these diseases, horses can present with Liver *Qi* Stagnation (insulin metabolism abnormalities) which then progresses to Spleen *Qi* Deficiency with Damp-Heat (obesity, laminitis, lethargy). This is followed by *Yin* Deficiency or *Qi-Yin* and last is *Yang* Deficiency (Box 24.5).

Diabetes: In Chinese medicine, there are three primary pathways that are considered to induce diabetes: imbalanced diet (particularly overeating), emotional stress (creating chronic Liver *Qi* Stagnation), overwork (damage to Kidney Essence). Box 24.6

Box 24.6

Lung Heat (Upper *Xiao*) – *Qing Fei San*/Red Lung[a]

Stomach Heat (Middle *Xiao*) – *Yu Nu Jian*/Jade Lady[a]

Kidney *Yin* Deficiency – *Zi Shen Ming Mu Tang*/Xiao Ke Fang[a]

Kidney *Qi-Yin* Deficiency – *Jiang Tang Cha, Yu Quan Wan*

Hypothyroid: The most common TCVM Patterns encountered in dogs that are treated with Chinese herbal medicine are *Yang/Qi* Deficiency (poor digestion, loose stools, cool extremities) and *Qi/Yin/*Blood Deficiency (lethargy, PU/PD, alopecia, cool feet). Herbal formulas may be combined to treat the dominant presenting patterns. For example: *Qi*-Blood Deficiency, one may use *Si Wu Tang* with *Si Jun Zi Tang* or could substitute *Lui Wei Di Huang* for *Si Wu Tang* if the *Yin* Deficiency is more pronounced than Blood Deficiency (Box 24.7) [1].

Box 24.7

Liver *Qi* Stagnation – *Si Hai Su Yu Wan*/Si Hai Formula[a]

Yuan Qi/Yang Qi Deficiency – *Xiao Ying San*/You Gui Wan

Qi-Yin Deficiency – *Jia Bing Fang*

Hyperthyroid: Inappropriate diet may be one of the leading causes of thyroid dysfunction in cats. It is also seen as a sequela to chronic illness. Chinese herbal medicine treatment is generally used as an adjunct to conventional treatment (Box 24.8). [1]

Box 24.8

Liver *Qi* Stagnation with Blood-Phlegm Stagnation – *Hai Zao Yu Hu Tang*/Sargassum Jade Pot[a]

Yin Deficiency with *Yang* Floating – *Jia Kang Fang*/Hyper Jia Bing[a]

Addison's Disease: Sudden collapse from hypoadrenocorticism is from a profound loss of *Yang* which results in death. During acute crash, treat with conventional medicine. When stable, can start a TCVM approach for maintenance (along with conventional drugs). The TCVM diagnosis for this condition is Kidney *Jing* Deficiency (Kidney *Yang* + Kidney *Yin*). There are two options for Chinese herbal medicine treatment: 1) *You Gui Wan* (morning) + *Zuo Gui Wan* (evening), 2) Epimedium powder[a] (tonifies everything, safe for long-term use as maintenance).

Gastrointestinal Disorders

(Web Cases 8–11)

Anorexia: Anorexia can be part of a multitude of conventional medical syndromes which create the loss of appetite or poor appetite. In TCVM, it can be divided into four primary patterns that may be treated with Chinese herbal medicine (Box 24.9).

Box 24.9

Stomach Cold – *Wei Chang He*/Happy Earth[a]
Stomach Heat – *Yu Nu Jian*/Jade Lady[a]
Food Stasis – *Bao He Wan*
Spleen *Qi* Deficiency – *Liu Jun Zi Tang*/Six Gentlemen, *Xiang Sha Liu Jun Zi Tang*/Eight Gentlemen[a]

Vomiting: Vomiting is caused by rebellious Stomach *Qi* or failure of Stomach *Qi* to descend. Similar to anorexia, it may be part of many diseases in companion animals. The most common causes are related to Food Stagnation, Liver *Qi* Stagnation and hypofunction of the Spleen and Stomach (Box 24.10) [4].

Box 24.10

Exogenous Pathogenic Factors (disrupt Stomach) – *Wei Chang He*/Happy Earth[a] or
Huo Xiang Zheng Qi (add *Ju Pi San* if severe stomach pain)
Food Stagnation – *Bao He Wan* (add Four Gentlemen if Spleen *Qi* Def)
Liver *Qi* Stagnation – *Chai Hu Shu Gan*/Liver Happy[a] (use *Xiao Yao San* if have diarrhea also)
Spleen *Qi* Deficiency – *Xiang Sha Liu Jun Zi Tang*/Eight Gentlemen[a] (add *Shen Ling Bai Zhu* if diarrhea)
Stomach *Yin* Deficiency – *Xiao Yao San* + *Er Chen Tang*/ Stomach Happy[a] (add Four Gentlemen if Spleen *Qi* Def)

Diarrhea: TCVM Patterns for diarrhea in horses are divided in five patterns while companion animals have four TCVM Patterns. The similarities between Chinese herbal medicine treatment of small and large animals and differences are included in Box 24.11.

Box 24.11

Cold-Damp (Horses) – *Ping Wei San*/Equine GI Formula[a]
Heat-Toxin/Damp-Heat (Horses) – *Yu Jin San*
Heat-Toxin/Damp-Heat (Dogs, Cats) – *Da Xiang Lian Wan*/Great Saussurea Coptis[a]
Liver *Qi* Stagnation (Horses) – *Xiao Yao San*
Liver-Spleen Disharmony (Dogs, Cats) – *Xiao Yao San*
Spleen *Qi* Deficiency (Horses, Dogs, Cats) – Shen Ling Bai Zhu
Kidney *Yang* Deficiency (Horses, Dogs, Cats) – *Si Shen Wan*/ Four Immortals[a]
Foal Diarrhea – *Wu Mei San*/ Mume Formula[a]

Abdominal Pain/Colic: This clinical condition is most common in horses but can occur in dogs. It results from *Qi*-Blood Stagnation in the abdomen and is divided into five TCVM Patterns (Box 24.12).

Box 24.12

Cold/*Qi* Stagnation – *Ju Pi San*
Damp-Heat Pattern – *Yu Jin San*
Bloat/Gaseous colic – *Xiao Zhang San*
Blood Stagnation – *Shao Fu Zhu Yu*
Food Stagnation – *Bao He Wan*

Impaction/Constipation: In TCVM, impaction and constipation belong to an obstruction syndrome. Constipation (dry hard feces with difficult defecation) is a clinical problem for cats and dogs while impaction (cecal and colonic) is a common cause of colic in horses. From a TCVM perspective, etiologies underlying the Large Intestine's decreased ability to move and eliminate feces include: Internal Heat, Internal Dryness (*Yin*-Blood Deficiency), *Qi* Deficiency (Box 24.13).

Box 24.13

Heat – *Da Cheng Qi Tang*
Qi Stagnation – *Xiao Zhang San*
Qi Deficiency – *Fan Xie Ye*
Yin/Blood Deficiency – *Dang Gui Cong Rong*

Musculoskeletal and Neurological Conditions

(Web Cases 12–15)

Bi Syndrome (Osteoarthritis and Muscle-Tendon Pain): In TCVM, the term *Bi* syndrome refers to pain and stiffness in the muscles, tendons, bones, and joints [3]. The root causes are related to the pathogens: Wind, Cold, Damp, Heat (Excess pattern). Bony *Bi* (chronic *Bi* syndrome) is a Kidney Deficiency pattern (*Qi, Qi/Yang, Yin, Qi/Yin*) which can be further complicated by pathogens (Box 24.14).

Box 24.14

Painful *Bi*/Cold *Bi* – *Du Huo Ji Sheng Tang*/Dok's Formula[a]/Equine *Du Huo*[a]
Fixed *Bi*/Damp *Bi* – *Yi Yi Ren San*/Coix Formula[a]
Kidney *Qi/Yang* Deficiency *Bi* – *Sang Ji Sheng San*/Loranthus[a]
Kidney *Yin/Qi* Deficiency *Bi* – *Di Gu Pi*
Kidney *Qi/Yang* Deficiency *Bi* – *Sang Zhi San*
Heat Bi (immune-mediated arthritis) – *Bai Hu Si Miao*/*Si Miao San*

Disc Disease and Spondylosis: These conditions fall under the general category of *Bi* syndrome. Acute disc disease with paralysis/paresis, use strong Blood-moving herbs. Chronic disc disease and spondylosis will also need to address the Deficiencies that will be present due to disease chronicity (Box 24.15).

Box 24.15

Wind-Cold-Damp – *Xiao Huo Luo Dan*
Blood Stagnation – *Da Huo Luo Dan*/Double P II[a]
Cervical Region – Double P II + *Jing Tong Fang*/Cervical Formula[a]
Thoraco-lumbar Region (*Qi/Yang* Deficiency) – Double P II + *Bu Yang Huan Wu*
Thoraco-lumbar (*Yin* Deficiency) – Double P II + *Di Gu Pi*
Heat Toxin (Discospondylitis) – *Qing Ying Tang*

Seizures: In TCVM, seizures belong to "Internal Wind" syndromes. They are commonly associated with Phlegm, Stagnation, Liver Blood/*Yin* Deficiency and disharmony of *Zang Qi* [3]. Commonly, two herbal formulas may need to be selected: Example – formula to address the Excess condition (i.e., *Di Tan Tang*) + formula for the Deficiency (i.e., *Yang Yin Xi Feng*) [5] (Box 24.16).

Box 24.16

Liver Blood Deficiency – *Bu Xue Xi Feng* (may add *Di Tan Tang*)
Liver/Kidney *Yin* Deficiency – *Yang Yin Xi Feng* (may add *Di Tan Tang* or *Ding Xian Wan*)
Kidney *Jing* Deficiency – Epimedium and *Di Tan Tang*

Liver/Kidney *Yin* Deficiency and Liver Blood Deficiency – *Tian Ma* Plus II (may add *Di Tan Tang*)
Obstruction by Wind-Phlegm – *Ding Xian Wan*
Liver *Qi* Stagnation with Internal Profusion of Phlegm-Fire – *Di Tan Tang* + *Long Dan Xie Gan*
Stagnation of Blood – Di Tan Tang + Tao Hong Si Wu/Stasis in Mansion of Mind[a]

Peripheral Nerve Paralysis: Peripheral nerve paralysis is characterized by *Qi* Deficiency and in some cases a local Stagnation (Box 24.17).

Box 24.17

Laryngeal hemiplegia – *Bu Zhong Yi Qi*
Facial paralysis – *Mian Tan Fang*/Facial P Formula[a]
Radial nerve paralysis – *Ba Zhen Tang*/*Qi* Performance[a]
Bladder atonia – *Jin Suo Gu Jing*

Head Trauma/Spinal Cord Injuries: These are related to severe acute trauma (e.g., falling, car accident, blows to the body, bite wounds). Chinese herbal strategies are to stop bleeding, relieve pain, control Heat/inflammation, tranquilize Liver *Yang*, tonify *Qi* and clear internal Wind (Box 24.18).

Box 24.18

Bleeding/Pain – *Yunnan Bai Yao* + *Shen Tong Zhu Yu*/Body Sore[a]
Qi-Blood Stagnation (head, coma) – *Nao Yu Fang*/Stasis in Mansion of Mind[a]
Qi-Blood Stagnation (spine, paresis) – *Da Huo Luo Dan*/Double P II[a]
Heat Toxin (inflammation brain/spine) – *Pu Ji Xiao Du Yin*
Internal Wind (seizures) – *Ling Jiao Gou Teng*
Qi/Yang Deficiency (with paresis) – *Bu Yang Huan Wu*

Neoplasia

(Web Case 16)

Chinese herbal medicine – Formulas for cancers are determined by the presenting TCVM Pattern(s) of the patient, as well as their general health, and conventional treatments they are undergoing [1]. Cancer is always considered a *Qi* Deficiency (usually accompanied by Blood Deficiency) which is complicated by severe *Qi*-Blood Stagnation with increasing severity to Blood Stasis. Herbal formulas chosen, therefore, should move Stagnation/address Stasis and provide support for the Deficiencies. Finally, one may add additional herbs/formulas to bring the main formula to a particular area of the body (transporter herb).

Formulating Cancer Protocols – Choose herbs and herbal formulas thoughtfully. It is important to address the specific TCVM Pattern(s) the patient is presenting, along with the type of cancer and the animal's quality of life. For example, a patient with bladder cancer showing signs of severe Damp-Heat in the lower-*Jiao* (straining, hematuria, Heat signs), may benefit from Stasis Breaker combined with *Long Dan Xie Gan* [1]. In contrast, a very elderly *Yin* Deficient animal; one might choose *Liu Wei Di Huang Wan* with *Shao Fu Zhu Yu Tang*. For bone cancer in an Excess pattern animal, one might choose Stasis Breaker (attack tumor/Blood Stasis), combined with *Wei Qi* Booster (Blood-*Qi* tonics, increase *Wei Qi*-immunomodulation) and half dose Bone Stasis (transporter). An older, Deficient pattern animal may need *Qi* and *Yin* tonics added along with milder cancer formulas (Box 24.19) [1].

Box 24.19

All Tumor Types
Tonify *Qi* and Blood – *Wei Qi* Booster[a]
Mild, softer mass, weak patient – Max's Formula[a]
Breaks Blood Stasis, large mass – Stasis Breaker[a]
Tumor Location/Transporter Herbal Formulas
Vascular/Heart/Blood tumors (i.e., Mast Cell Tumor) – *Xue Fu Zhu Yu Tang*
Lower abdomen masses – *Shao Fu Zhu Yu Tang*
Heart base mass – *Ge Xia Zhu Yu*
Kidney/Bladder – *Wu Ling San*
Sinus/Nasal – *Xin Yi San*
Any tumor with hemorrhage – *Yunnan Bai Yao*
Anus/Testes/Ovary/Uterus/Urethra – Prostate Invigorator[a]
Mammary gland – Breast Stasis Formula[a]
Brain – Stasis in the Mansion of the Mind[a]
Cervical region – Cervical Formula[a]
Disc (thoraco-lumbar) – Double P II[a]
Feet – Four Paws Damp Heat[a]
General head/Mouth – *Pu Ji Xiao Du Yin*
Liver – Artemisia Combination[a] or Liver Happy[a]
Lung/Lower Airway- Red Lung[a] or *Qing Fei San*
Osteosarcoma – Bone Stasis Formula[a]
Spleen/Stomach – Happy Earth[a]
Thyroid – Sargassum Jade Pot[a]

Ophthalmic Conditions

(Web Case 17)

Conjunctivitis, keratitis, keratoconjunctivitis sicca (KCS), anterior uveitis, equine recurrent uveitis (ERU): In TCVM, healthy vision depends on healthy Liver and Kidney Element function. Liver Blood and *Yin* moisten the eyes. Heat/Liver Fire can burn up the *Yin* and create redness, eyelid inflammation, or sclerosis of the lens. Blood and *Yin* Deficiency create dry, itchy eyes and can be involved with cataracts, glaucoma, and uveitis (Box 24.20) [1].

Box 24.20

Stagnation – *Ju Ming San*/ Haliotis[a], (keratitis/KCS, uveitis/ERU, chronic conjunctivitis)
Liver Heat with Stagnation – *Long Dan Xie Gan*, *Fang Feng San* (KCS, acute conjunctivitis, uveitis/ERU
Liver-Kidney *Yin* Deficiency – *Qi Ju Di Huang* (KCS, anterior uveitis, ERU, cataracts)
Blood and *Yin* Deficiency – *Ming Mu Di Huang*, *Qi Ju Di Huang*

Renal and Bladder Disorders

(Web Cases 18 and 19)

Chronic Renal Disease – The management of chronic renal disease in companion animals is not well-addressed by conventional medications and usually follows a rapid decline with poor quality of life. Chinese herbal medicine can make a significant impact on these patients' lives both in quality and length of life. The herbalist, in addition, to selecting Chinese herbal medicines that treat the TCVM Kidney Pattern should also select herbal medicines to address the other clinical signs presented by these animals such as vomiting, anorexia, or anemia (Box 24.21).

Box 24.21

Kidney *Qi* Deficiency – *Jin Gui Shen Qi*
Kidney *Yang* Deficiency – *You Gui Wan*
Kidney *Yin* Deficiency – *Zuo Gui Wan*, *Liu Wei Di Huang*
Kidney *Qi* and *Yin* Deficiency – *Xia Xiao Fang*/Rehmannia 11[a]

Urinary Tract Infection: Chinese herbal medicine is effective as a primary treatment or as an adjunct treatment along with antibiotics (Box 24.22).

Urinary Incontinence: Chinese herbal formulas are effective as primary treatment or as an adjunct treatment and can be used safely with conventional medications (Box 24.23).

Respiratory Conditions

(Web Case 20)

Nasal Discharge and Congestion: Chinese herbal medicine can be effective as a primary treatment or as an adjunct to conventional medications in more severe disease (Box 24.24).

Cough: Coughing is associated with a number of clinical conditions as well as TCVM Patterns. Wind-Cold is superficial and acute with clear nasal discharge, while Wind-Heat is becoming more invasive and accompanied by fever and loud cough. Lung-Heat has a chronic persistent cough and nasal discharge is thick/yellow. Phlegm-Damp has very little nasal discharge but has a cough that is loud and productive. Deficiency coughs include Lung *Yin* Deficiency (prolonged weak cough at night) and Lung *Qi* Deficiency (cough with weak voice, fatigue). Box 24.25

Summary

The clinical conditions and the Chinese herbal medicines that are listed in this chapter are just a small sample of the large number of single herbs/herbal formulas, both current and dating back 2,000 years, that are available to veterinarians integrating Chinese herbal medicine into their clinical practices. This interesting but complex area of veterinary medicine continues to grow as evidenced by the expanding number of excellent Chinese herbal courses both at the beginner and advanced levels that a clinician, who wants to enhance their knowledge and improve clinical outcomes, can attend. A list of textbooks is also provided under "recommended reading" that veterinarians, practicing Chinese herbal medicine, can consult for greater detail on the medical conditions and associated Chinese herbal medicines introduced to the reader in this chapter.

"Only when one refines the old and learns from the new can one become a real doctor"

Huang Di Nei Jing (*Yellow Emperor's Classic of Internal Medicine*)

Note

1 Chinese herbal formulas, Dr Xie's Jing Tang Herbal Inc, Ocala, FL USA.

Recommended Reading

1 Xie, H. and Preast, V. (2010). *Xie's Chinese Veterinary Herbology*, 559,563,568–569,570–574. Ames, IA: Wiley-Blackwell.

2 Xie, H. and Priest, V. (2008). *Chinese Veterinary Herbal Handbook*, 2e, 340–341. Reddick, FL: Chi Institute of Chinese Medicine.

3 Ma, A. (2016). *Clinical Manual of Chinese Veterinary Herbal Medicine*, 238,3,287. Gainesville, FL: Ancient Art Press.

4 Xie, H. and Preast, V. (2007). *Xie's Veterinary Acupuncture*, 276. Ames, Iowa: Blackwell Publishing.

5 Xie, H., Wedemeyer, L., and Chrisman, C. (2014). *Practical Guide to Traditional Chinese Veterinary Medicine, Small Animal Practice*, 80–95. Reddick, FL: Chi Institute Press.

6 Chen, J., Chen, T., Beebe, S., and Salewski, M. (2012). *Chinese Herbal Formulas for Veterinarians*. City of Industry, CA: Art of Medicine Press Inc.

7 Marsden, S. (2013). *Essential Guide to Chinese Herbal Formulas*. Yeppon, Australia: College of Integrative Veterinary Therapies (CIVT).

25

Case Based Approach to Integrative Veterinary Practice

Mitchell McKee

Introduction

American author and speaker Dale Carnegie once said, "Most of the important things in the world have been accomplished by people who have kept on trying when there seemed to be no hope left at all" [1]. Perhaps integrative medicine was born out of a similar desire; to keep trying and never give up. Such persistence has led to new technological advances that have enhanced our ability to diagnose and treat patients. Tried and true methods of old have emerged once again and are being utilized to improve treatment outcome and quality of life. No better time has ever existed to provide veterinary patients with the best integrative treatment options available.

Each veterinary patient is unique and often circumstances differ. The patient dictates the treatment more so than the practitioner. Integrative medicine allows the practitioner to provide individualized care instead of a one size fits all approach for common conditions.

Integrative Approach to Veterinary Medicine

Medical treatment of the clinical cases in this series embraces both conventional medicine and the principles of Traditional Chinese Veterinary Medicine (TCVM) to combine East and West into an integrative medical approach to small animal medicine. The clinical conditions are presented according to conventional diagnoses and the Five Element TCVM Pattern (Table 25.1).

Clinical Cases

Wood Element

Common Wood (liver) related conditions seen in practice include conjunctivitis, eye conditions (including immune-mediated), and cranial cruciate ligament disease.

Table 25.1 TCVM Five Element* attributes [2]. Xie H, Preast V 2013 / Chi University.

Element	Wood	Fire	Earth	Metal	Water
Organ	Liver	Heart	Spleen	Lungs	Kidney
Function	Maintain smooth flow of *Qi*	Governs blood and vessels	Transforms and transports food energy (*Qi*) and body fluids	Governs *Qi*	Governs bones and water pathway
	Store Blood	Houses *Shen* (spirit and mind)		Distributes food *Qi* and body fluids	Stores genetic material
Affected structures	Eyes	Heart	GI tract	Respiratory tract	Urinary tract
	Tendons	Mind		Skin	Bones
	Ligaments			Hair coat	

* Each element is listed with the associated organ, organ function, and corresponding affected structures. The table has been modified to include only those aspects of each element that apply to this case series and is not a full and complete representation of all known TCVM attributes.

Integrative Veterinary Medicine, First Edition. Edited by Mushtaq A. Memon and Huisheng Xie.
© 2023 John Wiley & Sons, Inc. Published 2023 by John Wiley & Sons, Inc.
Companion Website: www.wiley.com/go/memon/veterinary

Conjunctivitis, Keratoconjunctivitis Sicca (KCS), Pannus

Conjunctivitis, also known in TCVM as Heat/Fire in the Liver, is often caused by infection and inflammation resulting in Liver Heat Rising Upward toward the eyes. Chronic irritation can cause TCVM deficiencies, such as Liver *Yin* and Blood deficiencies, leading to KCS and pannus. Topical medications containing steroids, antibiotics, and tear stimulants have long been used to treat these conditions (Figure 25.1).

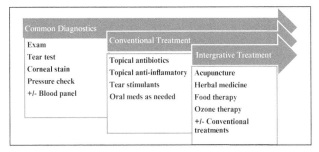

Figure 25.1 This flow chart demonstrates initial diagnostics with conventional treatment followed by the expanded treatment with improved outcomes available by using an integrative approach.

Case 1

Signalment: 10 yr. female spayed (FS) Shih Tzu

Conventional Diagnosis: KCS, severe conjunctivitis, partial response to therapy

TCVM Diagnosis: Liver *Yin* and Blood deficiency with Heat Fire Flaring Up

Integrative Treatment: Herbal therapy was added due to poor response to conventional treatment (Figure 25.2)

Outcome: Clinical signs resolved in 45 days. Schirmer's test normalized: OD 16 mm, OS 14 mm

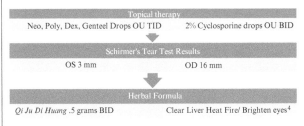

Figure 25.2 Case 1 Integrative Treatment.

Case 2

Signalment: 9 yr. male intact German Shepard (Figure 25.3)

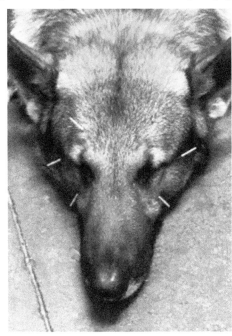

Figure 25.3 Picture of Case 2 during an acupuncture session for chronic superficial keratitis/pannus.

Conventional Diagnosis: Chronic superficial keratitis/pannus

TCVM Diagnosis: Liver *Yin* and Blood Deficiency with Liver Fire Flaring Up

Integrative Treatment: Topical, acupuncture, and herbal therapies (Figure 25.4)

Outcome: Eyes returned to normal in two weeks. Occasional flare ups were managed in similar fashion. Other supplements given by owner to address deficiency patterns.

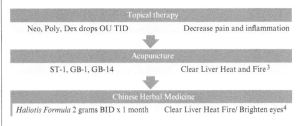

Figure 25.4 Case 2 integrative treatment.

Therapeutic Review

Table 25.2 lists common integrative therapy options for eye problems.

Table 25.2 Integrative therapies for common eye conditions. Adapted from [3]. Dewey C, Xie H, 2018; [4]. Xie H, 2011; [5]. Fowler M, Xie H, 2022.

Integrative treatment method	Integrative approach	Therapeutic results
Acupuncture	ST-1	Clears Liver Heat and Liver Fire
	GB-1	Expels Wind
	GB-14	Clears Heat
Herbal medicine	*Haliotis Formula*[a]	Clears Liver Heat
		Cools Blood
	Qi Ju Di Huang[a]	Brightens eyes
		Nourish *Yin*
Food therapy	Chicken egg white	Clear Liver Heat
	Celery	
	Collard greens	
	Chrysanthemum	
Ozone therapy	Subcutaneous (SQ)	Immune support
	Rectal	Anti-viral, anti-bacterial
	Topical	Anti-inflammatory

[a] Jing Tang Herbal, Reddick, FL.

Tendon/Ligament

Cranial cruciate ligament (CCL) problems can be associated with acute injury or weakened tendon strength over time. Radiographs along with the presence or absence of cranial drawer and tibial thrust are indicated for accurate assessment. Surgery, pain management, rehab, and physical therapy have proven beneficial to restore muscle strength, stability, and mobility.

Figure 25.5 compares conventional and integrative approaches to CCL disease while Table 25.3 further demonstrates an integrative treatment approach.

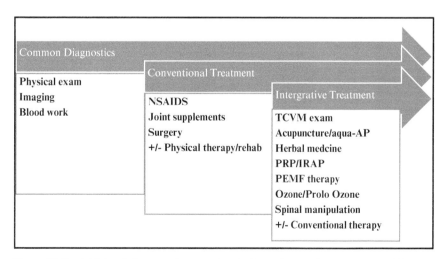

Figure 25.5 Additional therapeutics associated with an integrative approach to CCL disease are listed and compared to conventional therapy. PEMF= pulsed electromagnetic field; PRP= platelet rich plasma; IRAP= interleukin-1 receptor antagonist protein.

Case 3

Signalment: 11 yr MN mixed-breed canine

Conventional Diagnosis: Left CCL tear

TCVM Diagnosis: Liver *Yin* and Blood Deficiency with Local *Qi*/Blood Stagnation

Integrative Treatment: Conventional treatment initiated and combined with multiple integrative therapies (Figures 25.6 and 25.7)

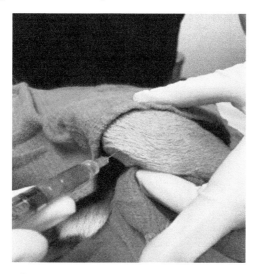

Figure 25.6 Mixed-breed canine with a left CCL tear which is undergoing stem cell therapy treatment.

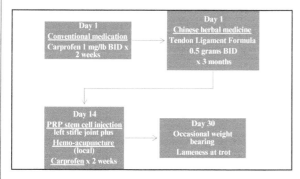

Figure 25.7 Flow chart demonstrating integrative treatment for Case 3.

Outcome: On Day 60 – no swelling, crepitation or lameness at walk or trot; by Day 90 the dog resumed normal activities. Similar cases treated with this protocol have either been prescribed PEMF loop therapy over the affected joint twice daily for 60 to 90 days or had ozone injected into the joint during the stem cell procedure. It is the author's experience that these patients have a shorter healing time closer to two months with return to normal function.

Therapeutic Review

Table 25.3 Integrative treatment options for cranial cruciate ligament disease. Adapted from [3]. Dewey C, Xie H, 2018; [4]. Xie H, 2011; [5]. Fowler M, Xie H, 2022.

Integrative treatment method	Integrative approach	Therapeutic results
Acupuncture	GB-34, BL-40	Treat stifle pain, tendon/ ligament disorder, rear limb pain
	ST-36, ST-35a, ST-35b	
	LIV-3	
	BL-60	Tonify Liver *Yin* and blood
		Aspirin point for any pain
Chinese herbal medicine	Tendon ligament formula	Nourish Liver *Yin* and Blood strengthen tendons/ligaments
		Moves Blood
		Resolves Stagnation
Platelet rich plasma/IRAP*	Joint injections	Stimulate healing
		Decrease pain
Ozone therapy Prolotherapy	SQ, rectal, or directly into joint	Stimulates healing
		Decrease inflammation
PEMF* therapy	Loop over affected limb or lounge to lay on	Stimulates healing
		Decreases pain
Spinal manipulation	Restrictions of spine and limbs	Decrease pain, Improve circulation Alleviate restrictions Decrease adhesions

* IRAP = interleukin-1 receptor antagonist protein, PEMF = pulsed electro-magnetic field.

Fire Element

The Heart (Fire Element) directs and propels the blood flow and houses the *Shen* [2]. The *Shen* represents the mind and/or spirit. When the *Shen* is normal, there is inner peace and normal mental health. Congestive heart failure and behavioral issues are common Fire Element problems seen in practice.

Congestive Heart Failure

Congestive heart failure patients should be assessed based on history, exam findings, blood chemistry analysis, and appropriate imaging to determine an accurate diagnosis before starting conventional medications (Figure 25.8).

Common underlying heart related TCVM patterns can include Heart *Qi, Yin,* and *Yang* deficiency. Patterns related to other elements such as the lungs and kidneys are often

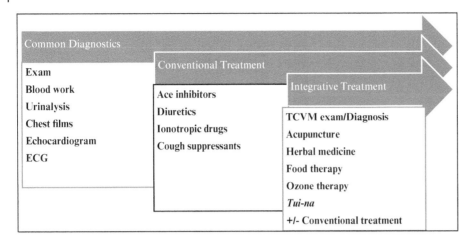

Figure 25.8   This flow chart demonstrates the important conventional diagnostics and treatment with therapy expansion available by using an integrative approach.

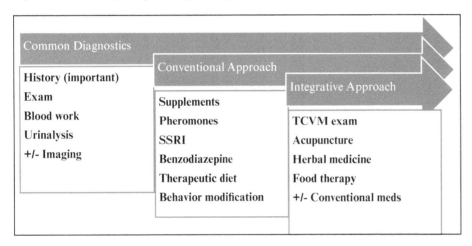

Figure 25.9   This flow chart lists conventional diagnosis and treatment of behavioral conditions as well as integrative therapies that can improve clinical outcomes. SSRI = serotonin reuptake inhibitors.

present and should be considered when developing an integrative treatment plan.

Behavioral Problems/Shen *Disturbance*

Anxiety, panic, aggression, noise aversions, fears, litter box issues, and other unusual behaviors can have multiple origins. Ongoing stress over time will adversely affect the Shen leading to Liver *Qi* Stagnation and Heart *Yin* and Blood deficiency. The addition of TCVM therapy can enhance treatment of these abnormal clinical behaviors (Figure 25.9).

Case 4

Signalment: 10 yr. FS Chihuahua (Figure 25.10)

Conventional Diagnosis: Congestive heart failure, collapsing trachea, progressive anxiety

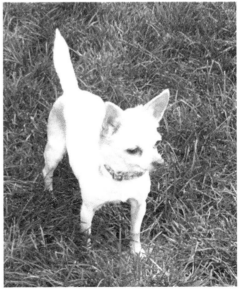

Figure 25.10   Case 4 patient.

Current Clinical History: Conventional medications no longer working: Lasix, Enalparil, Pimobendan, Hydrocodone, and Temaril P

TCVM Diagnosis: Heart *Qi/Yin* deficiency, Lung *Qi* deficiency, *Shen* Disturbance

Integrative Treatment: The successful integrative treatment used for this patient is presented in Figure 25.11.

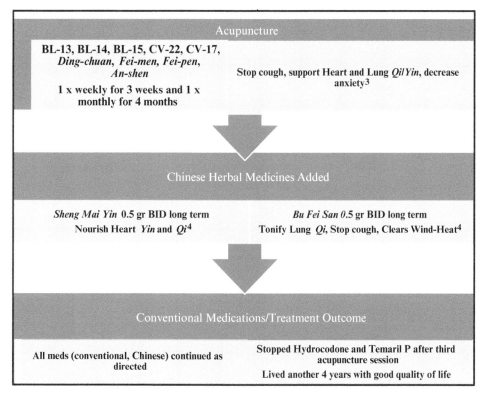

Figure 25.11 Integrative treatment of Case 4 combining conventional therapy, Chinese herbal medicine, and acupuncture.

Outcome: The lasix, enalapril, pimobendan, and both herbal supplements were continued long term with little to no cough noted. No dietary changes were made due to preexisting factors warranting a prescription urinary diet. The patient lived another four years past initiation of integrative care with good quality of life.

Case 5

Signalment: 6 yr. MN, 18 lb, DSH cat from a multi-pet household (2 cats, 6 dogs)

Clinical Signs: urinating outside the litter box, excessive drinking, hiding, easily agitated, aggressive toward other household pets.

Conventional Diagnostics: Normal blood panel, urinalysis, and imaging (all bloodwork/UA normal)

Conventional Diagnosis: Obesity (18 lbs), Inappropriate urination (behavior origin), Feline Lower Urinary Tract Disease (FLUTD)

TCVM Diagnosis: Liver *Qi* Stagnation (agitation, avoiding owner interaction), Heart *Yin* and Blood deficiency (excessive thirst), and *Shen* Disturbance (hiding under bed, anxiety, inappropriate urinations).

Integrative Treatment: Diet for weight loss and FLUTD, acupuncture BL-14, BL-44, BL-15, BL-45, *An-shen*, *Da-feng-men*, BL-18, BL-47, BL-19, BL-48 (1 x weekly for 4 weeks) plus Concentrated *Shen* Calmer[a] (x 3 months).

Outcome: After the first treatment the patient was more relaxed and stretched out on the floor to be petted. After the second session he began to interact with household pets in a friendly manner. After four acupuncture treatments all inappropriate urination and unwanted behavior had resolved.

Therapeutic Review for Integrative Therapies for Fire Element Clinical Cases (Table 25.4)

Table 25.4 Integrative treatment options for congestive heart failure and behavioral problems. Adapted from [3]. Dewey C, Xie H, 2018; [4]. Xie H, 2011; [5]. Fowler M, Xie H, 2022.

Integrative treatment method	Integrative approach	Therapeutic results
Acupuncture/Aqua-AP	BL-14, BL-43	Tonify Heart *Qi*, stop cough, *Shen* disturbance
	BL-15, HT-7	Tonify Heart *Qi, Yin* and Blood, *Shen* disturbance
	BL-18, BL-47	Liver *Qi* Stagnation, *Shen* disturbance
	CV-22, CV-17, *Ding-chuan, Fei-men, Fei-pen*	Cough, dyspnea, regulate *Qi*
	Da-feng-men, An-shen	*Shen* disturbance
Chinese herbal medicine	*Heart Qi* tonic	Tonify Heart *Qi*, moves Blood, Nourish *Yin* and *Qi*
	Sheng Mai Yin	Calms *Shen*
	Shen calmer	Nourish Heart Blood and *Yin* smooth Liver *Qi*
		Nourish Liver *Yin*
Food therapy	Salmon	Tonify Heart *Qi*
	Ground beef	
	Chickpeas	
	Chicken	
	Chicken egg yolk	
	Chicken egg white	
	Ground turkey	Tonify Heart *Yin*
	Lima bean	
	Blueberry	
	Watermelon	

Earth Element

Gastrointestinal problems are associated with the earth element and include vomiting, loose stools, lack of appetite, and weight loss. Symptoms vary and can be acute or chronic in nature.

Diarrhea – Acute

Diarrhea of acute onset with mucus and or blood is referred to as Spleen Damp Heat in TCVM. All parasites detected by fecal analysis should be treated appropriately. A common integrative approach to Spleen Damp Heat (blood or mucus containing stools) includes:

Aqua-acupuncture: GV 1 (stop diarrhea) [3]
Herbal Medicine: *Great Saussurea Coptis* 0.5 gr per 10lbs BW, BID x 5–7 days [4]
Ozone Therapy: Rectal at 35 micrograms/ml concentration @ 1 ml per pound body weight
Diet Modification: Ground turkey, white fish, brown rice, red beans, and pumpkin [5]
Conventional: Medications or prescription diets as needed

Diarrhea-Chronic

Chronic diarrhea such as IBD (inflammatory bowel disease) is more consistent with Spleen *Qi* Deficiency. A complete diagnostic work-up is essential for chronic cases including ultrasound and endoscopy. An approach similar to acute diarrhea plus recognition of the underlying pattern can lead to success. A fecal transplant can be considered for refractory cases to restore a healthy GI biome.

Acupuncture: SP-3, SP-6, SP-9, ST-36, LI-10 (points to tonify *Qi*) [3]

Herbal Medicine: *Shen Ling Bai Zhu* or *Xiang Lian San* (formulas for chronic diarrhea) [4]

Food Therapy: Chicken, sardines, oats, quinoa, green peas, lima beans, pumpkin, sweet potato to tonify *Qi* or prescription diet [5].

Ozone Therapy: Rectal or SQ

Conventional Medications: At full or reduced dosage.

Case 6

Signalment: 10 yr. FS Shih-Tzu (case 1 patient)

Clinical Signs: Loose stools with intermittent blood and mucus for 2 to 3 months. Metronidazole responsive until discontinued.

Conventional Diagnosis: IBD (unconfirmed)/antibiotic responsive diarrhea

TCVM Diagnosis: Spleen *Qi* deficiency with Damp Heat

Integrative Treatment and Outcome: Successful integrative treatment used for this patient is presented in Figure 25.12

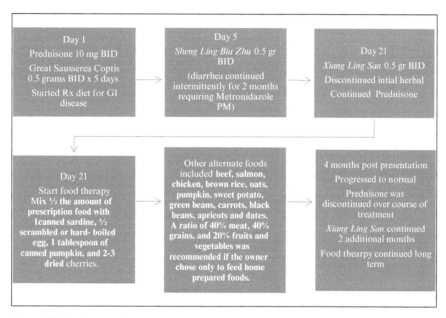

Figure 25.12   Integrative treatment plan and progress for Case 6.

Metal Element

The Metal Element (lung) governs respiration, helps distribute body fluids, and nourishes the skin and hair coat [2]. Common metal conditions seen in practice include coughing, upper respiratory tract infections, collapsing trachea, skin, and hair coat abnormalities.

Cough-Acute/Upper Respiratory

Tracheobronchitis, Kennel Cough, or other contagious and infectious coughs are secondary to exposure to pathogenic bacteria and viruses from a conventional perspective. The same can be said for cats and kittens that suffer from upper respiratory infections. From a TCVM perspective, pathogens such as Heat, Cold, Damp, and Dry can be causal factors. An appropriate integrative treatment plan should be based on history, physical exam, and diagnostic findings.

Case 7

Signalment: Four-month F DSH with recurrent mucopurulent nasal discharge.

Clinical History: Short term response to antibiotics, non-responsive to anti-viral medication.

Conventional Diagnosis: Chronic upper respiratory disease; Confirmed diagnosis after rhinoscopy: severe, chronic-active rhinitis with bony remodeling, reactive cartilage proliferation, granulation tissue and edema. No neoplasia or infectious agents were seen.

TCVM Diagnosis: Nasal Damp Heat

Integrative treatment: Prednisolone 2.5 mg × 7 days plus Ozone SQ 1 × /week for 3 weeks.

Outcome: The condition resolved during course of treatment. Two years without symptoms thus far.

Cough-Chronic

Chronic cough due to collapsing trachea is considered Lung *Qi* deficiency plus Local Stagnation. Conventional medications may be required on an ongoing basis. An integrative approach can help control symptoms and improve quality of life.

Table 25.5 lists integrative treatment options and therapeutic results for acute and chronic cough.

Case 8

Signalment: 10 yr. old MN mix breed canine (Figure 25.13)

Clinical Signs: Chronic harsh cough, labored breathing, worse with activity, partial response to medication

Conventional Diagnosis: Collapsing trachea (Figure 25.14)

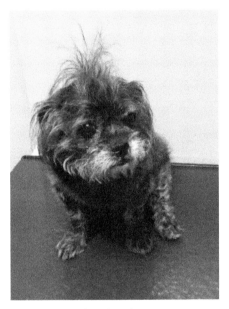

Figure 25.13   Case 8 patient.

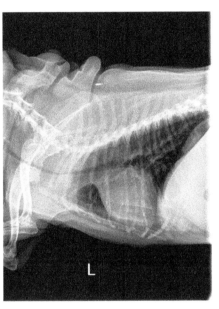

Figure 25.14   Left lateral radiograph demonstrates a narrowed portion of trachea in the lower neck area.

TCVM Diagnosis: Lung *Qi* deficiency with Local Stagnation

Integrative Treatment and Outcome: Case treatment and progress demonstrated in Figure 25.15

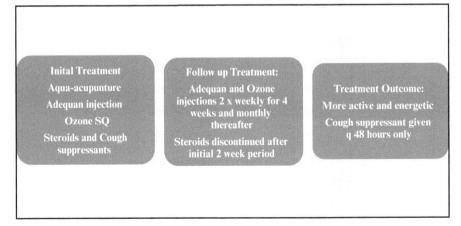

Inital Treatment
Aqua-acupunture
Adequan injection
Ozone SQ
Steroids and Cough suppressants

Follow up Treatment:
Adequan and Ozone injections 2 x weekly for 4 weeks and monthly thereafter
Steroids discontinued after initial 2 week period

Treatment Outcome:
More active and energetic
Cough suppressant given q 48 hours only

Figure 25.15   Case 8 integrative treatment and outcome.

Table 25.5 Integrative treatment options for acute and chronic cough Adapted from [3]. Dewey C, Xie H, 2018; [4]. Xie H, 2011; [5]. Fowler M, Xie H, 2022.

Integrative treatment method	Integrative approach	Therapeutic results
Acupuncture/aqua-acupuncture	*Ding-chuan*, CV-22, CV-17	Improve cough, dyspnea
	BL-13, LU-1, LU-7	Tonify Lung *Yin* and *Qi*
Chinese herbal medicine	*Zhi Sou San, Yin Qiao San*	Stop cough, clear Phlegm, Wind, Heat
	Bu Fei San	Tonify Lung *Qi*, stop cough
	Lily combination[a]	Nourish Lung *Yin*, cools Blood, Open the lungs
Tui-na	*An-fa, Rou-fa* at CV-22, CV-17, *Ding-chuan*	Stop cough
Ozone therapy	SQ	Anti-inflammatory
	Rectal	Anti-viral
		Anti-bacterial
		Immune support

[a] Jing Tang Herbal. Reddick, FL.

Skin Conditions

Skin disease is another common condition associated with the Metal element. Identifying the root cause and developing a treatment plan can be difficult, especially in chronic cases. An integrative approach can provide wadditional modalities to compliment or replace conventional therapies.

Case 9
Signalment: 11 yr. male Australian Shepard
Clinical Findings (dermatology): severe multifocal crusts, erosions/ulcerations-face, feet, tip of prepuce, ears, +/− anus
Conventional Diagnosis: Pemphigus foliaceus (biopsy confirmed)
Conventional Treatment (initial): Multiple topical therapies, Prednisone 20 mg tablets (30 mg BID with taper), topical med twice weekly, Silver Sulfadiazine ear medication, Atopica (cyclosporine) 50 mg capsules once daily (added after initial prednisone dose did not achieve remission).
TCVM Diagnosis: Blood stagnation
TCVM Treatment: *Mu Dan Pi* (conc. powder) − Cools blood, removes stagnation [4]
Integrative Treatment: Prednisone (10 mg EOD), Atopica (50 mg EOD), and herbal BID
Outcome: Condition stabilized with time to achieve lowest effective dose of immune suppressants − 18 months

Ear Conditions

Otitis externa is common in companion animals. In TCVM, otitis is referred to as Gallbladder Damp Heat due to the proximity of the ears to the Gallbladder Channel. The external pathogen Damp is hard to clear from the ears and becomes a contributing factor to treatment failure.

A recent study published in 2019 examined an integrative approach to treating non-complicated cases of canine otitis externa [7]. One group of twelve participants received conventional topical treatment only while the other group of twelve received conventional topical treatment plus twice daily, *Long Dan Xie Gan*, Chinese herbal medication. The group that received integrative therapy had a 90% treatment success rate verses a 30% success rate for topical therapy alone [7]. A flow chart demonstrates additional integrative therapies for the ears (Figure 25.16).

Water Element

Osteoarthritis, intervertebral disc disease, spondylosis, urinary tract disease, incontinence, renal failure, and congenital abnormalities are associated with the water element (kidney).

Urinary Tract Infection/Bladder Damp Heat

Urinary tract infections are referred to as Bladder Damp Heat in TCVM. A complete urinalysis with urine culture is essential for treatment success. Surgery may be indicated if uroliths are present. Antibiotics based on culture results, herbal medicine, ozone therapy, and food therapy can provide an integrated approach to treatment (Figure 25.17).

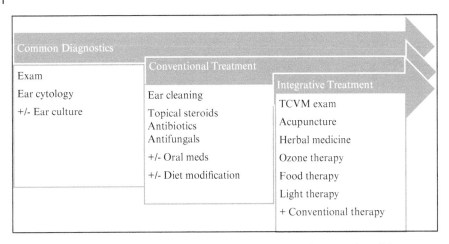

Figure 25.16 Flow chart for treatment of ear conditions using integrated medicine.

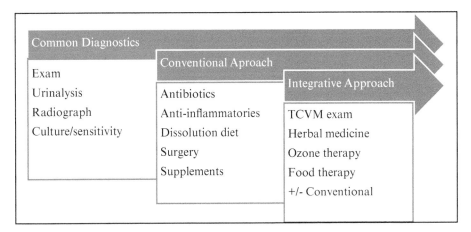

Figure 25.17 Flow chart for treatment of urinary tract infections using integrated medicine.

Table 25.6 lists TCVM integrative treatment options and therapeutic results for ear conditions.

Table 25.6 Summary of TCVM integrative treatment options for ear disease Adapted from [3]. Dewey C, Xie H, 2018; [4]. Xie H, 2011; [5]. Fowler M, Xie H, 2022.

Integrative treatment method	Integrative approach	Therapeutic results
Acupuncture	GB-2, TH-17, SI-19, BL-23	Clears Heat and Wind, benefits ears, *Qi*-Blood Stagnation in ears
Herbal medicine	Ear Damp Heat	Clears Heat and Damp Heat
		Cools Blood, calms Liver
	Long Dan Xie Gan	Clears Liver Heat
		Clears Damp Heat
		Drains Damp
		Soothes Liver *Qi*
		Nourishes Blood
Ozone therapy	SQ, rectal, topical, ear insufflation	Anti-inflammatory
		Antibacterial
		Immune system support
		Promote healing
Food therapy	Cod, egg whites, celery, collard greens, red beans	Clears Liver and Gallbladder Damp Heat

Case 10

Signalment: 9 yr. FS Shorkie (Figure 25.18)

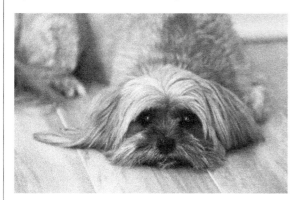

Figure 25.18   Case 10 patient.

Clinical Signs: Frequent urination, hematuria, straining to urinate

Conventional Diagnostics: A complete blood panel was normal. Red blood cells, white blood cells, excess protein, and bacteria were noted on urinalysis. Abdominal films revealed multiple large stones within the bladder (Figure 25.19).

Conventional Diagnosis: Urinary tract infection with uroliths

TCVM Diagnosis: Bladder Damp Heat

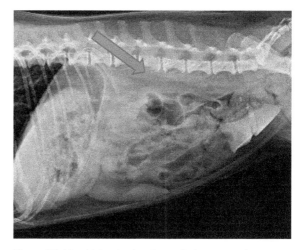

Figure 25.19   Abdominal radiograph demonstrating radiopaque uroliths (arrow).

Integrative Treatment: The patient was placed on antibiotics, a prescription urinary diet, and Chinese herbal medicine (Crystal Stone Formula[a]). Given patient discomfort, surgery was elected to remove the stones. Analysis confirmed the stones were 100% struvite. Two weeks post-op, urinalysis revealed a large amount of blood still present, few WBC, and no bacteria. The herbal formula, Eight Righteous[a], was added to clear the excess damp heat still present in the bladder. The flow chart below demonstrates treatment progression (Figure 25.20).

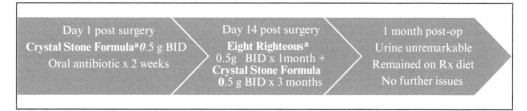

| Day 1 post surgery **Crystal Stone Formula**[a] *0*.5 g BID Oral antibiotic x 2 weeks | Day 14 post surgery **Eight Righteous**[a] 0.5g BID x 1month + **Crystal Stone Formula** 0.5 g BID x 3 months | 1 month post-op Urine unremarkable Remained on Rx diet No further issues |

Figure 25.20   Case 10 integrative treatment with clinical outcome.

Urinary Incontinence

Urine leakage on bedding or furniture is a common presenting complaint and often confused by clients as a urinary tract infection. These cases occur more often in spayed female patients and can require more than one medication to control. Multiple conventional factors have been attributed to this issue and can be neurologic in origin. Urinary incontinence from a TCVM standpoint can indicate a deficiency in Kidney *Qi*. Additional herbal supplements to support the kidney can be beneficial in controlling clinical signs.

Case 11

Signalment: 11 yr. FS Australian Shepard

Conventional Diagnosis: Nonresponsive urinary incontinence

Conventional Treatment: Current medications – Proin 50 mg BID plus Incurin SID

TCVM Diagnosis: Kidney *Qi* deficiency

Integrative Treatment: Add herbal medication (*Jin Suo Gu Jing*) -Tonify Kidney *Qi*, stop incontinence [4]

Outcome: Incontinence resolved; however, any attempt to modify or remove either conventional medication or the herbal medication resulted in treatment failure.

Bone and Joint Disease

Bone and joint disease is common among companion animals. Multiple TCVM deficiency patterns can occur such as Kidney *Yin* and *Qi* deficiency, Kidney *Yang* deficiency and Bony *Bi* syndrome. Several integrative therapeutic options are available and not limited solely to those listed in the flow chart (Figure 25.21).

Common Diagnostics

Exam
Blood work
Radiographs

Conventional Approach

Non-steroidals
Steroids
Joint injections
Rehab
Therapeutic diet
Joint supplement

Integrative Approach

TCVM exam
Acupuncture
Herbal medicines
Food therapy
Tui-na
Platelet Rich Plasma
Ozone therapy/prolotherapy
Spinal manipulation
PEMF therapy
+/- Conventional meds

Figure 25.21 Flow chart demonstrating additional therapeutics associated with integrative medicine.

Case 12
Signalment: 4 yr. MN Rottweiler (See below Figure)

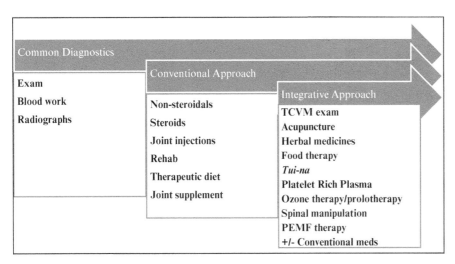

Conventional Diagnosis: Bilateral CCL tears plus repair, chronic neck, back, and elbow pain, no longer playful, painful when going up and down stairs.

Current Treatment: Rimadyl, tramadol, gabapentin, acetaminophen/codeine, joint supplements, adequan injections, previous stem cell therapy, and shockwave.

TCVM Diagnosis: Kidney *Yin* and *Qi* deficiency plus local *Qi*/Blood Stagnation of elbows, neck, and stifles.

Integrative Treatment: Acupuncture 1 x /week for 4 weeks + *Tui-na*, then monthly for 8 months. Add Chinese herbal medicines – Body Sore[a] and *Di Gu Pi* (2 gr. BID). Continue conventional medications as prescribed.

Outcome: Mobility improved with significant increase of activity levels after third acupuncture treatment. Tramadol was discontinued. The carprofen dose was reduced by half daily. Gabapentin was continued. The patient was maintained on the herbal formulas with good quality of life for three years from initial presentation. Details pertaining to the integrative treatment approach in this patient as well as optional therapies are listed in Table 25.7.

Therapeutic Review

Table 25.7 Integrative treatment options for bone and joint disease Adapted from [3].Dewey C, Xie H, 2018; [4]. Xie H, 2011; [5]. Fowler M, Xie H, 2022.

Integrative treatment method	Integrative approach	Therapeutic results
Acupuncture	BL-23, BL-54, BL-40, KID-3, *Shen-shu, Shen-peng, Shen-Jiao, Jian-jiao, Bai-hui*	Hip and pelvic limb problems, tonify Kidney *Yin, Qi, Yang*, back pain, Bony *Bi* syndrome, *Qi*-Blood Stagnation
Herbal medicine	Body sore[a]	Strengthens back, resolves pain, tonify Kidney *Yang* and *Yin*
	Hindquarter weakness[a]	Tonify Kidney *Qi* and *Yin*
		Strengthen back and rear limbs
	Di Gu Pi[a]	Tonify Kidney *Yin* and *Qi/Yang*
		Clears deficient
	Equine *Du Huo*[a]	Heat/Stagnation
		Nourish Blood
		Eliminates Wind, Cold, Damp
Food therapy	Dependent on pattern: lamb, venison, sweet potato, chicken, beef, oatmeal, turkey, duck, brown rice, green beans	Relieve Stagnation, nourish Kidney *Qi, Yin, Yang*
Tui-na	*Gun-fa, Rou-fa, Tui-fa*	Resolve Stagnation
		Improve circulation
Platelet Rich Plasma (PRP)	Joint injections	Stimulate healing, reduce pain, slow progression of disease
Ozone therapy	SQ, rectal, IV	Promote healing, decrease inflammation, oxygen to deficient tissues
Spinal manipulation	Limbs, neck, spine	Alleviate restrictions, decrease pain, prevent adhesions
Pulsed electro-magnetic field therapy (PEMF)	Loop or lounge	Decrease pain and inflammation

[a] Jing Tang Herbal. Reddick, FL.

Conclusion

The cases in this chapter were selected to demonstrate the ability of integrative medicine to compliment, replace, and reduce the need for conventional treatments. Integrative medicine provides practitioners with select tools with multiple options to prevent illness, restore health, and improve quality and longevity of life.

From a personal perspective, integrative medicine evokes memories of an old red toolbox; rusted, dented, scratched up, and covered in a layer of Tennessee dust (Figure 25.22). For years it sat atop a table at the old farmhouse and served as a catch all for whatever came out of a pair of overall pockets at the end of the day. No true order existed to its contents. No accurate inventory was ever known. New and old tools alike were mixed in somewhat chaotic harmony. Yet, time and time again, it held the right tool for the right job at just the right time.

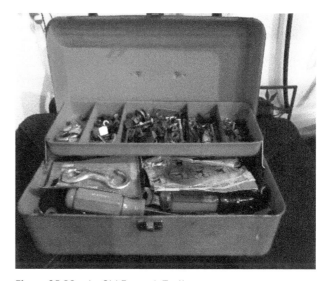

Figure 25.22 An Old Farmer's Toolbox.

References

1 Dale Carnegie Quotes. (2022). BrainyQuote.com, BrainyMedia Inc. https://www.brainyquote.com/quotes/dale_carnegie_100661 (accessed March 10, 2022).

2 Xie, H. and Preast, V. (2013). *Traditional Chinese Veterinary Medicine Fundamental Principles*, 2e. Reddick, FL: Chi Institute Press, 93–95.

3 Dewey, C. and Xie, H. (2018). *Clinicians Guide to Canine Acupuncture*. Reddick, FL: Chi Institute Press, 45, 103, 109, 114, 67, 24, 25, 120, 58, 68, 59, 69, 142, 143, 145, 149, 154, 155, 147, 127, 32, 33, 35, 10, 13, 1, 4, 104, 99, 51, 62, 71, 78, 62, 150, 151, 156, 134.

4 Xie, H. (2011). *Chinese Veterinary Herbal Handbook*, 3e. Reddick, FL: Jing Tang Publishing, 215, 117, 80, 54, 103, 272, 249, 107, 250, 264, 209, 62, 59, 239, 235, 253, 245, 246, 189, 136, 187, 86.

5 Fowler, M. and Xie, H. (2020). *Veterinary Medicine Food Therapy*. Reddick, FL: Chi University Press, 322, 343, 349, 375, 390, 294, 221, 223, 226.

6 Xie, H. and Ferguson, B. (2007). *Application of Tui-na in Veterinary Medicine*. Reddick, FL: Chi Institute Press, 91–93.

7 McKee, M. and Shiau, D. (2019). A randomized and controlled comparative study to determine the effectiveness of *Long Dan Xie Gan* in combination with osurnia for the treatment of acute canine otitis externa. *Am J Tradit Chin Vet Med* 14 (2): 13–22.

26

Clinical Application of Integrative Veterinary Medicine in Equine Practice

Amelia Munsterman

Introduction

Traditional Chinese Veterinary Medicine (TCVM) is now commonly integrated into the everyday diagnostic and therapeutic plans of equine practitioners. This integration can include the use of acupuncture points to help define disease or musculoskeletal disorders, but also for treatment once a diagnosis is made. Herbal therapies are also becoming mainstream, using more traditional combinations of Chinese herbal medicines in support of other therapeutic interventions. Combined with massage therapy and manipulative treatments, the full spectrum of TCVM is used to treat diseases in modern veterinary practice. This chapter will discuss four common issues seen by equine practitioners and the integrative approach to managing these conditions in horses.

Lameness

Lameness is one of the primary reasons that people seek alternative and complementary medicine in horses [1]. It is also the most researched of all conditions that affect the horse in the literature, and acupuncture is the most common alternative intervention that is sought. It has been shown that acupuncture can both change a horse's gait and reduce lameness scores, and recent publications using objective measures such as inertial sensors have confirmed these findings [2]. While encouraging, it is important to note when choosing acupoints for intervention that a standardized approach to therapy using a single formula for all causes of lameness has shown a poor outcome [3, 4]. This supports the use of tailored interventions and personalized medicine using pattern diagnosis to treat orthopedic disease.

Use of acupoint and Meridian (or *Jing-Luo*) sensitivity for identification of lameness is well described in TCVM literature and an established diagnostic tool [5, 6]. In this technique, acupoints are stimulated with a blunt instrument, and the response to an acupoint or select set of acupuncture points is used to guide/locate the source of lameness. Responses to the acupoint scan can be as subtle as a skin twitch, or can be more intense, such as biting or striking out. Recent research has corroborated the observations seen during acupoint scans and correlated them to other objective measures of lameness evaluation, lending support for the use of this diagnostic tool for identification of the site of orthopedic pain in horses. For example, in one report, sensitivity for acupoints that are representative of stifle pain were correlated with findings on ultrasound, radiographs and thermography, with a sensitivity of 88% and specificity of 57% for the presence of a stifle lesion [7]. In another study using acupoints to localize and identify lameness during a clinical examination, acupoints showed a sensitivity of 82% and specificity of 78%, with an overall accuracy of 80% [8].

Lameness is typically caused by a local *Qi* or blood stagnation, however there are other patterns that can be associated with acute and chronic arthritis and other musculoskeletal disorders [9]. The practitioner should use the scan, as well as a detailed history, motion palpation, physical exam, and a dynamic exam when formulating a treatment plan. Treatment using acupuncture will involve local acupoints in combination with acupoints along meridians that run through the affected structures and acupoints to treat the constitution and TCVM pattern(s). The addition of herbal medicine to move blood and *Qi* provides synergism to the acupuncture protocol.

In addition, *Tui-na* can be used to treat musculoskeletal injuries using targeted massage. For example, *Ca-fa*, a rubbing technique, can be used to warm arthritic joints. *Tui-fa*, or deep tissue massage, can loosen tissues, move *Qi* and improve circulation. *Ji-ya-fa* techniques, including *An-fa* or *Dian-fa* pressing techniques can treat acupoints or

Integrative Veterinary Medicine, First Edition. Edited by Mushtaq A. Memon and Huisheng Xie.
© 2023 John Wiley & Sons, Inc. Published 2023 by John Wiley & Sons, Inc.
Companion Website: www.wiley.com/go/memon/veterinary

Ah-shi points and relieve pain. *Gun-fa*, a rolling technique, can smooth joints and invigorate blood and is useful in arthritic patients. *Dou-fa*, a shaking technique, can loosen joints and reduce muscle atrophy while *Yao-fa*, or passive range of motion, is good at releasing joints and maintaining cartilage health.

One of the most frustrating musculoskeletal conditions that is presented to the equine veterinarian are horses that have developed laminitis. This debilitating disease is difficult to manage and can progress to the point that euthanasia is the only option. There are a number of publications that support the use of TCVM, and specifically acupuncture, as part of a multimodal therapeutic strategy for this disease; and the results are encouraging [10, 11]. While hemoacupuncture, dry needle acupuncture and electro-acupuncture have all been used for treatment of laminitis, in one report electro-acupuncture showed improved benefits compared to dry needle stimulation, which may require additional investigation [12]. In addition, low level laser therapy may improve outcomes in both acute and chronic cases of laminitis when applied at acupoints, and when treating wounds surrounding the hoof [13]. Acupuncture, *Tui-na*, food therapy and herbal medicines all may be used to help reduce pain and regain function in laminitis cases. It is important for each case to treat the TCVM pattern, rather than only the symptoms of laminitis, for best results.

Back pain is another condition that has been well-studied in regards to alternative interventions, including TCVM. Stimulation of acupuncture points appears to provide a significant improvement, allowing horses to return to athletic performance [14–19]. In one report, electro-acupuncture performed better than the conventional therapy using phenylbutazone when treating hoses with chronic thoracolumbar pain [18]. Interestingly, different types of acupoint stimulation, including laser, injection or needles, produced similar effects for back pain in horses in a different study [15]. Other therapeutic modalities, including chiropractic and massage, also have shown improved nociceptive thresholds compared to phenylbutazone and rest, with kinematic studies demonstrating that chiropractic therapies improve symmetry and thoracic extension [20, 21]. The evidence thus far is supportive for the use of alternative therapies in treatment of back pain in horses.

Gastrointestinal Disease

Colic is the second most common condition seen by equine practitioners and is a general term for any sign of abdominal pain. The causes of colic include parasympathetic dysfunction, obstructive lesions, inflammatory or infectious diseases, and strangulating lesions. It is important to obtain a thorough history to help narrow the list of suspected causes, and to assist in the approach to therapy, as the list of differentials is long. A thorough physical exam and work-up, including nasogastric intubation, trans-rectal palpation, and transabdominal ultrasonography is indicated, with a minimum hematology profile for assessment of hydration and serum electrolytes.

Most colic can be medically managed and should respond within 12–24 hours, as the cause is often a functional obstruction such as vagotonia ("gas colic") or an impaction caused by obstruction of the flow of ingesta. These diseases are commonly due to changes in the balance of the autonomic nervous system, systemic dehydration, or inappropriate feeds. In TCVM, these causes of colic can be due to *Qi*-Blood or liver *Qi* stagnation, which disrupt the normal transformation and transportation of food by the spleen and stomach [22]. Obstructive syndromes causing impactions are referred to as *Jie Zheng* in TCVM. Patterns associated with this syndrome can include excess or acute patterns such as food stagnation and excess heat, as well as deficiency patterns of spleen *Qi*, *Yin* and/or blood. It is well described in other species that acupuncture can improve and modulate gastrointestinal motility by somatoautonomic reflexes, modulation of the enteric nervous system, and direct stimulation of the brain to integrate the effects of the CNS on gastrointestinal function [23]. Therefore, an integrative approach to medical management of colic in the horse can be applied along with conventional treatments to improve and speed recovery.

Treatment of colic starts with pain management, followed by therapies that address the source of the colic signs. Conventional medications should be provided in an integrative approach, including non-steroidal medications and anti-spasmodic drugs (n-butyl scopolammonium bromide), along with judicious sedation for the exam and initial treatment. Fluid imbalances should be corrected, and feed should be withheld until the horse is passing feces and vital parameters are within normal limits. Treatment of concurrent issues, including intestinal parasites and gastric ulceration, is indicated with proper anthelmintics and proton-pump inhibitors. Dietary and lifestyle management changes are helpful to prevent recurrence.

As described, integrative therapies are useful in treatment of medical colic, and acupuncture is indicated at acupoints to treat the pattern. Acupuncture points for pain management can include ST-36 to move and support *Qi*, and LIV-3 to treat stagnation. Classical acupoints to treat colic include *Jiang-ya* over the tip of the alar cartilage and *Er-ding* at the ear base, and the horse's response to these acupoints can help to differentiate between surgical and medical causes of colic [22]. Herbal therapies such as *Wei Le San* or *Yu Nu Jian* for gastric ulcers, and the laxative/purgative *Fan Xie Ye* are alternatives to conventional medications used for these clinical conditions, and may be used alongside traditional therapies [24, 25]. Administration of senna as a laxative should be used with caution, as it can result in abdominal distension and increased discomfort when compared to other similar medications [26]. Long term herbal medicine support for the gastrointestinal system can be provided with the use of *Ma Wei Chang He* to strengthen spleen *Qi* and move stomach *Qi* [27]. Food therapy is very useful in horses with colic, to treat the TCVM pattern after colic and to prevent recurrence. Neutral grass hay is recommended for all horses after colic, which is slowly reintroduced starting at a quarter of the normal ration. Wheat bran or flax seed is useful for gas colic caused by stagnation or heat, and *Qi* can be supported with oats, rice bran, sweet potato, and carrots [28].

Wound Management

Injuries to skin, muscle and deeper tissues including bone, joints, or other synovial lined structures is a relatively common issue in equine practice. Wound healing occurs in four overlapping stages which include acute inflammation, debridement, proliferation with restoration of the injured tissues, and then maturation of the new tissues into a functional scar. Acupuncture and moxibustion have been shown to help improve acute wound management by reducing inflammation, accelerating fibroblast proliferation, and angiogenesis [29, 30]. Acupuncture is also useful in later stages, to activate and improve remodeling of scar tissue, especially when using the technique called "surround the dragon." [31] While formal research in horses for wound management using TCVM is sparse, one study in horses did note a reduction in excess granulation tissue and improvement in non-healing wounds using gold implants in the wound edges with the "surround the dragon" technique [32].

Common patterns found in horses with wounds include heat toxin causing stagnation of *Qi* and blood, or *Qi* and blood stagnation with *Yin* deficiency in acute wounds [33]. These horses will show signs of heat with a red tongue and rapid pulse. More chronic wounds will have a deficiency of *Qi* and blood, preventing proper contraction and epithelialization. Signs of deficiency will predominate, with pale tongue and weak pulses.

Treatment will center on proper wound management, including debridement, closure if possible, and assessment of additional structures involved. Bandages are important to keep the wound clean, reduce movement, prevent excess granulation tissue formation, and to allow for wound contraction. Wound salves can be selected, if desired, but must be based on the stage of healing as there is no single formula effective for all stages of healing. Early wound management may require hygroscopic dressings to remove edema, including sugar or honey. Honey is also useful for its antibacterial properties, and its ability to promote epithelialization and angiogenesis [34]. In horses with heat toxin, with a red tongue and fast pulse, *Jin Huang Gao*[1] can be used to relieve pain and reduce inflammation [35]. In the intermediate stages of wound healing, equine wounds are often quite productive, and an absorbent layer such as dressings containing calcium alginate will be required. As the wound begins to epithelialize, a non-stick dressing is required to prevent injury to the delicate fibroblasts.

Acupuncture can be used to treat the pattern for each stage of wound healing, and to help with pain management. Common acupoints to treat *Qi* stagnation (pain) include LIV-3 and LI-4. LI-4 can also be combined with LI-11 to clear heat and open the surface, along with GV-14, *Tai-yang, Er-jian, Wei-jian*, and *Wei-ben*. To treat phlegm and purulent discharge, SP-10 and BL-40 are indicated to cool the blood, and clear heat. Moxibustion can be used over the wound and coupled with the acupuncture needles is especially useful in early wound healing. To support and move *Qi*, ST-36 or LI-10 are used. Acupuncture points surrounding the wound are chosen to "surround the dragon," and in this technique, needles are placed at ≥2 cm intervals at a steep angle close to the wound edges.

Once epithelization is complete in wounds over joints or limbs, range of motion exercises should be started, with gradual increases in mobility and exercise based on a positive response to treatment. *Tui-na* massage techniques can be incorporated into the therapy, with use of gentle *Mo-fa* touch to improve circulation, *Tui-fa* pushing techniques to realign scar tissues and reduce nodules, and *An-fa* pressing techniques to relieve pain and move *Qi*. *Ba-shen-fa* can stretch joints, and vibrating techniques such as limb shaking with *Dou-fa* and *Zhen-fa* using vibrating massagers are helpful to invigorate *Qi*. If the horse is stalled for extensive periods to allow for wound management, spinal manipulation and close attention to the health of the other joints and tissues is indicated.

Fever of Unknown Origin

Fever is a common, non-specific clinical sign leading to veterinary evaluation and treatment. Fever is caused by the production and release of pyrogenic cytokines. These include IL-1, IL-6, TNF-alpha, leptin and substance P, that result in the release of prostaglandin E-2 (PGE-2) as part of the body's immune response to pathogens [36]. Any infectious or inflammatory disease can cause fever, and the most common sources of fever in horses include respiratory infections and enterocolitis. Other causes of fever can include stress, intense exercise and tissue damage due to trauma or myopathies. Fever should be differentiated from hyperthermia, where the body's temperature rises above the hypothalamic set point secondary to environmental changes or release of endocrine mediators. Non-steroidal anti-inflammatory medications are useful for fever but will be ineffective for hyperthermia. Glucocorticoids can be helpful in treating inflammation to reduce fever however they should be used with caution in the face of any infectious disease. In any fever, the practitioner must treat the primary disease to eliminate the cause of the inflammation.

In TCM, fever is not classified based on body temperature alone, but other factors that differentiate the fever further by the body part affected and the pattern diagnosis. Fever is also categorized by the time of day, whether it rises or falls, and the phases of the fever as it progresses and resolves over time [37]. In humans, 19 different types of fever have been described.

In TCVM, high fever is most commonly classified as excess heat and subcategorized based on the location [38]. Invasion into the superficial level of the body, or *Wei* stage, is classified as a wind-heat pathogen with a red tongue and fast pulse. With progression of heat into a deeper tissue or organ level, or *Qi* stage heat, the horse begins to show signs of dryness, with excess thirst, anorexia, dry feces, and concentrated urine. In addition to eliminating heat, treatment should focus on generating body fluids. As fever becomes more severe and the disease is progressing, heat can enter the *Ying* or blood stage. Coma or seizures may occur and signs of disseminated intravascular coagulopathies may develop, with a dark red tongue and thready pulse. Additional treatments should be selected in these cases with a neurologic component to subdue wind and calm *Shen*.

Acupuncture has been shown to be highly effective at treating fever and inflammation in animals as well as humans. While the pattern diagnosis must be addressed, *Jing*-well points can be selected in the horse to treat all heat patterns, as they connect the *Yang* and *Yin* meridians and can therefore move *Qi* and clear heat. Second-level *Shu*-transporting points are often chosen, as the *Ying*-spring points both control and can clear heat from the body. In rats, acupuncture using the second level points LIV-2, BL-66 and HT-8 was effective at reducing fever caused by injection of lipopolysaccharide, likely through inhibition of gene transcription for inflammatory mediators including IL-1b and IL-6 [39]. Additional points, such as LI-4 and LI-11 are used in horses to open the surface and clear heat. The effect of these points may be due to inhibition of PGE-2 in the inflammatory cascade, as electro-acupuncture at LI-11 has been shown to be effective at treating fever in an animal model [40]. GV-14 is also commonly recommended to clear heat, as it is the *Yang* gathering point. In a clinical trial in humans, GV-14 was effective at treating fever due to wind-heat, secondary to a common cold [41]. Classical points to clear heat that can be selected as part of the treatment protocol in horses include *Xiong-tang*, *Jing-mai*, *Tai-yang*, *Wei-jian*, and *Er-jian*.

There are six important herbs, which along with their derivatives, have been shown in the literature to effectively reduce fever in experimental animal studies and in clinical trials [36]. *Chai Hu* (Bupleurum) may provide its effects by inhibiting secretion of cAMP, reducing cytokine expression, and inhibiting the activation of the NF-kB pathway. *Huang Qin* (Scutellaria Radix) has two main active components, baicalin and bailalein, that have been shown to reduce fever by reducing free radicals, PGE-2 and cytokine production. *Huang Qin* can also prevent the activation of the NF-kB pathway. The essential oil of *Chuan Xiong* (Ligusticum) is also anti-pyretic, inhibiting the COX-2 pathway, cAMP production in the hypothalamus and reducing NF-kB activation. *Gui Zhi* (Cinnamomum) contains a compound called cinnamaldehyde that has central effects in the hypothalamus, reducing fever through molecular channels as well as reductions in PGE-2 production. *Lian Qiao* (Forsythia) extracts exert an antipyretic effect centrally through reductions in cAMP, PGE-2, and TNF-a along with suppression of the toll like receptor 4 pathway. Finally, *Jin Yin Hua* (Lonicera) has been commonly used to reduce fever in TCVM. In both in-vivo (mouse model) and in-vitro (herb extracted flavonoids) studies, *Jin Yin Hua* demonstrated protective activity against expression of LPS-induced lung inflammatory cytokines through decreased nuclear NF-κB binding activities; thereby inhibiting the expression of TNF-α, IL-1β and IL-6. In addition, it had the beneficial activity of increasing the expression of the anti-inflammatory cytokine, IL-10. [42]

Combinations of these herbs have been used in herbal formulas historically, and in modern times. A formula used in TCVM for fever is *Yin Qiao San*, used to dispel wind-heat, or heat in the *Wei* stage [43]. Clinical signs will include a cough, a red tongue with a yellow or white coating and a rapid, floating pulse. This herbal formula contains *Ban Lan Gen* (Isatis), *Bo He* (Mentha), *Dan Zhu Ye* (Lophatherum), *Gan Cao* (Glycyrrhiza), *Jie Gen* (Platycodon), *Jin Yin Hua* (Lonicera), *Jing Jie* (Schizonepeta), *Lian Qiao* (Forsythia), *Lu Gen* (Phragmites), and *Niu Bang Zi* (Arctium).

Bai Hu[2] is also used to clear heat and purge fire and is effective for *Qi* stage heat. Clinical signs will include a red tongue with yellow coating, and a slippery, strong pulse [44]. It contains *Gan Cao* (Glycyrrhiza), *Geng Mi* (non-glutinous rice), *Shi Gao* (gypsum), and *Zhi Mu* (Anamarrhena). A second formula specific in TCVM for *Qi* stage heat is *Bai Hu Si Miao*[3] used to eliminate wind-damp heat and resolve stagnation. It contains *Cang Zhu* (Atractylodes), *Chuan Niu Zi* (Cyanthula), *Gui Zhi* (Cinnamomum), *Hai Tong Pi* (Erythrina), *Huang Bai* (Phellodendron), *Shi Gao* (gypsum), *Yi Yi Ren* (Coix) and *Zhi Mu* (Anamarrhena).

Finally, *Qing Ying Tang* is an herbal formula indicated for heat in the *Ying* stage, to cool blood, and nourish *Yin*

[45] Clinical signs of heat in the *Ying* stage include pete-chia, tachypnea, a deep red tongue and thin, rapid pulse. It contains *Dan Shen* (Salvia), *Dan Zhu Ye* (Lophatherum), *Huang Lian* (Coptis), *Jin Yin Hua* (Lonicera), *Lian Qiao* (Forsythia), *Mai Men Dong* (Ophiopogon), *Mu Dan Pi* (Moutan), *Shen Di Huang* (Rehmannia) and *Xuan Shen* (Schrophularia).

Conclusion

Modern horse owners are often quite knowledgeable and accepting of the addition of integrative therapies for treatment of their horses and may ask for the addition of these treatments to the therapeutic plan prescribed by their veterinarian. There is support in the literature for the use of TCVM to treat many of the common problems affecting horses. This provides clinicians an evidence-based approach to both evaluate and treat disease. A plan that combines both complementary and conventional treatment allows the practitioner to provide the best of both worlds, for the best outcome for the horse.

Notes

1 Golden Yellow Salve, Jing Tang Herbal, Inc., Ocala, FL. USA.
2 White Tiger, Jing Tang Herbal, Inc., Ocala, FL. USA.
3 *Bai Hu Si Miao*, Jing Tang Herbal, Inc., Ocala, FL. USA.

References

1 Shmalberg, J., Xie, H., and Memon, M.A. (2019 October). Horses referred to a teaching hospital exclusively for acupuncture and herbs: a three-year retrospective analysis. *J Acupunct Meridian Stud* 12 (5): 145–150.

2 Dunkel, B., Pfau, T., Fiske-Jackson, A. et al. (2017 January). A pilot study of the effects of acupuncture treatment on objective and subjective gait parameters in horses. *Vet Anaesth Analg* 44 (1): 154–162.

3 Robinson, K.A. and Manning, S.T. (2015 December). Efficacy of a single-formula acupuncture treatment for horses with palmar heel pain. *Can Vet J* 56 (12): 1257–1260.

4 Labens, R., Schramme, M., Sampson Hale, J.M. et al. (2022). Effect of needle and extracorporeal shockwave stimulation of acupuncture points on equine chronic multilimb lameness using a single-formula approach. *VCOT Open* 05 (02): e83–e92.

5 Fleming, P. (2001). Diagnostic acupuncture palpation examination in the horse. In: *Veterinary Acupuncture: Ancient Art to Modern Medicine*, 2e (ed. A.M. Schoen), 433–441. St. Louis, MO: Mosby Inc.

6 Xie, H. and Preast, V. (2002). *Traditional Chinese Veterinary Medicine: Fundamental Principles*, 290–292. Reddick, FL: Jing Tang.

7 Mariani, L.P.R., Sampaio, F., Silveira, A.B. et al. (2019 October). Pressuring of acupoints as a complement to the diagnosis of stifle diseases in horses. *J Acupunct Meridian Stud* 12 (5): 151–159.

8 Le Jeune, S.S. and Jones, J.H. (2014). Prospective study on the correlation of positive acupuncture scans and lameness in 102 performance horses. *Am J Tradit Chin Vet Med* 9 (2): 33–41.

9 Xie, H. and Preast, V. (2007). *Xie's Veterinary Acupuncture*, 247–251. Ames, IA: Blackwell Publishing.

10 Steiss, J.E., White, N.A., and Bowen, J.M. (1989 April). Electroacupuncture in the treatment of chronic lameness in horses and ponies: a controlled clinical trial. *Can J Vet Res* 53 (2): 239–243.

11 Faramarzi, B., Lee, D., May, K., and Dong, F. (2017 August). Response to acupuncture treatment in horses with chronic laminitis. *Can Vet J* 58 (8): 823–827.

12 Aljobory, A.I., Jaafar, S.E., and Ahmed, A.S. (2021). Acupuncture and electroacupuncture in the treatment of laminitis in racing horses: a comparative study. *Iraqi J Vet Sci* 35 (1): 15–21.

13 Petermann, U. (2011). Comparison of pre- and post-treatment pain scores of twenty one horses with laminitis treated with acupoint and topical low level impulse laser therapy. *Am J Tradit Chin Vet Med* 6 (1): 13–25.

14 Klide, A.M. (1984). Acupuncture for treatment of chronic back pain in the horse. *Acupunct Electro-Ther Res* 9 (1): 57–70.

15 Klide, A.M. and Martin, B.B., Jr. (1989 November 15). Methods of stimulating acupuncture points for treatment of chronic back pain in horses. *J Am Vet Med Assoc* 195 (10): 1375–1379.

16 Martin, B.B., Jr and Klide, A.M. (1987 January–February). Treatment of chronic back pain in horses. Stimulation of acupuncture points with a low powered infrared laser. *Vet Surg* 16 (1): 106–110.

17 Martin, B.B., Jr and Klide, A.M. (1987 May 1). Use of acupuncture for the treatment of chronic back pain in horses: stimulation of acupuncture points with saline solution injections. *J Am Vet Med Assoc* 190 (9): 1177–1180.

18 Xie, H., Colahan, P., and Ott, E.A. (2005 July 15). Evaluation of electroacupuncture treatment of horses with signs of chronic thoracolumbar pain. *J Am Vet Med Assoc* 227 (2): 281–286.

19 Sheta, E., Farghali, H., Ragab, S. et al. (2019 October). Stimulation of bladder acupoints by cloprostenol for treating back soreness in athletic horses. *J Acupunct Meridian Stud* 12 (5): 166–171.

20 Gomez Alvarez, C.B., L'ami, J.J., Moffat, D. et al. (2008 March). Effect of chiropractic manipulations on the

kinematics of back and limbs in horses with clinically diagnosed back problems. *Equine Vet J* 40 (2): 153–159.

21 Sullivan, K.A., Hill, A.E., and Haussler, K.K. (2008 January). The effects of chiropractic, massage and phenylbutazone on spinal mechanical nociceptive thresholds in horses without clinical signs. *Equine Vet J* 40 (1): 14–20.

22 Xie, H. and Preast, V. (2007). *Xie's Veterinary Acupuncture*, 283–286. Ames, IA: Blackwell Publishing.

23 Yu, Z. (2020 June 21). Neuromechanism of acupuncture regulating gastrointestinal motility. *World J Gastroenterol* 26 (23): 3182–3200.

24 Ma, A. (2020). *Clinical Manual of Chinese Veterinary Herbal Medicine*, 5e. 271–275. Gainesville, FL: Ancient Art Press.

25 Munsterman, A.S., Dias Moreira, A.S., and Marqués, F.J. (2019 September). Evaluation of a Chinese herbal supplement on equine squamous gastric disease and gastric fluid pH in mares. *J Vet Intern Med* 33 (5): 2280–2285.

26 Ribeiro Filho, J.D., Alves, G.E.S., and Dantas, W.M.F. (2012). Treatment of experimental large colon impaction in horses: enteral and parenteral fluid therapy and senna (Cassia augustifolia Vahl). *Clínica Médica e Cirúrgica Animal* 59 (1): 32–37.

27 Ma, A. (2020). *Clinical Manual of Chinese Veterinary Herbal Medicine*, 5e. 245–247. Gainesville, FL: Ancient Art Press.

28 Ying, W. (2020). Food therapy for horses. In: *Integrative and Traditional Chinese Veteirnary Medicine Food Therapy: Small Animal and Equine* (ed. M. Fowler and H. Xie), 673–710. Reddick, FL: Chi University Press.

29 Park, S.I., Sunwoo, Y.Y., Jung, Y.J. et al. (2012). Therapeutic effects of acupuncture through enhancement of functional angiogenesis and granulogenesis in rat wound healing. *Evid Based Complementary Altern Med* 2012: 464586.

30 Kan, Y., Zhang, X.N., Yu, Q.Q. et al. (2019 April 25). Moxibustion promoted wound healing in rats with full-thickness cutaneous wounds. *Zhen Ci Yan Jiu* 44 (4): 288–292.

31 Rozenfeld, E., Sapoznikov Sebakhutu, E., Krieger, Y., and Kalichman, L. (2020 December). Dry needling for scar treatment. *Acupunct Med* 38 (6): 435–439.

32 Frauenfelder, H. (2008). The use of acupuncture beads to control exuberant granulation tissue in equine skin wounds: a preliminary study. *Equine Vet Educ* 20: 587–595.

33 Xie, H. and Preast, V. (2007). *Xie's Veterinary Acupuncture*, 319. Ames, IA: Blackwell Publishing.

34 Scepankova, H., Combarros-Fuertes, P., Fresno, J.M. et al. (2021 August 7). Role of honey in advanced wound care. *Molecules* 26 (16): 4784.

35 Ma, A. (2020). *Clinical Manual of Chinese Veterinary Herbal Medicine*, 5e. 365–366. Gainesville, FL: Ancient Art Press.

36 Ma, L.L., Liu, H.M., Luo, C.H. et al. (2021 March). Fever and antipyretic supported by traditional Chinese medicine: a multi-pathway regulation. *Front Pharmacol* 22 (12): 583279.

37 Yu, M.Z., Wang, Y.G., Ball, M. et al. (2010). Nineteen clinical features of fever in Chinese medicine. *J Tradit Chin Med* 30 (4): 302–304.

38 Xie, H. and Preast, V. (2007). *Xie's Veterinary Acupuncture*, 309–311. Ames, IA: Blackwell Publishing.

39 Son, Y.S., Park, H.J., Kwon, O.B. et al. (2002 February 8). Antipyretic effects of acupuncture on the lipopolysaccharide-induced fever and expression of interleukin-6 and interleukin-1 beta mRNAs in the hypothalamus of rats. *Neurosci Lett* 319 (1): 45–48.

40 Fang, J.Q., Guo, S.Y., Asano, K. et al. (1998 September–October). Antipyretic action of peripheral stimulation with electroacupuncture in rats. *In Vivo* 12 (5): 503–510.

41 Xiao, L., Jiang, G.L., Zhao, J.G. et al. (2007 March). Clinical observation on effects of acupuncture at Dazhui (GV 14) for abating fever of common cold. *Zhongguo Zhen Jiu* 27 (3): 169–172.

42 Hirsch, D., Shiau, D., and Xie, H. (2017). A randomized and controlled study of the efficacy of *Yin Qiao San* combined with antibiotics compared to antibiotics alone for the treatment of feline upper respiratory disease. *Am J Trad Chin Vet Med* 12 (2): 39–47.

43 Ma, A. (2020). *Clinical Manual of Chinese Veterinary Herbal Medicine*, 5e. 261–262. Gainesville, FL: Ancient Art Press.

44 Ma, A. (2020). *Clinical Manual of Chinese Veterinary Herbal Medicine*, 5e. 237–238. Gainesville, FL: Ancient Art Press.

45 Ma, A. (2020). *Clinical Manual of Chinese Veterinary Herbal Medicine*, 5e. 326–327. Gainesville, FL: Ancient Art Press.

Index

Integrative Veterinary Medicine, First Edition. Edited by Mushtaq A. Memon and Huisheng Xie.
© 2023 John Wiley & Sons, Inc. Published 2023 by John Wiley & Sons, Inc.
Companion Website: www.wiley.com/go/memon/veterinary